TRACHEOSTOMY
AND
VENTILATOR DEPENDENCY

Management of Breathing, Speaking, and Swallowing

TRACHEOSTOMY
AND
VENTILATOR DEPENDENCY

Management of Breathing, Speaking, and Swallowing

Donna C. Tippett, MPH, MA, CCC-SLP

Assistant Professor
Division of Audiology and Speech-Language Pathology
Department of Otolaryngology–Head and Neck Surgery
and
Assistant Professor
Department of Physical Medicine and Rehabilitation
Johns Hopkins University
Baltimore, Maryland

2000
Thieme
New York • Stuttgart

Thieme New York
333 Seventh Avenue
New York, NY 10001

Senior Medical Editor: Andrea Seils
Editorial Director: Ave McCracken
Director, Production and Manufacturing: Anne Vinnicombe
Marketing Director: Phyllis Gold
Sales Manager: Ross Lumpkin
Chief Financial Officer: Seth S. Fishman
President: Brian D. Scanlan
Cover Designer: Marsha Cohen
Compositor: Alexander Graphics
Printer: Maple-Vail

Library of Congress Cataloging-in-Publication Data

Tracheostomy and ventilator dependency : management of breathing,
   speaking, and swallowing / [edited by] Donna C. Tippett.
        p.   cm.
      ISBN 0-86577-774-8 (hard cover)
      1. Tracheotomy.   2. Artificial respiration.   3. Respirators
   (Medical equipment)   I. Tippett, Donna C.
      [DNLM: 1. Tracheostomy—rehabilitation.   2. Respiration,
   Artificial.   WF 490 T7589 1999]
   RF517.T734   1999
   617.5'33—dc21
   DNLM/DLC
   for Library of Congress   99-10470
                                                                  CIP

Important note: Medical knowledge is ever-changing. As new research and clinical experience
broaden our knowledge, changes in treatment and drug therapy may be required. The authors and
editors of the material herein have consulted sources believed to be reliable in their efforts to
provide information that is complete and in accord with the standards accepted at the time of
publication. However, in view of the possibility of human error by the authors, editors, or
publisher of the work herein, or changes in medical knowledge, neither the authors, editors,
publisher, nor any other party who has been involved in the preparation of this work, warrants
that the information contained herein is in every respect accurate or complete, and they are not
responsible for any errors or omissions or for the results obtained from use of such information.
Readers are encouraged to confirm the information contained herein with other sources. For
example, readers are advised to check the product information sheet included in the package of
each drug they plan to administer to be certain that the information contained in this publication is
accurate and that changes have not been made in the recommended dose or in the
contraindications for administration. This recommendation is of particular importance in
connection with new or infrequently used drugs.

Some of the product names, patents, and registered designs referred to in this book are in fact
registered trademarks or proprietary names even though specific reference to this fact is not always
made in the text. Therefore, the appearance of a name without designation as proprietary is not to
be construed as a representation by the publisher that it is in the public domain.

Printed in the United States of America
5 4 3 2 1

TNY ISBN 0-86577-774-8
GTV ISBN 3-13-108571-1

Listen to the Exhortation of the Dawn!
Look to this Day!
For it is Life, the very Life of Life.
In its brief Course lie all the
Varieties and Realities of your Existence:
The Bliss of Growth,
The Glory of Action,
The Splendour of Beauty;
For Yesterday is but a Dream
And Tomorrow is only a Vision;
But Today well lived makes
Every Yesterday a Dream of Happiness,
And every Tomorrow a Vision of Hope.
Look well therefore to this Day!
Such is the Salutation of the Dawn!

Sir William Osler

Contents

Contributors

John R. Bach, MD
Vice Chairman and Professor
Department of Physical Medicine and
    Rehabilitation
Professor, Department of Neurosciences
Director of Research and Associate Medical
    Director
Department of Physical Medicine and
    Rehabilitation
Co-Director, Jerry Lewis Muscular Dystrophy
    Association Clinic
University Hospital
Newark, New Jersey
and
Medical Director
Center for Ventilator Management
    Alternatives
Kessler Institute for Rehabilitation
West Orange, New Jersey

Beth C. Diehl, RNC, MS, CCRN, NNP
Case Manager, Neonatal ICU
Johns Hopkins Hospital
Baltimore, Maryland

Louella K. Dorsey, RN, MSN, CRRN
Clinical Nurse Specialist
Kennedy Krieger Institute
Faculty Associate
Johns Hopkins University School of Nursing
Baltimore, Maryland

Lynn E. Driver, MS, CCC-SLP
Speech-Language Pathologist
Division of Speech-Language Pathology
Department of Physical Medicine and
    Rehabilitation
C.S. Mott Children's Hospital
University of Michigan Health Systems
Ann Arbor, Michigan

Glendon M. Gardner, MD
Senior Staff, Otolaryngologist
Department of Otolaryngology–Head and
    Neck Surgery
Henry Ford Hospital
Detroit, Michigan

Michael C. Iannuzzi, MD
Senior Staff, Pulmonologist
Division of Pulmonology and Critical Care
    Medicine
Department of Otolaryngology–Head and
    Neck Surgery
Henry Ford Hospital
Detroit, Michigan
and
Associate Professor
Case Western Reserve University Medical
    School
Cleveland, Ohio

Yuka Ishikawa, MD
Clinical Supervisor
Department of Pediatrics
National Yakumo Hospital
Department of Pediatrics
Sapporo University of Medicine
Hokkaido, Japan

Charnan L. S. Koller, RN, BA, CRRN
Lead Nurse Clinician
Kennedy Krieger Institute
Baltimore, Maryland

Barbara J. de Lateur, MD
Professor and Director
Department of Physical Medicine and
    Rehabilitation
Johns Hopkins University School of Medicine
Baltimore, Maryland

Mark J. McGinley, MBChB
Department of Pulmonary and Critical Care
University of Maryland School of Medicine
Baltimore, Maryland

Alice K. Silbergleit, PhD, CCC-SLP
Senior Staff, Speech-Language Pathologist
Division of Speech-Language Sciences and
*   Disorders*
Department of Neurology
Henry Ford Hospital
Detroit, Michigan
and
Assistant Professor
Case Western Reserve University Medical
*   School*
Cleveland, Ohio

Kenneth H. C. Silver, MD
Chief and Associate Professor
Division of Rehabilitation Medicine
Department of Neurology
University of Maryland School of Medicine
Baltimore, Maryland

Dean S. Tippett, MD
Chief, Division of Neurology
Co-Director, Ethics Committee
St. Agnes Hospital
Clinical Associate Professor
Department of Neurology
University of Maryland School of Medicine
Baltimore, Maryland

Donna C. Tippett, MPH, MA, CCC-SLP
Assistant Professor
Division of Audiology and Speech-Language
*   Pathology*
Department of Otolaryngology–Head and
*   Neck Surgery*
Assistant Professor
Department of Physical Medicine and
*   Rehabilitation*
Johns Hopkins University School of Medicine
Baltimore, Maryland

Lura Vogelman, MA, CCC-SLP
Clinical Specialist and Faculty Member
Loyola Speech and Hearing Center
Loyola College of Maryland
Baltimore, Maryland

Foreword

This book has been eagerly anticipated by those who manage patients who require tracheostomy and the use of a ventilator. It is both theoretical and practical and, as such, provides the background information and the detail needed for hands-on management. The book contains a number of special features such as chapters on ethical issues, pediatric considerations, and post-hospitalization care. The multiple figures, illustrations, and case studies facilitate understanding of the chapter concepts. The sections on clinical competencies assist readers in fulfilling the requirement of healthcare organizations that clinical competencies exist to assess and measure staff performance. The extensive citations increase reader knowledge about previous and current research, and facilitate easy access to research to support their clinical practices. The broad scope of information covered by experts facilitates understanding of management of tracheostomy and ventilator dependency without having to consult multiple references. Finally, it is especially appropriate that this book has been dedicated to Doctor Arthur A. Siebens, who spent much of his professional life developing singular expertise in and unfailing compassion for the care of these patients.

Barbara J. de Lateur, MD

Preface

The concept for this book originated from my experiences working in the Johns Hopkins rehabilitation unit at the Good Samaritan Hospital in Baltimore, Maryland. Dr. Arthur A. Siebens, founder and director of rehabilitation medicine at Johns Hopkins and Good Samaritan Hospitals, developed many innovative programs at "Good Sam," including a rehabilitation program for individuals with tracheostomy and ventilator dependency. Perhaps because of his own unique and varied medical background, which encompassed professorships in rehabilitation medicine and surgery, pediatrics, and physiology, Dr. Siebens strove to apply basic science to the care of his patients, and encouraged the participation of individuals from a variety of disciplines in the evaluation and treatment of those with tracheostomy and ventilator dependency. His goal was the exchange of information and ideas to make life better for his patients. No idea—even the unconventional (those who knew Dr. Siebens would say especially the unconventional!)—was dismissed without consideration. The questions of patients, their families and caregivers, and staff did not go unaddressed. Everyone was a valued member of the team. Dr. Siebens' patients were as devoted to him as he was to them. Evidence of this is that many individuals with complex medical problems and significant functional deficits returned to Dr. Siebens over the course of several years, some traveling great distances and overcoming many difficulties to keep their outpatient appointments. The careers of those who worked with Dr. Siebens grew in this environment of academic inquiry, respect, thoughtful consideration, and excellent patient care. I am a grateful beneficiary of Dr. Siebens' influence.

This book, which is dedicated to Dr. Siebens, addresses basic and clinical concepts in the management of individuals with tracheostomy and ventilator dependency. It includes contributions from individuals from the disciplines of neurology, nursing, otolaryngology, pediatrics, pulmonary and critical care, rehabilitation medicine, and speech-language pathology. The contributors are experts in their fields; their outstanding and diverse work enhances this book's worth.

Chapter 1 covers the structure and function of the human respiratory system, including airway anatomy, pulmonary circulation, respiratory musculature, pulmonary mechanics, airway defenses and clearance, ventilation, and gas exchange. Chapter 2 addresses the pathophysiology of respiratory insufficiency, respiratory complications, and respiratory failure in individuals with tracheostomy and ventilator dependency, and approaches to avoid these complications, such as noninvasive ventilatory support. The evolution of mechanical ventilation is described in Chapter 3. Chapter 4 is an overview of technical issues pertaining to tracheostomy and mechanical ventilation, including the components of tracheostomy cannulas, forms of ventilatory support, specialty tracheostomy tubes, and indications for tracheotomy and for adjusting ventilator settings. Communication options with tracheostomy and ventilator dependency are presented in Chapter 5, including nonoral options, cuff deflation, and speaking valves. Management of swallowing disorders is the focus of Chapter 6. The effects of tracheostomy on swallowing, use of bedside and radiographic swallowing examinations, and value of cuff deflation and valving to promote safer swallowing are presented. The special concerns of the pediatric population are considered in Chapter 7, covering such topics as anatomy and physiology of respiration unique to pediatric patients, respiratory management in children, and the impact of tracheostomy and ventilator dependency on the development of oral communication, feeding, and swallowing. Chapter 8 is designed to provide information about post-hospitalization care. Medical stability, community re-entry, caregiver education, equipment needs, and financial planning are reviewed. Ethical concerns are examined in Chapter 9, including the very difficult situation of a competent patient who wishes to discontinue ventilatory support. When appropriate, case studies are provided throughout the book to illustrate chapter principles.

This book is primarily intended for speech-language pathologists, especially those who work in highly sophisticated and technologically advanced environments. Other audiences include students and practitioners in nursing, occupational therapy, physical therapy, respiratory therapy, and in the medical specialties of neurology, otolaryngology, pediatrics, pulmonary and critical care, and rehabilitation medicine. The intention of the text is to bring the reader from an understanding of respiratory anatomy and physiology through the care of individuals with tracheostomy and ventilator dependency. This melding of basic and clinical concepts is vital for the comprehensive care of individuals with tracheostomy and ventilator dependency.

Donna C. Tippett, MPH, MA, CCC-SLP

Acknowledgments

The efforts of many contributed to the development of this book. My heartfelt gratitude is extended to my family, patients, friends, and colleagues in the Department of Otolaryngology–Head and Neck Surgery and Department of Physical Medicine and Rehabilitation, Johns Hopkins University; Department of Rehabilitation Services and the Shock Trauma Center, University of Maryland; and Good Samaritan Hospital, Baltimore, Maryland.

1

Structure and Function of the Respiratory System

MARK J. MCGINLEY AND KENNETH H.C. SILVER

The primary function of the lung is the removal of carbon dioxide from and the supply of oxygen to circulating blood. Gas exchange occurs by interfacing air and blood over the large surface area of pulmonary vasculature and respiratory mucosa. A number of body systems play a role in this process. In addition to the pulmonary system, the nervous system controls ventilation, the musculoskeletal system provides the mechanical support and undertakes the work of breathing, and the circulatory system directs blood through respiratory exchange surfaces.

The lung also has secondary functions, some of which have only recently been described. For example, the lung is the source of angiotensin I converting enzyme (ACE), which converts angiotensin I to angiotensin II (a potent vasoconstrictor) (1). Additionally, a number of vasoactive substances (endogenous molecules that have the capacity to cause vasodilation or vasoconstriction of the pulmonary vascular bed, thus fundamental to the regulation of vascular tone) are completely or partially inactivated during passage through the lung, e.g., bradykinin, serotonin, and the prostaglandins E1, E2, and F2 (2). Although of vital importance, these secondary lung functions will not be discussed further.

This chapter provides a basic review of the structure and function of the human respiratory system, emphasizing airway anatomy, pulmonary circulation, respiratory musculature, pulmonary mechanics, airway defenses and clearance, ventilation, and gas exchange. Where relevant, the effects of tracheostomy and ventilator dependency on respiratory system structure and function are highlighted.

Tracheostomy and Ventilator Dependency: Management of Breathing, Speaking, and Swallowing. Edited by Donna C. Tippett, MPH, MA, CCC-SLP. Thieme Medical Publishers, Inc. New York © 2000.

Upper Airway

The upper airway, which is illustrated in Figure 1–1, consists of the nasal passages, the sinuses, the pharynx, the epiglottis, and the larynx. Its function is to conduct air to the lower airway; protect the lower airway from foreign material; and warm, filter, and humidify the inspired air.

The structure of the nose with its two nasal cavities, turbinates, and rich vascular supply, provides maximum contact between inspired air and the nasal mucosa. The nose clears debris from the inspired air in two ways. The hairs at the entry of the nostril trap particulate matter. Subsequently, the nasal cilia sway together in waves to move trapped particles posteriorly (3). This function is of great physiologic importance. For example, the ability of the nose to filter out inhaled microbes likely plays an important role in preventing lower respiratory tract infections, as is demonstrated by the increased risk of pneumonia in tracheo-stomized patients (4). *Resistance* is generally defined as that property of the airways that impedes flow and is primarily dependent on the diameter of the airway. The resistance to airflow in the nose is normally 50% of the total airway resistance, which becomes physiologically important with exercise (hence the change to mouth breathing in this circumstance) and with nasal obstruction by polyps and rhinitis (5). The vascular mucosa and the large surface area of the turbinates are ideally suited for the function of warming and humidification of inspired air. Air is heated approximately to body temperature on passage through the nose while its relative humidity is raised to 95%.

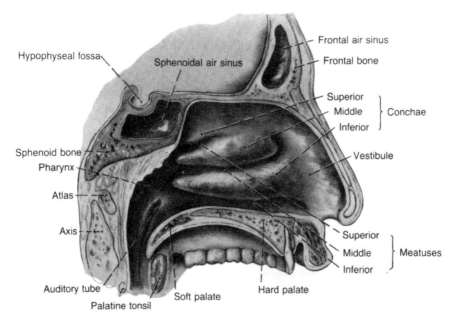

Fig. 1–1. Lateral view of nasal cavity with nasal septum removed. Reprinted, with permission, from Jacob, Francone, and Lassow (75).

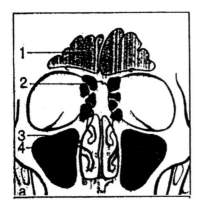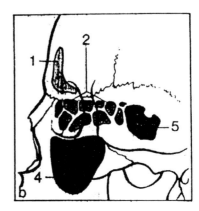

Fig. 1–2. Nasal sinuses. **a:** Frontal section. **b:** Sagittal section. *(1)* Frontal sinus; *(2)* Ethmoid sinus; *(3)* Maxillary ostium; *(4)* Antral cavity; *(5)* Sphenoid cavity. Reprinted, with permission, from Becker, Naumann and Pfaltz (76).

The sinuses are cystic airspaces in the skull (Fig. 1–2) that produce mucus for the nasal cavity, regulate the temperature of the inspired air, and act as resonance chambers for the voice. They are divided into two groups: the paranasal and the mastoid sinuses. The paranasal sinuses include the frontal, ethmoid, sphenoid, and maxillary sinuses. All are lined with ciliated, mucus-producing cells and have small pathways that communicate with the nasal cavity, the pathway meatus lying underneath the nasal turbinates. Occlusion of the meatus causes fluid to accumulate in the sinuses, potentially leading to sinusitis. The mastoid sinus communicates with the middle ear which explains why otitis media can progress to the serious complication of mastoiditis.

Air passes from the nasal cavity into the space behind the nasal cavity and the mouth called the *pharynx*. The pharynx extends to the point where the airway (larynx) and the esophagus divide. There are three divisions of the pharynx: the nasopharynx, the oropharynx, and the hypopharynx (or laryngeal pharynx). The nasopharynx begins at the base of the nasal cavities and extends to the soft palate. It contains the euststachian tubes and the lymphoid mass known as the adenoids. The eustachian tubes form a connection with the middle ear. The eustachian tube is about 4 cm in length and is normally collapsed. It is usually stretched open during yawning and swallowing due to the action of the tensor veli palatini muscle (6). Blockage of the eustachian tube, due to infection or mucosal edema, impairs the drainage of the middle ear and thus facilitates the development of otits media. The oropharynx extends from the soft palate and uvula to the level of the epiglottis. Part of the oropharynx can be seen with the mouth open and the tongue depressed. The palatine and lingual tonsils are contained within the oropharynx. The hypopharynx contains the larynx.

The larynx contains the vocal folds which permit phonation (Fig. 1–3). They also serve a sphincter function, assisting in the prevention of aspiration. The principal cartilages of the larynx are the thyroid, arytenoid, and cricoid. The cricoid cartilage lies directly below the thyroid and is attached to it by the cricothyroid membrane. The arytenoid cartilages serve as an attachment site for the vocal fold

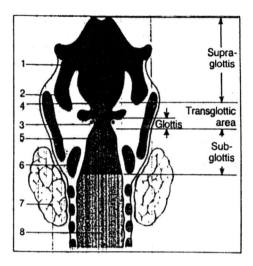

Fig. 1–3. Compartments and individual structures of the larynx. *(1)* Aryepiglottic fold forming the boundary between the larynx and the hypopharynx; *(2)* Piriform sinus which belongs to the hypopharynx; *(3)* Vocal ligament; *(4)* Anterior commissure; *(5)* Thyroid cartilage; *(6)* Cricoid cartilage; *(7)* Thyroid gland; *(8)* Trachea. Reprinted, with permission, from Becker, Naumann, and Pfaltz (77).

ligaments. They swing in and out from a fixed point, thus opening and closing the space between the vocal folds. This to and fro action permits variation in the pitch of sound. All the intrinsic muscles of the larynx, except the cricothyroids, are supplied by the recurrent laryngeal nerves. The long intrathoracic course of the left recurrent laryngeal nerve, which hooks around the aorta and runs up the mediastinum between the trachea and the esophagus, makes it vulnerable to involvement by thoracic neoplasms and compression by an aortic aneurysm. The space between the vocal folds is called the *glottis*. Air has to flow through the glottis in order to create sound. Bypassing the glottis by means of a tracheostomy prevents phonation unless the external opening of the tracheostomy is occluded and air is once again directed up through the glottis (see Chapter 5). The epiglottis is an integral part of the laryngeal structure. It is a leaf-shaped cartilaginous structure extending from the base of the tongue and attached to the thyroid cartilage by ligaments. It projects upward and posteriorly. During swallowing the epiglottis flaps down to direct swallowed material into the esophagus, contributing to protection of the laryngeal opening.

Lower Airway

The structures from the trachea to the distal alveolar sacs form part of what is collectively known as the lower airway. Its function is to conduct air, provide mucociliary defense, and, most importantly, perform gas exchange.

Conducting Zone

The first 16 divisions of the tracheobronchial tree do not partake in gas exchange and are commonly referred to as the *conducting zone*. The volume of gas in this zone is approximately 150 ml and is known as the *anatomic dead space*. Anatomic dead space begins at the nose and ends at the level of the respiratory bronchioles. This area is termed *dead space* as it receives ventilation that is wasted, i.e., does not participate in gas exchange.

The trachea extends from the cricoid cartilage in the larynx to the point where it divides into the right and left mainstem bronchi, (i.e., the carina). The lining of the trachea consists of ciliated epithelium and mucus-producing goblet cells (7). The anterior portion of the trachea is made up of C-shaped rings of cartilage, and the posterior portion (membranous trachea) is composed of smooth muscle and lies anterior to the esophagus.

The surgical creation of an opening in the trachea is called a *tracheotomy*. The stoma that remains is referred to as the *tracheostomy*. This is a well-established surgical procedure and was performed at the time of the ancient Egyptians over 3,000 years ago (8). Trendelenburg, in 1869, was the first to describe the use of a tracheostomy tube with an inflated cuff for assisting ventilation during human anesthesia (9). In the past, tracheostomy was indicated mainly for emergency airway problems. Today, however, the most common type of patient receiving a tracheostomy is the patient requiring prolonged ventilation because of neuromuscular disorders, chronic obstructive lung disease, edematous lung injury, multiorgan failure, or recalcitrant pneumonia (10). Controversy exists over the optimum time to convert an endotracheal tube to a tracheostomy. In general, if the anticipated need for an artificial airway is less than 10 days, the translaryngeal route is preferred. If an artificial airway is needed for more than 21 days, then tracheostomy is the preferred route of ventilation (11).

Tracheostomy tubes are either disposable or nondisposable (Jackson stainless steel tracheostomy tube). The disposable tubes are made of polyvinyl chloride and are either cuffed or uncuffed. A fenestration can be placed in the tube, allowing exhaled air to pass over the vocal folds permitting speech. Most cuffs are the high-volume–low-pressure type. Inflating the cuff establishes a seal, which permits positive pressure ventilation and theoretically prevents aspiration. Cuff pressures should not exceed 30 mm Hg as pressures in excess of this have a significantly higher risk of obstructing tracheal capillary blood flow (11), which can lead to necrosis of tissue and the development of a tracheoesophageal fistula. One of the physiologic consequences of a tracheostomy is that the dead space volume is reduced by approximately 60% (12). Tracheal mucocilary clearance is depressed following tracheostomy (13), permitting pathogenic bacteria to bind more avidly to the tracheal mucosa (14). Patients with tracheostomies develop more serious local infections, such as infections with *Pseudomonas* and other enteric gram-negative bacilli (4). In the majority of cases, these infections resolve with appropriate local care, but antibiotics may be necessary on occasion.

The divisions of the tracheobronchial tree with its respective bronchopulmonary segments are schematically depicted in Figure 1–4.

The angle formed by the take-off of the right mainstem bronchus is much less acute than is the case on the left. This angulation results in a greater incidence of aspiration into the right lung, and the accidental intubation of the right mainstem bronchus when an endotracheal tube is advanced too far into the airway. After penetrating the lung the right mainstem bronchus divides into three lobar bronchi that supply the upper, middle, and lower lobes of the right lung. The two lobar divisions of the left mainstem bronchus supply the two lobes of the left lung, i.e., the upper and the lower. As the bronchi continue to bifurcate and trifurcate, they begin to loose their cartilage and become known as bronchioles,

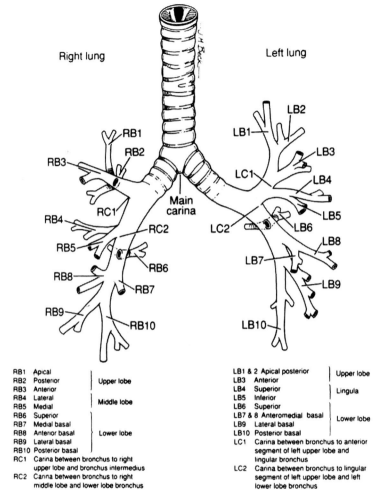

Fig. 1–4. Normal (upright) anatomy of the tracheobronchial tree in an adult human. Reprinted, with permission, from Prakash (78).

which consist primarily of connective tissue and smooth muscle. Bronchioles are held open due to the radial traction from the elastic forces of the lung tissue. The destruction of the supporting elastic tissue of the lung, which occurs with emphysema, reduces the outward radial traction on the small airways. This results in air trapping and obstruction of the outflow of air from the lungs.

Respiratory Zone

As one continues more distally along the bronchial tree, alveolar buds begin to appear on the walls of the bronchioles, marking the beginning of the respiratory bronchioles. The respiratory bronchiole gives rise to alveolar ducts which, in turn, give rise to the alveolar sacs, which are composed of numerous individual alveoli. The structures from the respiratory bronchiole to the distal alveolus form a functional unit known as the *acinus*. The acinus is the primary gas-exchanging unit of the lung and collectively the acini form the respiratory zone of the lung. The distance from the terminal bronchiole to the most distal alveolus is only about 5 mm, but the respiratory zone constitutes most of the lung, its volume being about 3,000 ml (15).

There are approximately 300 million alveolar–capillary units in adult lung (16). The total surface area of the lung parenchyma is 50 to 100 square meters, about the size of a tennis court. The alveoli are surrounded by capillaries so dense that, when fully recruited, they form almost a complete sheet of blood. Small holes, known as *pores of Kohn*, are present in the walls of the alveoli and permit the even distribution of gas among the alveoli of an alveolar sac (17).

The alveolar epithelium is made up of two cell types. Type 1 alveolar cells are squamous epithelium one cell layer thick. They promote gas exchange and prevent the leakage of fluid into the alveolus. Type 2 cells produce surfactant, a lipoprotein that reduces the surface tension within the alveolus. Surfactant prevents the alveoli from collapsing, especially during expiration (18). Surface tension is due to the liquid lining the alveoli. This liquid develops a cohesive force that tends to collapse the alveoli, particularly at smaller lung volumes. Surfactant makes it easier to expand the lung, thereby reducing the work of breathing (18). A deficient amount of surfactant production, due to lung immaturity, is responsible for the neonatal respiratory distress syndrome, in which the alveoli collapse during expiration and dramatically increase the work of breathing.

The alveolus also contains a fluctuating population of large mononuclear cells called *alveolar macrophages*. In addition to secreting numerous cytokines (a family of small cellular molecules that modulate the expression of the body's immune response), they ingest foreign materials that have evaded the cough reflex and the mucociliary clearance system (19).

Airway Innervation

The tracheobronchial tree is innervated by both sympathetic and parasympathetic nerve fibers. Acetylcholine is the principal chemical mediator secreted by the parasympathetic nervous system. In the lung, the vagus nerve is the source of parasympathetic nerve supply. Stimulation of the vagus nerve causes bronchoconstriction via the action of acetylcholine. The sympathetic fibers originate from the postganglionic branches of the second to fifth thoracic ganglia of the sympathetic trunk. Sympathetic receptors are primarily beta-2 receptors. When these adrenergic receptors are stimulated by catecholamines or beta-2 agonist medications, the result is bronchodilation (20). Alternatively, bronchodilation can be achieved by blocking the effects of the vagus nerve with an anticholinergic medication, e.g., ipratropium bromide, which is commonly used in the treatment of emphysema.

Circulation

Bronchial

The lung has a dual blood supply, i.e., the bronchial and the pulmonary circulation. The bronchial circulation is a division of the systemic circulation and as such transports blood under high pressure. The bronchial arteries supply blood to the bronchi and bronchioles as far as the distal portion of the terminal bronchioles. These arteries arise from the aorta, and not infrequently from the intercostal arteries, traverse the bronchi, and drain into the pulmonary veins (21).

Pulmonary

The pulmonary circulation is a low pressure system with a mean pulmonary artery pressure of 15 mm Hg, in contrast to the systemic circulation with a mean arterial pressure of 100 mm Hg. The pulmonary circulation begins in the main pulmonary artery, which receives unoxygenated blood from the right side of the heart. The main pulmonary artery divides into the left and right pulmonary arteries, and they in turn divide with each division of the airway, until they finally terminate in a capillary network surrounding the individual alveoli. The now oxygenated blood flows into pulmonary veins, which eventually form the four large pulmonary veins that drain into the left atrium. Vasomotor tone plays an important part in the local regulation of blood flow in relation to ventilation (22). One example of active control is hypoxic pulmonary vasoconstriction. The smooth muscle in the walls of small pulmonary arteries contracts when exposed to an environment of alveolar hypoxia. The precise mechanism of this response is unknown, but since it occurs in excised isolated lungs, it clearly does not depend on central nervous system control (23). In addition, excised segments of pulmonary artery can be shown to constrict if their environment is made hypoxic, suggesting a local action of the hypoxia on the artery itself (23). Hypoxic pulmonary vasoconstriction has the effect of directing blood flow away from hypoxic regions of the lung. Other things being equal, this will reduce the amount of ventilation–perfusion mismatching in a diseased lung and minimize the fall in the arterial partial pressure of oxygen (PaO_2).

Lymphatic

Lymph is the tissue fluid that enters the lymphatic vessels. Lymphatic channels are present in the pleura and the peribronchial and perivascular spaces, forming networks around the structures that they accompany in the thoracic cavity. The channels contain valves that promote unidirectional lymph flow. Lymph flows from the periphery toward the main lymphatic channels along the bronchial tree, toward the lymph nodes clustered about each hilus. It then flows to either the thoracic duct or the right lymphatic duct that drains into the left and right subclavian veins, respectively. The function of the lymphatic system is to maintain fluid homeostasis and provide immunologic defense (24). Filtering is performed in the lymph nodes before the lymphatic fluid is returned to the general circulation, thereby protecting the body from dissemination of foreign material. Aggregates of lymphoid tissue are known to exist in the airways and are referred to as bronchus-associated lymphoid tissue or BALT. Lymphocytes in these aggregates are principally B cells that express mainly Ig A immunoglobulins (25). Ig A is the predominant immunoglobulin in seromucous secretions such as saliva and tracheobronchial secretions. It provides a form of local immune defense by binding to a foreign antigen, thus facilitating the clearance of that antigen from the tracheobronchial tree.

Pleura

The lungs and the thoracic cavity are lined by the pleura, a continuous sheet of elastic and collagenous fibers that consists of two layers: the visceral and the parietal pleura. The visceral pleura envelops the surface of the lungs, lung fissures, and the hilar bronchi and vessels. The parietal pleura lines the inner surface of the thoracic cavity and has nerve receptors for pain. A mucous solution is produced by the cells of the pleura which allows for the smooth movement of the surfaces over one another. There is a net negative pressure of about –5 mm Hg within the pleural space due to the inward elastic recoil force of the lungs and the outward opposing tendency of the thoracic cage. The pleural space is essentially a potential space between the two pleural surfaces. If excessive fluid (pleural effusion) or air (pneumothorax) accumulate in this space, lung expansion may be inhibited. The right and left parietal and visceral pleura are entirely separate, allowing pleural space disease (e.g., pneumonic pleural effusion) to exist in one hemithorax and be absent in the other.

Muscles of Respiration

Inspiratory Muscles

The principal muscle of inspiration is the diaphragm, which together with some of the accessory muscles of respiration, are illustrated in Figure 1–5.

The muscular portion of the diaphragm attaches to the xiphoid process, the costal margins of the lower six ribs, and the vertebral column. Neural control of the diaphragm is via the phrenic nerve. Phrenic motor neurons lie in the cervical spinal cord segments C3–C5 in humans (26), hence the common mnemonic "3,4,5 keeps the diaphragm alive." Spinal cord lesions above the level of C6 damage all or part of the diaphragmatic neural supply, thus giving rise to a quadriplegia with a much higher likelihood of requiring external ventilatory support in the form of either mechanical ventilation or phrenic nerve electrical pacing. Spinal cord injuries at the C6 level or below spare diaphragmatic function, and are thus highly unlikely to result in the need for ventilatory assistance, despite varying degrees of intercostal muscle paralysis. Breathing is endurance work, and the muscle fiber composition of the diaphragm is well suited to the task. Approximately 55% of the fibers of the human diaphragm are of the slow twitch type, which are highly resistant to fatigue. A further 25% are relatively resistant to fatigue and the remaining 20% of the fibers are of the fast twitch glycolytic variety which fatigue quickly (26). When high-resistance workloads, which require strength, not endurance, are placed on the diaphragm, the muscle fibers may fatigue rapidly if energy demands exceed supply.

In the resting position, the diaphragm is dome shaped. On inspiration, the diaphragm contracts, flattening the dome. This action increases the superior–inferior dimension of the thoracic cavity, forces the abdominal contents downward, and

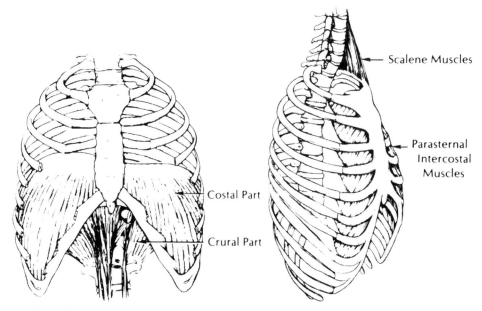

Fig. 1–5. Principal inspiratory muscles in the adult human. The left panel shows the diaphragm at the full expiratory position. The right panel shows the external (parasternal) intercostal and scalene muscles. Only the left-sided scalene muscle is shown. The sternocleidomastoid muscles are not depicted. Reprinted, with permission, from Rochester and Esau (79).

elevates the ribs; the chest and abdomen expand outward in a synchronous manner. Patients with severe weakness of the diaphragm are breathless and have paradoxical, or dyssynchronous, inward motion of the anterior abdominal wall during inspiration when supine (27). Paradoxical breathing also refers to the opposite finding of abdominal expansion while the chest exhibits an inward, or "caving in," motion during inspiration. This can be seen in quadriplegics injured between C6 and upper thoracic levels who retain diaphragmatic expansion, but lack intercostal muscle control.

The hyperinflated state of emphysema results in a flattening of the diaphragm and shortening of the length of its muscle fibers. This places the diaphragm at a mechanical disadvantage, reducing its force-generating capacity. This also explains why patients with severe emphysema may demonstrate a paradoxical pattern of breathing. Improvement of diaphragmatic curvature is one of the proposed mechanisms underlying the new lung volume reduction surgery for emphysema (28).

The external intercostal muscles have a lesser role in the act of inspiration. These muscles arise from the lower border of the first 11 ribs and have fibers that extend downward and forward to the upper border of the rib below. On inspiration, the external intercostal muscles contract, elevating the ribs and increasing the anterior–posterior dimension of the thoracic cavity.

The sternocleidomastoid muscle and the scalene muscles are collectively referred to as the *accessory muscles of respiration*. These muscles contribute to inspiration when breathing requires increased effort, e.g., running in a marathon or an attack of asthma. During inspiration the scalene muscles, which extend from the cervical vertebrae to the first two ribs, contract to elevate the first two ribs. The sternocleidomastoid muscle, which extends from the jawline to the sternum, assists in elevating the sternum. The action of these muscles therefore further increases the anterior–posterior diameter of the thorax.

Expiratory Muscles

Expiration during normal quiet breathing is a passive activity that occurs because of relaxation of the inspiratory muscles and the recoil of the lung parenchyma. The internal intercostal muscles also arise from the first 11 ribs, however their fibers are directed downward and backward to the upper border of the rib below. During forceful expiration (e.g., blowing out a candle), the internal intercostal muscles contract, decreasing the anterior–posterior diameter of the thorax by pulling the ribs downward and inward (7). Abdominal muscles that may be recruited for increased effort expiration include the internal and external oblique muscles, the rectus muscle, and the transversus abdominis muscle. When contracted, these muscles force the diaphragm upward and depress the lower ribs, decreasing the superior–inferior dimension of the thorax.

Respiratory Muscle Strength

The measurement of maximal inspiratory pressure (MIP) and maximal expiratory pressure (MEP) is commonly used to obtain a measure of global respiratory muscle strength. Several neurologic diseases are known to cause respiratory muscle weakness (e.g., mysthenia gravis, Guillain-Barré syndrome, acute poliomyelitis), and the clinical suspicion can be readily confirmed by the measurement of MIP and MEP.

MIP is the greatest subatmospheric pressure that can be generated during inspiration against an occluded airway and is normally measured at residual volume (RV) (Fig. 1–6). MEP is the highest pressure that can be developed during a forceful expiratory effort against an occluded airway and is usually measured at total lung capacity (TLC) (Fig. 1–6). The normal adult can generate inspiratory pressures in excess of -80 cm H_2O (29). The normal adult MEP values exceed $+100$ cm H_2O (29). Due to the effort dependence of both MIP and MEP, it is essential to instruct the subject carefully in the performance of the maneuver when testing.

The strength of the diaphragm muscle can be measured by calculating the difference in pressure generated in the stomach and esophagus, situated on opposite sides of the diaphragm. This value is the transdiaphragmatic pressure (P_{di}) and is measured by the insertion of a transnasal gastric and esophageal balloon (each attached to separate pressure transducers) and, as such, is more invasive than the measurement of MIP and MEP. It is, however, subject to the same patient effort and cooperation as required in the measurement of the maximal respiratory pressures (30).

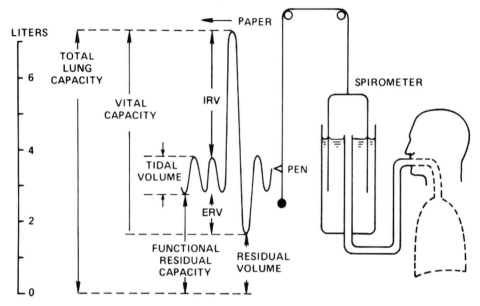

Fig. 1–6. Spirometric tracing illustrating the major divisions of lung volumes. Reprinted, with permission, from West (15).

Pulmonary Mechanics

Air flows from a region of higher pressure to one of lower pressure. Normal breathing in humans is accomplished by active contraction of the inspiratory muscles that enlarge the thorax. Expansion of the chest wall pulls on the lungs, enlarging the alveoli, alveolar ducts, and smaller airways. The negative pressure that is generated in the alveoli causes air to flow into mouth, nose, trachea, and alveoli. The active muscular contraction provides the force necessary to over-come the (1) elastic recoil of the lungs and the chest wall and (2) frictional resis-tance to airflow through the airways.

Elastic Recoil of the Lungs

A characteristic of the lung is that it tends to recoil inward, away from the chest wall; if the thorax is opened, the lung collapses. The chest wall, however, has an inherent tendency to recoil outward.

The elastic recoil of the lung is due to the connective tissue—elastin and collagen—that compose the lung parenchyma. A component of the lung's elastic recoil is also due to the surface tension generated at the air–liquid interface in the alveoli. At functional residual capacity (FRC), the chest wall is at a lower volume than its resting volume. If the thorax is opened, the chest wall volume expands by about 600–1,000 ml (31). The tendency of the lung to recoil away from the chest wall gives rise to a negative pleural pressure (Ppl). This is measured indirectly by measuring esophageal pressure with the use of an esophageal balloon. Tubing with a balloon at the tip is inserted, via the nose, into the distal esophagus. The balloon

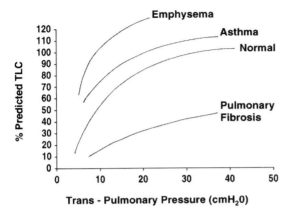

Fig. 1–7. Static pressure–volume relationship of the lungs in a healthy individual and in patients suffering from pulmonary fibrosis, asthma, and emphysema. The slope of the curve represents the compliance of the lung, and the position of the curve represents the elastic recoil of the lung.

is inflated with 3 cc of air and connected to a pressure transducer. When the patient inspires, the negative pleural pressure is transmitted to the esophageal balloon, and a negative deflection is registered on the graph paper.

The force that stretches the lung during inspiration is called the *transpulmonary pressure* and is simply the alveolar pressure minus the pleural pressure. The degree of stretch is indicated by the change in volume. The relationship of the change in lung volume to the change in transpulmonary pressure ($\Delta V/\Delta P$) under static conditions (i.e., a few seconds are allowed for measurements to be taken at points of no flow) is known as the compliance of the lung. The relationship between pressure and volume exhibits hysteresis, i.e., the relationship is not the same during inflation and deflation. Pressure/volume curves are usually measured during deflation from TLC. Various pathologic conditions such as acute respiratory distress syndrome (ARDS), pneumonia, pulmonary edema, pulmonary fibrosis, pneumothorax, and hemothorax lead to low compliance or stiff lungs. Pathologic conditions that affect total compliance generally fall into three categories: disease of the lung interstitium, disease of the intrapleural space, and disease of the chest wall. In patients with emphysema the compliance is high and the compliance curve is shifted upward and to the left, indicating a marked loss of elastic recoil (Fig. 1–7). In patients with pulmonary fibrosis, the compliance curve is shifted downward and to the right, indicating a significant increase in elastic recoil (Fig. 1–7).

Elastic Recoil of the Chest Wall

The elastic recoil of the chest wall is difficult to measure in the clinical setting as patients often find it difficult to relax completely. It can be assessed most accurately when the patient is paralyzed, and, therefore, this measurement tends to be obtained infrequently and usually in the research setting. The chest wall progressively stiffens with age. Obesity decreases chest wall compliance, and skeletal abnormalities of the spine that can produce deformities of the thoracic cage, such as kyphoscoliosis and ankylosing spondylitis, are also associated with extreme chest wall stiffness.

Resistance to Airflow

Resistance is a measurement of the opposition to the flow of gases through the airways. There are two types of resistance: tissue and airway. Tissue resistance, which is caused by the tissue friction during inspiration and expiration, normally makes up about 20% of total resistance. Airway resistance (Raw) is the opposition to flow of gases caused by friction between the walls of the airway and the gas molecules, as well as viscous friction between the gas molecules themselves.

Resistance is pressure divided by flow. Using Poiseuille's equation, resistance (R) can be expressed as follows:

$$R = 8nl/\pi r^4$$

where r is the radius of the tube, n is the viscosity of the gas, and l is the length of the tube. It follows that changes in the size of the airway radius will have a dramatic effect on airway resistance, i.e., resistance is increased 16-fold if the radius is halved. Airway resistance can be calculated from measurements of alveolar pressure and flow. Flow is measured with a pneumotachometer (a flow-sensing device), and alveolar pressure with a body plethysmograph (an air-tight box that measures changes in pressure and volume). The units of airway resistance are cm $H_2O/L/s$. Factors that affect airway resistance include airway length, radius, and flow rate. If the length of the airway is increased, resistance to flow increases. There is a direct relationship between flow rate and resistance, in that the higher the flow rate, the higher the resistance. A common example of increased airway resistance is an asthma attack, where bronchospasm dramatically reduces the radius of the airway, thus increasing resistance and reducing the flow of air.

Ventilation

The principal function of the lung is to exchange gas between the blood and the atmospheric air. This exchange of gases is achieved through the process of ventilation. The different volumes of the lung and how they contribute to gas exchange is central to understanding the process of ventilation.

Spirometry

The subdivisions of the lung may be measured using a spirometer. It is usual for volumes of gas/air to be expressed as volumes at body temperature and pressure saturated with water vapor (BTPS).

The terms commonly used to describe the subdivisions of the lung are indicated in Figure 1–6. It should be noted that there are four primary lung volumes, which do not overlap each other. Combinations of two or more lung volumes are termed *capacities*.

The following definitions are relevant:

TIDAL VOLUME (VT)

The volume of gas moved into or out of the lung in a single normal inspiration or expiration. It averages 500 ml or 5–8 ml/kg*. It represents the volume reaching the alveoli, about 350 ml, plus the volume in the conducting airways, known as the anatomic dead space, which is about 150 ml or 2 ml/kg.

INSPIRATORY RESERVE VOLUME (IRV)

The volume of air that can be inspired at the end of a normal tidal inspiration. The IRV is called on when increased tidal breathing is necessary, as in exercise. A normal value for an adult male would be 3,000 ml*.

EXPIRATORY RESERVE VOLUME (ERV)

The maximal volume of gas that can be exhaled after a normal exhalation. A normal value for an adult male would be 1,200 ml*.

RESIDUAL VOLUME (RV)

The volume of gas remaining in the lungs after a maximal expiration. This volume cannot be measured directly using spirometry. It is obtained indirectly, i.e., the functional residual capacity is calculated using a gas dilution technique, and the RV is derived using the formula RV = FRC − ERV. A normal value for an adult male would be 1,300 ml*. A high residual volume is indicative of air trapping and is a common finding in emphysema.

VITAL CAPACITY (VC) = IRV + VT + ERV

The volume of gas that can be exhaled after the deepest possible inspiration. This measurement can be obtained at the bedside with a handheld spirometer in a cooperative patient. A normal value for an adult male would be 4,700 ml*. This value is commonly decreased in patients with respiratory muscle weakness.

FUNCTIONAL RESIDUAL CAPACITY (FRC) = ERV + RV

The volume of air remaining in the lungs at the end of normal expiration. A normal value for an adult male would be 2,500 ml*.

TOTAL LUNG CAPACITY (TLC) = IC + FRC

The maximal volume of air in the lungs after a maximal inspiration. TLC is the sum of all lung volumes. A normal value for an adult male would be 6,000 ml*. This value is commonly reduced in patients with interstitial lung disease, e.g., pulmonary fibrosis.

RV, FRC, and TLC cannot be measured directly using a spirometer because they include air that cannot be expelled from the lungs. FRC is the most frequently indirectly measured capacity. Because the subject is in a resting position where the tendency of the chest wall to spring out is equally balanced by the tendency of the lungs to collapse inward and away from the chest wall, no effort is required to reach and maintain this position. To measure the absolute gas volume in the lungs, one of four methods may be used: closed-circuit helium equilibration, open-circuit nitrogen washout, whole body plethysmography or, less commonly, radiologic techniques. While these methods are commonly used in clinical practice, the specifics of the different methods are beyond the scope of this chapter.

---

*These are average volumes. There is a range of normal values that vary by age, body size, build, and sex. Volumes are about 25% less in women (32).

Two basic types of lung dysfunction can be defined by spirometry: obstructive patterns and restrictive patterns (33). The primary criterion for airflow obstruction is a lower than expected ratio of the forced expiratory volume in one second to the forced vital capacity (FEV_1/FVC). FEV_1 is the volume of gas that is exhaled in the first second of a forced exhalation from a starting point of maximal inspiration. FVC is the maximum volume of gas that can be expired, when the subject tries as forcefully and rapidly as possible, after a maximal inspiration to total lung capacity. The impairment of the FEV_1 is used to grade the severity of the obstructive defect (33). The FEV_1/FVC ratio tends to be normal or greater than expected in restrictive lung disease, but the FVC is typically decreased. The primary criterion, however, for diagnosing restrictive lung disease is the TLC (33). The amount of reduction in the TLC is used to grade the severity of the restrictive defect (33).

Alveolar Ventilation

Functionally, ventilation may be divided into the alveolar ventilation and dead space ventilation. Alveolar ventilation is that volume of gas that participates in gas exchange in the lungs. Dead space ventilation is that volume of the lungs that is ventilated but not perfused by pulmonary/capillary blood flow and, therefore, cannot partake in gas exchange. Dead space ventilation can be further subdivided into anatomic dead space, consisting of air passages proximal to the respiratory bronchioles and alveolar dead space, consisting of alveoli that have no blood flow but receive normal ventilation. These two components, the anatomic dead space and the alveolar dead space, form the physiologic dead space.

When the ventilation/perfusion ratios are similar throughout the lungs, as in normal subjects, an alveolar ventilation at rest of about 4 L/min is usually adequate (34). However, alveolar ventilation can be considered adequate only if it maintains the partial pressure of the respiratory gases leaving the lung within physiologic limits. Thus, the only satisfactory measure of effective alveolar ventilation in many clinical situations is the arterial carbon dioxide tension. Some causes of alveolar hypoventilation include depression of the respiratory center by drugs; hypoventilation associated with obesity (Pickwickian syndrome); diseases of the brain stem such as cerebral vascular accident; abnormalities of the spinal cord conducting pathways such as high cervical trauma; diseases of the nerves to respiratory muscles, for example, the Guillian-Barré syndrome; and diseases of the myoneural junction such as myasthenia gravis.

Maximal Voluntary Ventilation

Maximal voluntary ventilation (MVV) is the largest volume of air that can be breathed into and out of the lungs during a 10- to 15-s interval with voluntary effort (34). It is recorded in liters per minute, BTPS, by extrapolating the 10- to 15-s accumulated volume to 1 min. Normal MVV values in healthy young men average between 150 and 200 L/min (34). The MVV is a test of the overall function of the respiratory system and is routinely reported in a standard pulmonary function test. It is analogous to a sprint, in that you are trying to determine the limits of the respiratory system via the use of a brief maximal effort. It is influenced by the status of the respiratory muscles, the compliance of the lung–thorax system, the condition of the ventilatory control mechanisms, and the resistance offered by the airways and tissues. The MVV maneuver is largely dependent on subject effort and cooperation. Low MVV values should always be scrutinized to ascertain whether the reduction is a result of obstruction, muscular weakness, defective ventilatory control, or poor subject performance. An indirect index of subject effort may be obtained by multiplying the FEV_1 by a factor of 35 (34). For example, a subject with an FEV_1 of 2 L might be expected to ventilate about 70 L/min (35 × 2 L) during the MVV test. If the measured MVV is much less than 70 L/min, then subject effort may be suspect.

Control of Ventilation

Breathing is controlled by feedback mechanisms between receptors in the lung and periphery, and the respiratory center in the human brain stem. Simply stated, the respiratory center is stimulated by a fall in the blood pH or a rise in the $PaCO_2$ or a fall in the PaO_2. A more in-depth discussion of this topic can be found in the article by Gautier (35). The factors controlling ventilation fall into the broad categories of humoral and mechanical factors.

Humoral

Chemical signaling to the respiratory center comes from two distinct areas, namely, central and peripheral chemoreceptors.

Central Chemoreceptors

These chemoreceptors are located in the medulla and are primarily influenced by the hydrogen ion concentration (pH) of the cerebrospinal fluid (CSF). A decrease in the pH acts as a strong stimulus to increase the rate and depth of ventilation (36). The key determinant of the CSF pH is the partical pressure (P) of CO_2. An increase in the PCO_2 results in a maximal increase in the hydrogen ion concentration (decrease in pH) of the CSF because it lacks the protein buffers found in the blood.

Patients with severe emphysema commonly display a blunted respiratory drive to $PaCO_2$, and their drive tends to be preferentially driven by the PaO_2. This has important clinical implications because trying to normalize their PaO_2 with high oxygen flow rates, may have the deleterious effect of reducing ventilatory drive and result in worsening respiratory acidosis ($\uparrow Pa\,CO_2 : \downarrow pH$) and may even cause apnea and death.

Another clinical application of this physiologic principle is the apnea test used to diagnose brain death. If the brain is dead, then the respiratory center in the medulla will not respond to rising levels of $PaCO_2$. Patients are preoxygenated and then disconnected from the ventilator, while simultaneously provided oxygen at 8–12 L/min. The patient is then observed for evidence of spontaneous respiration. After 10 min, an arterial blood gas is drawn to ensure that the $PaCO_2$ is greater than 60 mm Hg. The patient is said to be apneic if the $PaCO_2$ is >60 mm Hg and there is no respiratory movement. The apnea test is only one of several tests used to confirm brain death and cannot be interpreted in isolation.

Peripheral Chemoreceptors

These chemoreceptors are found in the aortic arch and at the bifurcation of the carotid arteries, and are extremely sensitive to decreases in blood oxygen tension (37). Hypoxemia increases the activity of the peripheral receptors, leading to an increase in the rate and depth of ventilation. The peripheral chemoreceptors also respond to increases in $PaCO_2$ and hydrogen ion concentration with an increase in ventilation, but to a lesser degree than the central receptors.

Mechanical

STRETCH RECEPTORS

Stretch receptors are located in the bronchial smooth muscle. When stimulated by lung hyperinflation, impulses are sent to the respiratory center, via the vagus nerve, to limit further inflation and increase expiratory time. This is known as the Hering-Breuer inflation reflex. The Hering-Breuer deflation reflex initiates inspiratory activity at very low lung volumes. These reflexes represent the body's way of preventing over-distention of the lung, while at the same time avoiding atelectasis from breathing at abnormally low lung volumes.

IRRITANT RECEPTORS

Activity of the irritant receptors, which lie between the epithelial cells of the airway, is mediated via the vagus nerve (38). When stimulated by inhaled particles, such as cigarette smoke, or cold air, the reflex response is bronchoconstriction, cough, and increased respiratory rate. This reflex assists in clearing the irritant and reducing total exposure to the irritant

J-RECEPTORS

Juxtacapillary receptors, or J-receptors, are located in the alveolar walls near pulmonary capillaries. They are also innervated by the vagus nerve and when stimulated cause rapid, shallow breathing that may deteriorate to apnea with intense stimulation (39). Their role in normal pulmonary function is unclear. Stimulants include fluid in the alveoli and distention of the pulmonary capillaries, conditions that are present in ARDS, left heart failure, and pulmonary edema.

Gas Exchange

The blood–gas barrier is extremely thin, less than 0.5 μm over much of its extent, whereas its surface area is extremely large, approximately 70 square meters. Fick's law of diffusion states that the amount of gas that moves across a tissue sheet is proportional to the area but inversely proportional to the thickness. The structure of the lung is, therefore, ideally suited for its gas-exchanging function.

Both oxygen and carbon dioxide readily diffuse across the alveolar–capillary membrane. Carbon dioxide diffuses 20 times more readily than oxygen; factors that adversely affect diffusion are therefore less likely to affect the diffusion of carbon dioxide than that of oxygen. Gas exchange is completed by the time the red blood cell is only one-third of the way along the capillary, about 0.3–0.4 s. Because the red blood cell is in the capillary for almost a full second at rest, there is an enormous reserve time for gas exchange to occur. Patients with diseases that adversely affect diffusion, for example, pulmonary fibrosis with its thickened alveolar–capillary membrane, can have normal diffusion at rest but with exercise exhibit a fall in the oxygen saturation of hemoglobin (40). This is because the increase in cardiac output that occurs with exercise decreases the transit time of the red blood cell in the pulmonary capillaries, thus preventing the complete loading of oxygen.

An important concept in any discussion of gas exchange is that of partial pressure. The partial pressure of a gas is found by multiplying its concentration by the total pressure in the atmosphere. For example, dry air has 20.9% oxygen. The partial pressure of oxygen (PO_2) in dry air at sea level, where the barometric pressure is 760 mm Hg, is therefore $20.9/100 \times 760 = 159$ mm Hg. As can be seen from Figure 1–8, the differing partial pressures of gases in the venous and systemic

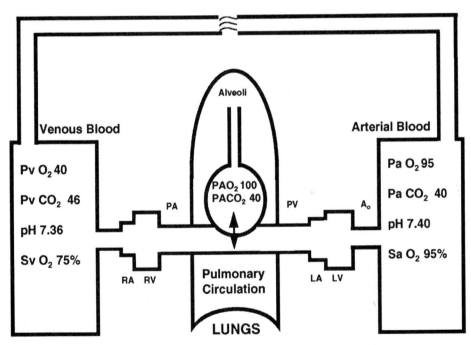

Fig. 1–8. Schematic representation of the partial pressures of gases in the arterial, venous, and pulmonary circulations. RA, Right atrium; RV, Right ventricle; PA, Pulmonary artery; PV, Pulmonary vein; LA, Left atrium; LV, Left ventricle; A_o, Aorta; Pv O_2, Venous blood partial pressure of oxygen (mm Hg); Pv CO_2, Venous blood partial pressure of carbon dioxide (mm Hg); Pa O_2, Arterial blood partial pressure of oxygen (mm Hg); Pa CO_2, Arterial blood partial pressure of carbon dioxide (mm Hg); PAO_2, Alveolar partial pressure of oxygen (mm Hg); $PACO_2$, Alveolar partial pressure of carbon dioxide (mm Hg); Sv O_2, Oxygen saturation of hemoglobin in venous blood; Sa O_2, Oxygen saturation of hemoglobin in arterial blood.

circulation establish a diffusion gradient whereby gases travel from an area of high to low partial pressure. In a state of normal ventilation and perfusion, the PaO_2 is approximately 100 mm Hg, and the $PaCO_2$ is close to 40 mm Hg.

The venous blood from the bronchial circulation drains directly into the pulmonary veins, which contain oxygenated blood on its way to the left side of the heart and the systemic circulation. This has the net effect of decreasing the partial pressure of oxygen in the systemic arteries relative to that of the alveolus. This alveolar–arterial gradient (A-a gradient), called the *anatomic shunt*, is normally 10 mm Hg in young healthy individuals (41). This is an anatomic shunt because deoxygenated blood is shunted across to the left side of the heart due to the anatomic drainage pattern of the bronchi. Numerous disease states can increase the A-a gradient above the normally accepted value of 10 mm Hg.

Ventilation/Perfusion Relationships

The ratio of alveolar ventilation ($\dot{V}$) to pulmonary blood flow ($\dot{Q}$) determines the composition of the gas leaving the lung. Ideally, each alveolus would be matched to well-perfused capillaries, leading to a $\dot{V}/\dot{Q}$ ratio of 1.0. However, ventilation and perfusion are not equally distributed throughout the lung. For example, due to gravitational forces, perfusion is greater at the base than at the apex of the lung. Regional differences in $\dot{V}$ and $\dot{Q}$ result in relatively greater ventilation than perfusion at the apex of the lung, making the $\dot{V}/\dot{Q}$ ratio high (3.0). Perfusion, however, is relatively greater than ventilation at the bases, making the $\dot{V}/\dot{Q}$ ratio low (0.6) (42).

Ventilation/Perfusion Inequalities

LOW V/Q (SHUNT)

There are two types of shunt, anatomic and physiologic. Anatomic shunt (see above) represents about 2% of the cardiac output that normally bypasses the pulmonary arterial system and drains directly into the pulmonary venous system. Physiologic shunt occurs when pulmonary blood flow is adequate but there is inadequate alveolar ventilation. In effect, perfusion is wasted. A common example of a physiologic shunt is that of pneumonia where large numbers of alveoli are filled with inflammatory and infective material and, therefore, unable to partake in gas exchange. An important diagnostic feature of a shunt is that the PaO_2 does not rise to the expected level when a patient is given 100% oxygen to breathe (43). This is because the shunted blood, which bypasses ventilated alveoli, is never exposed to the higher alveolar PO_2. Its addition to end-capillary blood continues to depress the arterial PO_2.

HIGH V/Q (DEAD SPACE)

In this situation alveolar ventilation is normal but the alveoli are poorly perfused; in effect, ventilation is wasted. This results in increased dead space ventilation. Examples of physiologic dead space ventilation include pulmonary embolism, and decreased pulmonary perfusion, as in low cardiac output or acute pulmonary hypertension; and mechanical ventilation with large tidal volumes or pressures that overdistend the alveoli to such a degree that alveolar pressure exceeds capillary pressure. Increased dead space ventilation increases the $PaCO_2$ because the blood carrying the CO_2 back from the tissues does not interface with the alveolus. Increased dead space ventilation demands an increased minute ventilation (respiratory rate × tidal volume) and, therefore, an increase in the work of breathing if a normal $PaCO_2$ is to be maintained.

Oxygen Transport in the Blood

Oxygen is transported in the blood in two ways: dissolved in the serum and in combination with the heme moieties of hemoglobin. The oxygen dissolved in the serum is measured as the PaO_2. The PaO_2 constitutes only 2 to 3% of the total oxygen transported in the blood. The overwhelming majority of the oxygen transported to the cells is in combination with hemoglobin and is measured as the percentage of O_2 saturation (Sa O_2). For example, an O_2 saturation of 80% means that 80% of the total hemoglobin is saturated with oxygen. It reflects a relationship between the amount of oxygen that is carried and the amount that can be carried. Each gram of hemoglobin can transport 1.34 ml of O_2 per 100 ml of blood (44). In a healthy individual with a hemoglobin concentration of 15 g/dl, the blood is capable of carrying 20.10 ml of oxyhemoglobin per 100 ml of blood. Blood is able to transport large amounts of O_2 because this forms an easily reversible combination with hemoglobin (Hb) to give oxyhemoglobin:

$$O_2 + Hb \rightleftharpoons HbO_2$$

The relationship between the partial pressure of oxygen and the number of Hb binding sites that have O_2 attached can be expressed graphically in the oxyhemoglobin dissociation curve which is depicted below in Figure 1–9.

The characteristic sigmoidal shape of the oxygen dissociation curve has several advantages. The fact that the upper portion is flat means that a fall of 20–30 mm Hg in arterial PO_2 in a healthy subject with an initially normal value, e.g., 100 mm Hg, will result in only a minor reduction in arterial oxygen-carrying capacity. It also illustrates that achieving a saturation above 96% has little effect on the

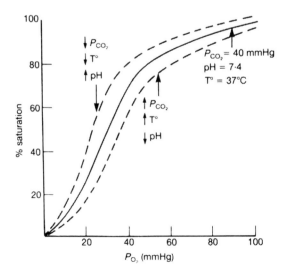

Fig. 1–9. The oxyhemoglobin dissociation curve, illustrating shifts from the normal position (solid black line) due to changes in temperature ($T°$), partial pressure of carbon dioxide (PCO_2) and pH. Reprinted, with permission, from Bray, Cragg, and Macknight (80).

oxygen-carrying capacity of the blood. The lower oxygen tension found in the distal tissues is associated with the steep part of the oxygen dissociation curve and reflects the ability of Hb to release oxygen readily in the hypoxic environment where it is needed most.

The affinity, or strength of the bond, between Hb and O_2 is affected by various physiologic states that cause the curve to shift to the right or to the left. Factors causing a shift of the curve to the left (increased oxygen affinity for hemoglobin; oxygen less readily given up in the tissues) include decreased hydrogen ion content, alkalemia, and decreased body temperature. Factors that cause the curve to shift to the right (decreased oxygen affinity for hemoglobin; oxygen more readily given up in the tissues) include increased PCO_2, acidemia, and increased body temperature.

Airway Defense

Quantitative cultures of saliva in healthy adults yield approximately 10^8 bacteria per ml (45). It is therefore not surprising that bacterial infections are a common occurrence in aspiration disorders. The respiratory system has numerous levels of defense which serve as protection against injury and infection.

Mucociliary Clearance

In a recent review article, Wanner and colleagues (46) highlighted the defensive properties of the mucociliary apparatus and described three major functions. First, it serves as a mechanical barrier by trapping particles in the surface liquid covering the airway epithelium and clearing them from the tracheobronchial tree by ciliary action. Second, the surface liquid acts as a chemical screen, i.e., oxygen radicals produced by cells in the mucociliary layer are toxic to foreign microbes. Third, the surface liquid provides a biological barrier function by allowing the inflammatory cells lining the airways to interact with microorganisms, thereby preventing them from adhering to and migrating through the airway epithelium.

The lower respiratory tract is lined by a ciliated epithelium extending from the proximal trachea to the terminal bronchioles. The cilia beat continuously moving mucus from the terminal bronchioles upward to the pharynx. The cilia conduct their power stroke when they are fully extended and attached to the surface layer of mucus. The recovery stroke takes place by a bending motion, which allows the cilia to remain in the nonviscous periciliary fluid (47). This is analogous to the freestyle swimming stroke, when the body is propelled through the water with the fully extended arm that recovers by a bending motion through the less viscous air. The ciliated epithelium is covered by surface liquids which classically have been divided into two layers: the periciliary layer (or sol phase) close to the cell surface and the mucus layer (or gel phase) on top of the sol phase. Respiratory mucus is produced by both submucosal glands and goblet cells. Figure 1–10 is a schematic representation of the mucociliary clearance anatomy.

Submucosal glands are found only in cartilaginous airways. The submucosal glands are primarily under parasympathetic nervous control, whereby cholinergic

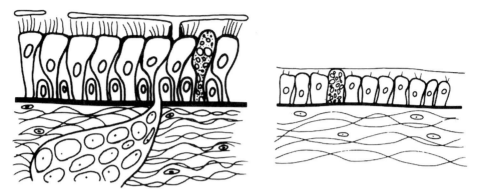

Fig. 1–10. Schematic representation of the normal adult mucociliary apparatus in central (left panel), e.g., trachea and peripheral (right panel), e.g., terminal bronchiole airways. The components of the apparatus in the central airways are, from top to bottom, the mucus layer (gel), periciliary fluid layer (sol), surface epithelial layer consisting of ciliated and nonciliated cells and submucosal gland. In comparison, there is no mucus layer, no submucosal glands, and the epithelium is flat and less densely ciliated in the peripheral airway. Reprinted, with permission, from Wanner, Salathe, and O'Riordan (46).

stimulation causes increased mucus secretion (48). Goblet cells seem to secrete on direct stimulation (49). The presence of a layer of mucus on the surface of the larger airways appears to be essential for the efficient removal of dust particles. Mucus is, however, absent in the more peripheral/distal airways of humans.

The airway fluid is mandatory for mucociliary transport. Without this fluid layer the cilia would be unable to beat and move the mucus upward toward the larger central airways. In cystic fibrosis, a defective protein, the cystic fibrosis transmembrane conductance regulator (CFTCR), is responsible for abnormalities of chloride permeability, which ultimately diminishes the periciliary fluid layer (50). The end result is a defective mucociliary clearance system and recurrent bacterial respiratory tract infections.

In addition, the fluid contains secretory Ig A immunoglobulins, lysozyme, peroxidase, and lactoferrin, all of which assist in the protection of the tracheobronchial tree (46). Ig A forms an immunologic barrier. Its importance can be appreciated from the fact that patients with a deficiency in Ig A (plus an Ig G subclass) show increased susceptibility to infections and an impairment of lung function (51). As secretory Ig A production is intimately linked to epithelial cell function, destruction of the mucosa can be expected to be associated with a decrease in bronchial Ig A concentration. Lysozyme, which is mainly produced by the submucosal glands, is directly bactericidal (52). Lactoferrin is primarily bactericidal to gram-negative bacteria (52,53), but more importantly, it traps iron ions, which are a growth requirement for many bacteria (53,54). Furthermore, it protects the epithelium by scavenging reactive oxygen species.

Pulmonary Macrophage

The pulmonary macrophage (PM) constitutes the largest single cell population in normal bronchoalveolar lavage (BAL) fluids and is the principal phagocytic cell in the distal airways (45). The PM plasma membrane contains a number of specific receptors, including complement and Ig G, that assist in the ingestion of foreign microorganisms. In addition, PMs release a number of cytokines that attract poly-morphonuclear leukocytes providing a second line of defense for the distal airways (45). PMs are required to bind, process, and present antigens in an immunogenic form to T-cells. Interleukin 1 (IL-1), which is produced by PMs, activates T-cells and attracts the influx of more T-cells from the circulating blood (55). In the presence of activated T-cells, B-cells transform into plasmacytes and secrete antibodies (55). The absence of bacteria in the bronchi is evidence that these anti-bacterial mechanisms are effective and continuously operative (56). Studies referred to by Laurenzi and Guarneri (57) support the view that substances which implant on the bronchial tree are cleared by the mucociliary apparatus and those that deposit in the alveoli are phagocytosed (ingested) by the pulmonary macrophage.

Defensive Reflexes

When atmospheric irritants are inhaled or gastric contents are aspirated, sensitive nerve endings in the upper airways—pharynx and larynx—trigger a number of powerful protective responses. Once this first line of defense has been breached and the irritant agents have passed through the larynx to the lower respiratory tract, additional sensory nerves are stimulated to evoke further defensive reflexes. In humans it is difficult to distinguish the reflex contribution of sensitive nerves in the lower airways from that of nerves in the larynx and above. If the stimulus is acute and severe, the immediate effects are likely to be coughing, gasping, bronchospasm, an increase in airway secretions, bradycardia, and hypotension. The afferent pathways are carried by the vagus nerve (58).

The pharynx serves multiple physiologic roles. It serves as a conduit for air going to and from the lungs and for food and fluid going to and from the stomach. The three categories of material that can be aspirated into the lungs are orally ingested material, oral or upper airway secretions, and regurgitated stomach contents. Traditionally, the major mechanisms protecting the lung from aspiration are cough, reflex laryngeal closure, and swallowing. Protection of the airway from aspiration depends on both mechanical and reflex mechanisms. During swallowing, the glottic aperture undergoes a cephalad and anterior motion, which combined with the posterior motion of the tongue effectively covers the glottic opening. In adults, ventilation and deglutition are mutually exclusive acts. The fact that 26 muscles are involved in the stabilization and closure of the upper airway is a measure of the complexity of this process (59).

Cough is a common protective reflex that can occur on a voluntary or involuntary basis. Involuntary coughing appears to be an entirely vagal phenomenon and is provoked by stimulation of vagally innervated structures such as the oropharynx, the larynx, the lower respiratory tract, and the tympanic membrane (60). Voluntary coughing can be initiated by both a wide variety of inflammatory or mechanical changes in the airways and the inhalation of a large number of chemical and mechanical irritants (60). The two primary functions of the cough reflex are to prevent foreign material from entering the lower respiratory tract and the removal of foreign material and excessive secretions from the lower respiratory tract. In otherwise healthy appearing individuals, a chronic cough is most likely to be due to one of four disorders: postnasal drip syndrome, asthma, gastroesophageal reflux, and chronic bronchitis (61).

Aspiration

Pulmonary aspiration is defined as penetration of material from the oropharynx into the larynx below the true vocal folds. Aspiration of pharyngeal secretions has been shown to occur, particularly during sleep, in healthy individuals without deleterious consequences (62,63). Sequalae of aspiration can include transient hypoxemia, chemical pneumonitis, mechanical obstruction, bronchospasm, pulmonary infection, and death. It has been shown that aspiration of the gastric contents produces a marked desquamation of the tracheal epithelium (64), facilitating pulmonary infection. Aspiration is a common complication in patients with artificial airways (65). It has been well documented that a significant number of chronically ventilated patients aspirate silently (66). Using videofluoroscopy, Elpern and colleagues (67) evaluated 83 medically stable tracheostomy patients admitted to a chronic ventilator unit. They found that 50% aspirated a food bolus and that 77% of the aspirators were silent aspirators. Airway desensitization from prolonged intratracheal intubation may contribute to the prevalence of silent aspiration (aspiration without cough).

Glottic reflexes are less sensitive in experimental animals with a tracheostomy (68). Although videofluoroscopy is the most commonly used imaging modality in the assessment of swallowing pathology, scintigraphy has been shown to provide additional useful information. Muz and colleagues in a study of head and neck cancer patients showed that scintigraphy was able to document distal airway penetration not detected on videofluoroscopy (69). In a more recent study, Silver and Van Nostrand demonstrated the utility of scintigraphy in quantifying the magnitude of aspiration, the rate of clearance of aspirated material, and used these findings to formulate a dysphagia treatment plan (70). Muz and colleagues (71) studied aspiration of food scintigraphically in 18 tracheostomized patients. These patients were studied twice, once with the tracheostomy tube occluded and again with it open. All the patients aspirated with an open tube, but only half did so when the tube was occluded. Occlusion of the tracheostomy tube had no significant effect on the oral transit time or the pharyngeal transit time, and, therefore, these factors were not thought to be responsible for the difference in aspiration rates.

Ikari and Sasaki (72) postulate that the subglottic pressure is the key for an intact glottic closure reflex. Dettlebach and colleagues (73) were able to significantly reduce the amount of aspiration in 11 tracheostomized patients by installing a one-way speaking valve [Passy-Muir valve (PMV)], thus providing some support for the subglottic pressure theory. Eibling and Gross (74) measured subglottic air pressure and airflow during swallowing in tracheostomized patients with and without a Passy-Muir valve. Using a pneumotachometer, they clearly demonstrated that attaching a PMV to a tracheostomy restores the subglottic pressure peak that occurs with swallowing. These data taken together suggest that closing the tracheostomy opening should restore this pressure and thereby reduce the degree of aspiration.

Summary

The basic structure and function of the respiratory system are discussed in this chapter, with particular attention to the physiologic effects of tracheostomy and ventilator dependence. Hopefully, this chapter provides clinicians with a better understanding of essential pulmonary anatomy and physiology, thus facilitating the optimal care for this unique and growing population of patients.

References

1. West JB. Ventilation, blood flow and gas exchange. In: Murray JF, Nadel JA, eds. *Textbook of respiratory medicine.* Vol. 1. Philadelphia: WB Saunders, 1994:67.
2. Hassoun PM, Fanburg BL, Junod AF. Metabolic functions. In: Crystal RG, West JB, eds. *The lung: scientific foundations.* New York: Raven Press, 1991:313–328.
3. Brain JD, Valberg PA, Sneddon S. Mechanisms of aerosol deposition and clearance. In: Moren F, Newhouse MT, Dolovich MB, eds. *Aerosols in medicine. principles, diagnosis and therapy.* Amsterdam: Elsevier, 1985:123.
4. Niederman MS, Ferrante RD, Zeigler A, et al. Respiratory infections complicating long-term tracheostomy. The implication of persistent gram-negative tracheo-bronchial colonization. *Chest* 1984;85:39.
5. McLean JA. Rhinomanometry and experimental nasal challenges. In: Settipane GA, ed. *Rhinitis.* Providence: Oceanside Publications, 1991:101.
6. Simkins CA. Functional anatomy of the eustachian tube. *Arch Otolaryngol* 1943;38:476.
7. Williams PL, Warwick R. *Gray's anatomy.* Edinburgh: Churchill Livingstone, 1980:1247;547.
8. Alberti PW. Tracheostomy versus intubation: a 19th century controversy. *Ann Otol Rhinol Laryngol* 1984;93:333.
9. Trendelenburg F. Beitrage zur den Operationen an den Luftwagen 2. Tamponade der Trachea. *Arch Klin Chir* 1871;12:121–133.
10. Heffner JE. Medical indications for tracheostomy. *Chest* 1989;96:186.
11. Lewis RJ. Tracheostomies: indications, timing and complications. *Clin Chest Med* 1992; 13:137–149.
12. Bates DV. *Respiratory function in disease.* Philadelphia: WB Saunders, 1989:26.
13. Grillo H. Congenital lesions, neoplasms and injuries to the trachea. In: Sabiston DC, Spencer FC, eds. *Gibbon's surgery of the chest.* Philadelphia: WB Saunders, 1983:273.
14. Price DG: Techniques of tracheostomy for intensive care unit patients. *Anaesthesia* 1983;38:902.
15. West JB. Ventilation, blood flow and gas exchange. In: Murray JF, Nadel JA, eds. *Textbook of respiratory medicine.* Vol. 1. Philadelphia: WB Saunders, 1994:52–53.
16. Schreider JP, Raabe OG. Structure of the human respiratory acinus. *Am J Anat* 1981;162:221–232.
17. Cordingley JL. Pores of Kohn. *Thorax* 1972;27:433.
18. King RJ. Pulmonary surfactant. *J Appl Physiol* 1982;53:1.
19. Wright SD, Detmers PA. Receptor-mediated phagocytosis. In: Crystal RG, West JB, eds. *The lung: scientific foundations.* New York: Raven Press, 1991:539–551.
20. Gustafsson B, Persson CGA. Effect of different bronchodilators on airway smooth muscle responsiveness to contractile agents. *Thorax* 1991;46:360–365.
21. Liebow AA. Patterns of origin and distribution of the major bronchial arteries in man. *Am J Anat* 1965;117:19.
22. Dawson CA. Role of pulmonary vasomotion in physiology of the lung. *Physiol Rev* 1984;44:544–616.
23. Lloyd TC. Pulmonary vasoconstriction during histotoxic hypoxia. *J Appl Physiol* 1965;20:488–490.
24. Yoffey JM, Courtice FC. *Lymphatics, lympha and the lymphomyeloid complex.* New York: Academic Press, 1970:294.

25. Bienenstock J, Mc Dermott MR, Befus AD. The significance of bronchus-associated lymphoid tissue. *Clin Respir Physiol* 1982;18:153–177.

26. Rochester DF. The diaphragm: contractile properties and fatigue. *J Clin Invest* 1985;75:1397–1402.

27. Mier-Jedrzejowicz A, Brophy C, Moxham J, et al. Assessment of diaphragm weakness. *Am Rev Respir Dis* 1988;137:877–883.

28. Cooper JD, Trulock EP, Triantafillou AN, et al. Bilateral pneumectomy (volume reduction) for chronic obstructive pulmonary disease. *J Thorac Cardiovasc Surg* 1995;109:106–119.

29. Wilson SH, Cooke N, Edwards R, et al: Predicted normal values for maximal respirtaory pressures in Caucasian adults and children. *Thorax* 1984;39:535.

30. De Troyer A, Estenne M. Limitations of measurement of transdiaphragmatic pressure. *Thorax* 1981;36:169–174.

31. Bates DV. *Respiratory function in disease*. Philadelphia: WB Saunders, 1989:29.

32. Society AT. Lung function testing: selection of reference values and interpretative stratagies. *Am Rev Respir Dis* 1991;144:1202.

33. Crapo RO. Pulmonary function testing. *N Engl J Med* 1994;331:25–30.

34. Ruppel G. *Manual of pulmonary function testing*. St Louis: Mosby, 1994:43–81.

35. Gautier H: Control of the pattern of breathing. *Clin Sci* 1980;58:343–348.

36. Bruce EN, Cherniack NS. Central chemoreceptors. *J Appl Physiol* 1987;62:389–402.

37. Mc Donald DM. Peripheral chemoreceptors: structure–function relationships of the carotid body. In: Hornbein TF, ed. *Regulation of breathing*. New York: Marcel Decker, 1981:105–319.

38. Sant'Ambrogio G. Nervous receptors of the tracheobronchial tree. *Annu Rev Physiol* 1987;49:611–627.

39. Coleridge JCG, Coleridge H. Afferent vagal C fiber innervation of the lungs and airways and its functional significance. *Rev Physiol Biochem Pharmacol* 1984;99:1–110.

40. Cherniack RM. Pulmonary ventilation, circulation and gas exchange. *Sem Resp Med* 1983;4:197–206.

41. Lilienthal JL, Riley RL, Premmel DD, et al. An experimental analysis in man of the oxygen pressure gradient from alveolar air to arterial blood during rest and exercise at sea level and at altitude. *Am J Physiol* 1946;147:199–216.

42. West JB. *Ventilation/bloodflow and gas exchange*. Oxford: Blackwell Scientific Publications, 1985:1–113.

43. Gold WM. Pulmonary function testing. In: Murray JF, Nadel JA, eds. *Textbook of respiratory medicine*. Vol. 1. Philadelphia: WB Saunders, 1994:846.

44. Cherniack RM. *Pulmonary function testing*. Philadelphia: WB Saunders, 1977:89.

45. Fick RB. Cell-mediated antibacterial defenses of the distal airways. *Am Rev Resp Dis* 1985;131:S43–S47.

46. Wanner A, Salathe M, O'Riordan TG. Mucociliary clearance in the airways. *Am J Resp Crit Care Med* 1996;154:1868–1902.

47. Satir P. How cilia move. *Sci Am* 1974;231:44–63.

48. Reid L. Natural history of mucus in the bronchial tree. *Arch Environ Health* 1973;10:265.

49. Phipps RJ, Richardson PS. The effects of irritation at various levels of the airway upon tracheal mucus secretion in the cat. *J Physiol (Lond)* 1976;261:563.

50. Riordan J, Rommens JM, Kerem BS, et al. Identification of the cystic fibrosis gene; cloning and characterization of complementary DNA. *Science* 1989;245:1066–1073.

51. Bjorkander J, Bake B, Oxelius V, et al. Impaired lung function in patients with Ig A deficiency and low levels of Ig G2 or Ig G3. *N Engl J Med* 1985;313:720–724.

52. Ellison RT, Giehl TJ. Killing of gram-negative bacteria by lactoferrin and lysozyme. *J Clin Invest* 1991;88:1080–1091.

53. Yamauchi KM, Tomita M, Giehl T, et al. Antibacterial activity of lactoferrin and a pepsin-derived lactoferrin peptide fragment. *Infect Immun* 1993;61:719–728.

54. Bullen JJ. The significance of iron in infection. *Rev Infect Dis* 1981;3:1127–1138.

55. Goodman JW. The immune response. In: Stites DP, Terr AI, eds. *Basic and clinical immunology*. Norwalk, CT: Appleton and Lange, 1991.

56. Laurenzi GA, Potter RT, Kass EH. Bacteriologic flora of the lower respiratory tract. *New Engl J Med* 1961;265:1273.

57. Laurenzi GA, Guarneri JJ. A study of the mechanisms of pulmonary resistance to infection: The relationship of bacterial clearance to ciliary and alveolar macrophage function. *Am Rev Respir Dis* 1966;93:134–141.

58. Coleridge JCG, Coleridge HM. Lower respiratory tract afferents stimulated by inhaled irritants. *Am Rev Respir Dis* 1985;131:S51–S54.

59. Proctor DF. The naso-oro-pharyngo-laryngeal airway. *Eur J Respir Dis* 1983;128:89–96.

60. Korpas J, Tomori Z. *Cough and other respiratory reflexes.* Basel: Karger, 1977.

61. Irwin RS, Corrao WM, Pratter MR. Chronic persistent cough in the adult: the spectrum and frequency of causes and successful outcome of specific therapy. *Am Rev Respir Dis* 1981;123:413–417.

62. Huxley EJ, Viroslav J, Gray WR, et al. Pharyngeal aspiration in normal adults and patients with depressed consciousness. *Am J Med* 1978;64:564–568.

63. Crausaz FM, Favez G. Aspiration of solid food particles into lungs of patients with gastroesophageal reflux and chronic bronchial disease. *Chest* 1988;93:376–78.

64. Wayne JW, Ramphal R, Hood CI. Tracheal mucosal damage after aspiration. *Am Rev Respir Dis* 1981;124:728.

65. Elpern EH, Jacobs ER, Bone RC. Incidence of aspiration in tracheally intubated adults. *Heart Lung* 1987;16:527–531.

66. Splaingard ML, Hutchins B, Sulton LD, et al. Aspiration in rehabilation patients: videofluoroscopy vs bedside clinical assessment. *Arch Phys Med Rehabil* 1988;69:637–640.

67. Elpern EH, Scott MG, Petro L, et al. Pulmonary aspiration in mechanically ventilated patients with tracheostomies. *Chest* 1994;105:563–566.

68. Sasaki C, Suzuki M, Horiuchi M, et al. The effect of tracheostomy on the laryngeal closure reflex. *Laryngoscope* 1977;87:1428–1433.

69. Muz J, Mathog RH, Miller PR, et al. Detection and quantification of laryngotracheopulmonary aspiration with scintigraphy. *Laryngoscope* **1987;97:1180–1185.**

70. Silver KH, Van Nostrand D. The use of scintigraphy in the management of patients with pulmonary aspiration. *Dysphagia* 1994;9:107–115.

71. Muz J, Hamlet S, Mathog R, et al. Scintigraphic assessment of aspiration in head and neck cancer patients with tracheostomy. *Head Neck* 1994;16:17–20.

72. Ikari T, Sasaki C. Glottic closure reflex: control mechanisms. *Ann Otol Rhinol Laryngol* 1980;89:220–224.

73. Dettelbach MA, Gross RD, Mahlmann J, et al. The effect of the Passy-Muir valve on aspiration in patients with tracheostomy. *Head Neck* 1995;17:297–302.

74. Ebling DE, Gross RD: Subglottic airway pressure: a key component of swallowing efficiency. *Ann Otol Rhinol Laryngol* 1996;105:253–258.

75. Jacob SW, Francone CA, Lassow WJ: *Structure and function in man.* Philadelphia: WB Saunders, 1982:445.

76. Becker W, Naumann HH, Pfaltz CR. Nose, nasal sinuses and face: applied anatomy and physiology. In: Buckingham RA, ed. *Ear, nose and throat diseases. a pocket reference.* Second edition. New York: Thieme, 1994:175.

77. Becker W, Naumann HH, Pfaltz CR. Larynx, hypopharynx and trachea: applied anatomy and physiology. In: Buckingham RA, ed. *Ear, nose and throat diseases. a pocket reference.* Second edition. New York: Thieme, 1994:389.

78. Prakash UBS: *Bronchoscopy.* New York: Raven Press, 1994:2.

79. Rochester DF, Esau SA. The respiratory muscles. In: Baum GL, Wolinsky E, eds. *Textbook of pulmonary diseases.* Vol. 1. Boston: Little, Brown and Company, 1994:74.

80. Bray JJ, Cragg PA, Macknight ADC, et al. *Lecture notes on human physiology.* Cambridge: Blackwell Scientific Publications, 1989:490.

2

Respiratory Insufficiency: Pathophysiology, Indications, and Other Considerations for Intervention

JOHN R. BACH AND YUKA ISHIKAWA

This chapter considers the mechanisms by which conventionally managed patients with any combination of weak inspiratory, expiratory, and throat muscles develop respiratory complications and respiratory failure. The means by which these complications can be avoided, hospitalizations eliminated, and tracheostomy avoided are presented.

Ventilation Versus Oxygenation Failure

Most bodily functions tend to plateau by age 19 years and diminish thereafter. Pulmonary function is no exception. Normally, the vital capacity (VC) (the maximum volume of air that one can inhale with one breath) plateaus at 19 years of age and thereafter decreases by 1% per year in men and 1.2% per year in women throughout life (1). Likewise, the ability to cough, or peak cough flows (PCF), plateau at 12–18 L/s then decrease to as little as 6 L/s in healthy elderly individuals. For those with lung disease or neuromusculoskeletal conditions, pulmonary function can plateau prematurely, and its rate of decline can greatly exceed normal (Fig. 2–1).

Although there may be significant overlap, particularly in the elderly, respiratory pathology can be categorized as intrinsic versus mechanical. People with obstructive lung diseases like chronic obstructive pulmonary disease, cystic fibrosis, and bronchopulmonary dysplasia have intrinsic lung disease, whereas people with restrictive lung diseases like neuromuscular diseases, spinal cord injury, and pulmonary fibrosis have essentially mechanical lung impairment. Those with in-

Tracheostomy and Ventilator Dependency: Management of Breathing, Speaking, and Swallowing. Edited by Donna C. Tippett, MPH, MA, CCC-SLP. Thieme Medical Publishers, Inc. New York © 2000.

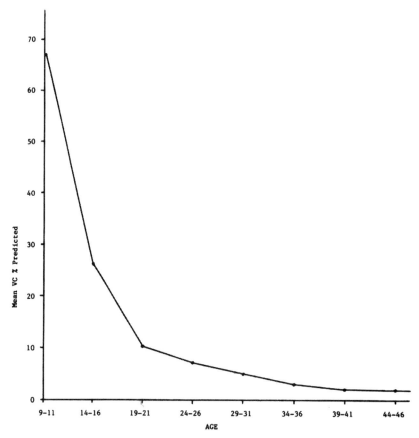

Fig. 2–1. Deterioration of vital capacity as a function of age for 29 Duchenne muscular dystrophy ventilator users. Reprinted, with permission, from Bach, Alba, Pilkington, and Lee (49).

trinsic disease have significant ventilation-perfusion mismatching that results primarily in impaired oxygenation of the blood. These patients are normocapnic or hypocapnic, often with severe hypoxemia. Significant hypercapnia occurs only during episodes of acute respiratory failure or with end-stage disease. On the other hand, those with mechanical dysfunction of the lungs or chest wall with respiratory muscle dysfunction develop global alveolar hypoventilation (GAH). For these patients hypercapnia usually precedes significant hypoxia or oxyhemoglobin desaturation. Ventilatory dysfunction, therefore, causes the abnormality in blood oxygenation and it should be corrected to normalize blood oxygen levels.

Despite the contrasting pathophysiology in intrinsic and mechanical conditions, there is a common tendency to manage ventilatory dysfunction like oxygenation impairment with the administration of oxygen, by intermittent positive pressure breathing (IPPB) treatments or bi-level positive airway pressure at inadequate pressures to assist inspiratory muscle function adequately, by continuous positive airway pressure (CPAP), and by over-medication, especially during respiratory tract infections. Indeed, for individuals with impaired oxygenation or ventilatory dysfunction, effective noninvasive methods of respiratory muscle rest and airway secretion clearance are underutilized as are other rehabilitation modalities in general (2). For both groups this leads to unnecessary dyspnea and hospitalizations (3), overreliance on intubation and tracheostomy (4), excessive physical deconditioning, and restriction in activities of daily living.

Pathophysiology

Restrictive Pulmonary Syndromes

Individuals with restrictive pulmonary syndromes have a reduction in VC. Restriction can be due to a combination of respiratory muscle weakness, paralysis, and mechanical factors involving the chest wall and lungs. Mechanical problems associated with chronic alveolar hypoventilation include thoracic deformities such as those which occur in the presence of scoliosis, morbid obesity, the use of improperly fitting thoracolumbar braces (used to hinder the development of scoliosis), and sleep associated hypopharyngeal collapse (obstructive sleep apnea) or other upper airway narrowing (5). Acute conditions that decrease pulmonary function, such as bronchial mucus plugging, pulmonary infiltrations, pleural diseases, pneumothoraces, and other respiratory complications, can exacerbate hypercapnia by making it more difficult to ventilate the lungs. It can result in acute respiratory failure when some combination of hypoventilation and ventilation-perfusion mismatching cause the patient to decompensate and develop severe blood gas disturbances.

For individuals with restrictive disorders who do not receive deep mechanically assisted insufflations, a rapid, shallow breathing pattern and inability to take occasional deep breaths can lead to microatelectasis in as little as 1 h (6). The long-term inability to take deep breaths, or chronic hypoinflation, leads to chronic microatelectasis and permanent loss, or for children, underdevelopment of lung tissues as well as decreased chest wall elasticity (7,8) and decreased pulmonary compliance (7,9,10). When the lungs and chest walls are not fully expanded by the taking or receiving of deep volumes of air, the lung tissues and the articulations of the spine and rib cage become tight and stiff. This occurs very much in the same way that skeletal articulations become stiff and contracted when they are not put through their full range of motion at least several times a day. Thus, decreased pulmonary compliance results initially from microatelectasis and ultimately from increased stiffness of the chest wall and lung tissues themselves (8). Pulmonary deterioration is exacerbated by suboptimal treatment of acute respiratory tract infections that lead to repeated pneumonic processes, pulmonary scarring, and further loss of elasticity. The presence of scoliosis exacerbates the loss of compliance which, in turn, increases the work of breathing.

Inadequacy of inspiratory muscle function can be the result of any combination of primary neuromuscular dysfunction, thoracic cage deformity, loss of respiratory exchange membrane and decreased pulmonary compliance, obstructive airway disease, or severe sleep disordered breathing. The atelectasis and increased work of breathing associated with respiratory muscle dysfunction lead to GAH (5).

Hypercapnia is likely when the VC falls below 55% of predicted normal and it is insidiously progressive (11). This results directly from the resort to shallow breathing to avoid overloading inspiratory muscles (12) and can, in itself, decrease respiratory muscle strength (13,14). The risk of pulmonary morbidity and mortality from acute respiratory failure correlates with increasing hypercapnia (15,16). Hypoxia and hypercapnia are exacerbated when intrinsic lung disease, scoliosis, sleep disordered breathing, or obesity complicate inspiratory muscle weakness. When not corrected by appropriate use of inspiratory muscle aids, the hypercapnia triggers the kidneys to retain bicarbonate ions (a compensatory metabolic alkalosis) (5). As the levels of blood bicarbonate increase, bicarbonate levels also increase in the brain. This, in turn, depresses the ventilatory response to hypoxia and hypercapnia. This permits worsening of GAH, and may decrease the effectiveness of the nocturnal use of inspiratory muscle aids once instituted (5); however, effective use of inspiratory muscle aids, even though often becoming necessary 24 h a day, can normalize blood carbon dioxide levels. This in turn neutralizes blood acidity and thereby relieves the strain on the heart muscle that would otherwise occur in the presence of acidic or hypoxic blood (17).

Individuals with restrictive pulmonary syndromes experience weakness of expiratory as well as inspiratory muscles. Indeed, the former is usually more marked than the latter (11,18). Expiratory muscle weakness decreases PCF. PCF is also decreased by any inspiratory muscle weakness that decreases the inspiratory capacity below 2.5 L (19), bulbar muscle weakness that impairs the retention of an optimal breath with a closed glottis or leads to aspiration of food or saliva, upper airway obstruction whether from tracheal stenosis, laryngeal muscle incompetence or postintubation vocal fold adhesions or paralysis, lower airway obstruction from concomitant obstructive pulmonary disease, or any other impediment to the generation of optimal cough airflows such as the presence of a foreign body somewhere in the airway. These individuals have difficulty clearing secretions, particularly during upper respiratory tract infections, when their spontaneous or assisted PCF does not exceed 5 L/s. They require an indwelling tracheostomy tube when PCF can no longer exceed 3 L/s at any time (20). In this case, mucus plugging can lead to ventilation-perfusion imbalance, gross atelectasis, airway collapse, pulmonary infiltrates and scarring, and eventually cardiopulmonary arrest. The cough reflex is also suppressed during sleep, and it is during sleep that mucus plugs may be more likely to cause sudden hypoxia and acute respiratory failure. Many patients with myopathic disease, such as Duchenne muscular dystrophy, also have varying degrees of cardiomyopathy that render them susceptible to hypoxia-triggered arrhythmias and cardiac decompensation.

Smoking, the presence of an endotracheal cannula, or profuse production of airway mucus for any other reason increases the tendency to develop chronic mucus plugging. For individuals managed conventionally, that is, without manually assisted coughing and assisted ventilation methods, chronic mucus plugging often leads to repeated intubation, bronchoscopy, and possibly permanent tracheostomy. The latter also reduces PCF; and failure of suction catheters to enter the left mainstem bronchus during routine suctioning can also lead to increased morbidity.

The first significant chronic blood gas abnormalities seen in individuals with restrictive pulmonary syndromes due to Duchenne muscular dystrophy, and probably in other neuromuscular conditions, usually occur during rapid eye movement sleep as short periods of hypercapnia and eventually hypoxemia (21). These periods gradually extend throughout most of sleep before significant blood gas disturbances occur with the person awake (22,23). As noted, the ventilatory responses to hypoxia and hypercapnia are diminished during sleep (24), and since the threshold for arousal is lower to hypoxia and higher to hypercapnia, more severe and prolonged blood gas alterations can occur without arousing the individual. Unless treated, this may result in increased risk of cardiac arrhythmia and cor pulmonale. For those who have arterial blood carbon dioxide tensions ($PaCO_2$) of greater than 50 mm Hg when awake, nocturnal oxyhemoglobin saturation (SaO_2) below 85% can occur (25). Increasing $PaCO_2$ and decreasing arterial oxygen tensions (PaO_2) cross at about 60 mm Hg—a point at which it is tempting, but an error, to provide supplemental oxygen. Supplemental oxygen administration normalizes SaO_2, but only at the expense of worsening hypercapnia, and causes coma or death from carbon dioxide narcosis. Oxygen levels should be stabilized by normalizing lung ventilation rather than by exacerbating lung underventilation.

Nocturnal blood gas alterations ultimately extend to 24 h a day as GAH. Waking hypercapnia tends to occur as a resort to shallow breathing to avoid respiratory muscle fatigue (26) when the VC falls below 40% (27) to 55% (11) of predicted normal. Severe carbon dioxide retention itself has been demonstrated to decrease muscle strength further (28). Normocapnic hypoxemia is also common (16) and may be due to decreased total oxygen diffusion across a diminished respiratory exchange membrane from microatelectasis or pulmonary fibrosis. Ventilatory insufficiency progresses insidiously, and the risk of acute respiratory failure increases with the loss of pulmonary volumes.

Obstructive Pulmonary Disease

Chronic obstructive pulmonary disease (COPD) affects 10 to 40% of all Americans, and is the fifth leading cause of death in the United States. It is likely to become increasingly prevalent with the increasing life expectancy of the general population (29).

Chronic bronchitis, emphysema, asthmatic bronchitis, and cystic fibrosis, the most common causes of COPD, usually have significant elements of both airway obstruction and disease of the lung tissues themselves. Emphysema and chronic bronchitis often result from a combination of genetic predisposition and environmental factors which include allergic reversible bronchoconstriction (asthma), respiratory infections, chemical inflammation (cigarette smoke, asbestoses), and, occasionally, metabolic abnormalities (e.g., alpha1-antitrypsin deficiency).

Cigarette smoking is the most common primary cause of COPD and lung cancer. One in 15 smokers will succumb to lung cancer. Depending on the amounts smoked, smokers are also up to 25 times more likely to die of COPD than nonsmokers (30); and all one-pack-a-day smokers would eventually develop emphy-

Table 2–1.   Signs and symptoms of alveolar hypoventilation.

Fatigue
Morning headaches
Frequent sleep arousals with dyspnea and tachycardia
Hypersomnolence
Difficulty with concentration
Frequent nightmares
Nightmares concerning breathing
Signs and symptoms of cor pulmonale
Lower extremity edema
Irritability, anxiety
Nocturnal urinary frequency
Polycythemia (documented Hct >50)
Impaired intellectual function
Nausea
Drop in grades at school
Depression
Decreased libido
Excessive weight loss
Muscle aches
Memory impairment
Poor control of upper airway secretions
Obesity

sema. On the average, 30- to 35-year-olds who smoke 10 to 20 cigarettes per day die five years sooner than do nonsmokers (31). Smoking cessation has been associated with improvement in symptoms (32) and pulmonary function (33), decreased risk of respiratory tract infections (34), and a long-term reduction in rate of loss of forced expiratory volumes (35).

Emphysema is characterized by distention of air spaces distal to terminal nonrespiratory bronchioles with destruction of alveolar walls. This occurs because of the unimpeded action of neutrophil-derived elastase at the bases of the lungs. This enzyme punches holes in biologic membranes to allow neutrophil entry. Alpha1-antiprotease normally protects the lungs by inactivating neutrophil-derived elastase, but it is destroyed by cigarette smoke and other toxins. This results in chronic inflammation and impairment of mucociliary clearance (36). Ultimately, there is loss of lung recoil, excessive airway collapse on exhalation, and chronic airflow obstruction.

Chronic bronchitis and cystic fibrosis are characterized by enlargement of tracheobronchial mucous glands and chronic mucus hypersecretion and chest infections. Of those with chronic bronchitis, 10% have an element of reversible bronchospasm. Unlike asthmatic bronchitis, however, most chronic bronchitis is irreversible; there is a lack of bronchial hyperreactivity; and there is a lack of responsiveness to bronchodilators (37). Mucus hypersecretion occurs, however, in both reversible and irreversible bronchitis, blocking airways, and setting the stage for recurrent infection, and airway and alveolar damage.

The respiratory muscles of COPD patients often become inadequate to handle the high ventilation levels needed to oxygenate the blood in the face of decreased respiratory exchange membrane surface area. Malnutrition is also commonly present and leads to respiratory muscle atrophy. Hypercapnic COPD patients have also been shown to have weaker respiratory muscles than normocapnic patients (38,39).

Indications for Intervention

The indication for introducing ventilatory assistance is symptomatic hypercapnia, whether hypercapnia is nocturnal-only or around-the-clock, or whether the patient has primarily obstructive or restrictive lung disease. The symptoms of chronic alveolar hypoventilation or hypercapnia are listed in Table 2–1.

Irrespective of the extent or duration of ventilatory insufficiency, ventilatory support can always be provided as well by a noninvasive means as by delivering intermittent positive pressure ventilation (IPPV) via an indwelling tracheostomy tube for individuals without severe intrinsic lung disease who have functional pharyngeal musculature (Table 2–2). However, individuals with primarily obstructive or intrinsic lung disease often require supplemental oxygen therapy

Table 2–2. Common conditions leading to chronic alveolar hypoventilation and functional pharyngeal musculature.

Neurological disorders
  Disorders of anterior horn cells like poliomyelitis, the spinal muscular atrophies, and
    motor neuron diseases
  Neuropathies involving the phrenic nerve including postsurgically associated with
    cardiac hypothermia, traumatic, radiation-induced, familial, paraneoplastic,
    infectious, autoimmune, Guillian-Barré syndrome, and idiopathic
  Multiple sclerosis
  Friedreich's ataxia
  Myelopathies of rheumatoid, infectious, spondylitic, vascular, traumatic, or idiopathic
    etiology
  Tetraplegia associated with pancuronium bromide, botulism

Myopathies
  Muscular dystrophies
    Duchenne and Becker dystrophinopathies
    Limb-girdle, Emery-Dreifuss, facioscapulohumeral, congenital, childhood autosomal
      recessive, and myotonic muscular dystrophy
    Congenital, metabolic, toxic, and inflammatory myopathies
    Myasthenia gravis

Sleep disordered breathing including obesity hypoventilation, central and congenital
    hypoventilation syndromes, and hypoventilation associated with diabetic
    microangiopathy, or familial dysautonomia
  Kyphoscoliosis
  Associated with lung resection
  Chronic obstructive pulmonary disease

which renders nocturnal noninvasive IPPV less effective (40), and the hypercollapsibility of their lower airways can render noninvasive airway secretion elimination methods ineffective. Specifically, those with GAH on the basis of respiratory muscle weakness who can generate over 160 L/min of PCF or for whom over 160 L/min of PCF can be generated by manually assisted coughing do not require tracheostomy tubes for long-term ventilatory support (41).

Noninvasive IPPV, including mouthpiece and nasal IPPV, are described in Chapter 3 and elsewhere (42).

The neurophysiologic mechanisms by which nasal IPPV can be effective during sleep include mechanical sealing of the oropharynx by the soft palate or lip closure to prevent excessive insufflation leakage and decreases in SaO_2. This does not appear to occur in a timely manner when patients receive supplemental oxygen. We speculate that this can be explained by failure of central mediated activity to decrease insufflation leakage when SaO_2 is maintained within normal limits by oxygen supplementation. Further evidence that corroborates this is that nasal IPPV is less effective in the acute setting for ventilator users who receive oxygen supplementation, particularly during sleep (5,43).

Thus, when SaO_2 is maintained within normal range by noninvasive methods of assisted ventilation and coughing, acute respiratory failure is avoided and neither hospitalization nor tracheostomy are needed even though individuals often become ventilator dependent around-the-clock. Indeed, patients are often much better cared for at home than in any hospital because hospitals often do not have the portable ventilators and other equipment to permit optimal use of noninvasive ventilation and it is very difficult for hospital nurses to provide manually assisted coughing and mechanical insufflation–exsufflation every 10–15 min or so as needed during severe chest colds whereas a devoted family member or care provider is often more than willing to do so.

Further, virtually no one with functional pharyngeal musculature who uses tracheostomy IPPV needs to use an inflated cuff out of the acute care setting (44). Despite these facts, physicians often fail to permanently deflate tracheostomy cuffs (44). This impairs swallowing and oral communication and eliminates the many options that can facilitate oral communication with a deflated cuff or cuffless tracheostomy tube (see Chapter 5).

Chronically hypoxic and hypercapnic individuals with intrinsic or obstructive lung disease benefit from oxygen administration and may benefit from IPPV; however, the prognosis is very poor whether the person is using invasive or noninvasive IPPV. Despite oxygen administration, a trial of nocturnal nasal IPPV is warranted when symptoms of hypercapnia are suspected.

Ventilators

Until 1978, most ventilators for long-term use were pressure-cycled ventilators. The pressures were set on these machines, and the volumes that they delivered varied with the airway resistance on a breath by breath basis. Typically, the pressures were set at about 20 cm H_2O. When the airway was obstructed by secretions, food, or spasm, the delivered air quickly reached the set pressure limit, and little air was delivered. Likewise, when there was a leak in the system, the ventilators increased their output to attempt to reach the set pressures. These ventilators had few or no alarms and when volume-triggered ventilators became available in 1978, they quickly became the most popular ventilators for home mechanical ventilation.

Today, tracheostomy IPPV is most commonly delivered via volume-triggered ventilators. Likewise, volume-cycled ventilators should also be used for all but small children with ventilatory insufficiency due to paralytic conditions. The volume, rate, high and low pressure alarms, and flow rates are typically set on these ventilators. When delivered volumes are increased, the flow rates must be increased or else there will not be sufficient time for the patient to exhale. Volume-triggered ventilators can usually provide synchronized intermittent mandatory ventilation (SIMV), assist-control ventilation, positive end-expiratory pressure (PEEP), pressure-assist ventilation, and supplemental oxygen. When the SIMV mode is set at a particular volume and rate, the ventilator delivers the set volume at the indicated rate and the patient breathes on his or her own between the assisted breaths, that is, he or she breathes through the circuit unaided until the ventilator delivers the next volume. SIMV should not be used with portable volume ventilators because of the resistance (obstruction) to unaided breathing through the ventilator circuitry between ventilator-delivered volumes.

With assist-control mode, each breath that the patient initiates is assisted by a set volume, and a backup rate can be adjusted to deliver the set volume even if the patient does not trigger the machine with his or her own efforts. Thus, volume-triggered ventilators deliver set volumes of air irrespective of airway resistance. Therefore, when the airway is obstructed by mucus, food, or spasms, the airway pressure can increase considerably, but the delivered volumes are not diminished. Likewise, if a leak is created in the system, the pressures fall and the ventilator does not increase the delivered volumes to compensate for the leakage.

Volume-triggered ventilators have both high and low pressure alarms. Among other things, the high pressure alarm permits them to also be used in a pressure-assist mode, a manner similar to that of pressure-triggered ventilators. That is, when the high pressure alarm is set to any desired amount (e.g., 20 cm H_2O) and the delivered volumes are set very high (e.g., 1,500 ml) the amount of air delivered to the patient's lungs will be a function of the set pressure. Once the quantity of air creates pressure in the lungs that equals that which is set on the ventilator, the rest of the as yet undelivered 1,500 ml of air is then vented to the atmosphere.

Pressure support ventilation, now available on certain portable volume ventilators, supplements each breath with the volume of air required to attain a set pressure. This approach is very similar to that of using a pressure-triggered ventilator. When pressures are set at about 20 cm H_2O, essentially full ventilatory support is provided. Pressure support is often provided in conjunction with assist-control mode ventilation, PEEP, and supplemental oxygen when attempting to wean patients from ventilators. This often unnecessarily complicated approach is suboptimal for weaning most patients with paralytic conditions (Table 2–2) because the ventilatory support is not controlled by the patient but by the machine and, as a result, there is a tendency for overventilation and inspiratory muscle deconditioning (45). The use of noninvasive respiratory muscle aids can be more effective than the pressure support, PEEP, supplemental oxygen combination by permitting the individual to control his or her own assisted ventilation and thereby avoiding hyperventilation and deconditioning (45).

Continuous positive airway pressure is most often delivered by CPAP machines. Its use is essentially to splint open the airways of sleeping individuals with obstructive sleep apnea syndrome. It is much like breathing with one's head outside of a speeding car. It fills the lungs with air; however, exhaling against a constant flow is unnecessary and uncomfortable for those with paralytic ventilatory insufficiency. Further, it does not assist inspiratory muscle function, and the increases in thoracic pressure that it causes can result in hemodynamic disturbances. Nevertheless, it is often used for individuals with obesity-hypoventilation syndrome despite the fact that simply splinting open their airways is rarely adequate because even with open airways the inspiratory muscles are not up to the task of ventilating the lungs. Bi-level positive airway pressure is more useful for people with inspiratory muscle weakness.

Bi-level positive airway pressure permits the independent adjustment of the inspiratory (IPAP) and expiratory airway pressures (EPAP). Thus, an IPAP of 12 cm H_2O can be delivered along with an EPAP of 7 cm H_2O. This has the effect of providing a pressure-assist of 12 minus 7, or 5 cm H_2O. This is often adequate for assisting ventilation for individuals with mild nocturnal alveolar hypoventilation due to mild inspiratory muscle weakness, but as weakness progresses, bi-level positive airway pressure becomes inadequate. Even when used at maximum IPAPs and minimum EPAPs, bi-level positive airway pressure spans are limited to under 35 cm H_2O and thus cannot deliver the large volumes of air required for the deep breaths needed for effective assisted coughing. Thus, bi-level positive airway pressure should not be used as a substitute for volume-cycled ventilators for adolescents or adults with chronic alveolar hypoventilation.

Swallowing and Speech Considerations

Individuals using bi-level positive airway pressure often complain of gagging as high flows reach the posterior pharynx when air leakage out of the mouth causes the machines to suddenly increase air delivery to compensate the leak. Flow rates cannot be adjusted on bi-level positive airway pressure machines. Likewise, the continuous delivery of air during both inspiratory and expiratory cycles makes swallowing very difficult if not impossible for individuals using nasal CPAP or bi-level positive airway pressure. Those who require 24-h ventilatory support should be switched to using volume-triggered ventilators during daytime hours and particularly during mealtimes. Likewise, nasal IPPV should not be used during waking hours except when the patient's lips or neck are too weak to grab a mouthpiece or the person is in bed. IPPV delivered via a mouthpiece held near to the mouth is the ideal method of ventilatory support for 24-h ventilator users during meals and during waking hours, in general. The individual takes a deep insufflation, then chews and swallows, and may repeat the process about six to eight times per minute.

Although there is no difficulty speaking when one uses mouthpiece IPPV and the increased volumes can greatly increase voice volume, speech during nasal

IPPV requires some attention. When individuals attempt to speak during the delivery of nasal IPPV, the transient glottic closure needed to generate consonant sounds causes high pressure in the eustachian tubes, and with it, sudden ear pain. Individuals quickly learn not to speak during these nasal insufflations. Once learned the patient can air stack using a mouthpiece or nasal IPPV, and the deep volumes permit many individuals to shout.

Although it is usually unnecessary to resort to tracheostomy for long-term ventilatory support or airway secretion elimination, because most clinicians suffer from intubation and tracheostomy paradigm paralysis (46), patients continue to be managed in this manner. Likewise, tracheostomy cuff inflation is not always needed to provide IPPV effectively or eliminate aspiration of food or upper airway secretions (44). Continuous cuff inflation is only indicated for those with severely paralyzed pharyngeal and laryngeal musculature. For most others who can articulate words, even those who tend to aspirate food, cuff deflation should be maintained at all times. The patient learns to use his or her glottis to control how much of the ventilator-delivered volume directly crosses the vocal folds (insufflation leakage) and how much initially enters the lungs before being exhaled out of the tracheostomy tube or out the upper airway for those using one-way tracheostomy tube valves or expiratory valve caps. Ventilator-delivered volumes are specifically set high enough to provide adequate leak for effective insufflation leakage speech and alveolar ventilation. A secondary benefit of this approach is that the upward airflows carry away airway debris and secretions that would otherwise stagnate on the cuff. If the leak is too little for effective speech despite delivered volumes that are high enough to hyperventilate the patient, then if any cuff is present it should be removed or else a smaller diameter tracheostomy tube should be placed with or without a cuff. If the leak is too great for adequate alveolar ventilation, then a wider diameter tracheostomy tube should be placed. Periods of cuff deflation often need to be increased as tolerated. This is because the tracheal walls are irritated and often irreparably damaged by cuff inflation and, with the cuff deflated, the high airflow pressures against them can cause discomfort.

Although, for individuals who are usually maintained with cuff deflation, there is a tendency to inflate the cuff overnight or during meals, both are usually unnecessary (5). Since cuff inflation hampers swallowing, it should be avoided if at all possible. Oximetry can be used to screen for food aspiration during meals. By blocking airways that feed large areas of respiratory exchange membrane, aspiration of airway secretions or food can cause a decrease from normal SaO_2. This must be quickly reversed by expelling the aspirated material. It is our clinical impression that chronic aspiration that does not result in a decrease in SaO_2 from a normal baseline is not associated with a high risk of respiratory complications, whereas aspiration associated with a long-term decrease in SaO_2 from normal levels is associated with a high risk of recurrent pneumonias. Any desaturations caused by food aspiration should be immediately reversed by performing mechanical insufflation–exsufflation via the indwelling tracheostomy tube. For most individuals, cuff inflation is only indicated during mechanical insufflation–exsufflation.

Summary

Thus, the use of inspiratory and expiratory muscle aids, rather than tracheo-stomy, facilitates speech, swallowing, quality of life, and survival with less risk of pulmonary complications and hospitalizations. Individuals with experience in using both invasive and noninvasive alternatives invariably prefer the latter (47); and noninvasive alternatives are much less expensive than the invasive options (48). Despite this, it has been more lucrative to place a tracheostomy tube than to take one out, perform bronchoscopy rather than eliminate bronchial mucus by insufflation–exsufflation, and hospitalize patients in intensive care rather than treat them at home with an oximeter, ventilator, and an insufflator–exsufflator. Recognition of the potential to save healthcare dollars and maintain quality of life by supporting the training and equipping of patients so that they can stay healthy and remain home will spare these individuals otherwise inevitable acute respiratory failure.

References

1. Bach JR. Pulmonary assessment and management of the aging and older patient. In: Felsenthal G, Garrison SJ, Steinberg FU, eds. *Rehabilitation of the aging and elderly patient*. Baltimore: Williams & Wilkins, 1993:263–273.
2. Bach JR. Ventilator use by muscular dystrophy association patients: An update. *Arch Phys Med Rehabil* 1992;73:179–183.
3. Bach JR, Rajaraman R, Ballanger F, Tzeng AC, Ishikawa Y, Kulessa R, Bansal T. Neuromuscular ventilatory insufficiency: The effect of home mechanical ventilator use vs. oxygen therapy on pneumonia and hospitalization rates. *Am J Phys Med Rehabil* 1998;77:8–19.
4. Bach JR, Ishikawa Y, Kim H. Prevention of pulmonary morbidity for patients with Duchenne muscular dystrophy. *Chest* 1997;112:1024–1028.
5. Bach JR, Alba AS. Management of chronic alveolar hypoventilation by nasal ventilation. Chest 1990;97:52–57.
6. Miller WF. Rehabilitation of patients with chronic obstructive lung disease. *Med Clin N Am* 1967;51:349–361.
7. De Troyer A, Deisser P. The effects of intermittent positive pressure breathing on patients with respiratory muscle weakness. *Am Rev Respir Dis* 1981;124:132–137.
8. Estenne M, De Troyer A. The effects of tetraplegia on chest wall statics. *Am Rev Respir Dis* 1986;134:121–124.
9. De Troyer A, Borenstein S, Cordier R. Analysis of lung volume restriction in patients with respiratory muscle weakness. *Thorax* 1980;35:603–610.
10. Gibson GJ, Pride NB, Newsom-Davis J, Loh LC. Pulmonary mechanics in patients with respiratory muscle weakness. *Am Rev Respir Dis* 1977;115:389–395.
11. Braun NMT, Arora MS, Rochester DF. Respiratory muscle and pulmonary function in polymyositis and other proximal myopathies. *Thorax* 1983;38:616–623.
12. Begin P, Grassino A. Inspiratory muscle dysfunction and chronic hypercapnia in chronic obstructive pulmonary disease. *Am Rev Respir Dis* 1983;143:905–912.
13. Rochester DF, Braun NMT. Determinants of maximal inspiratory pressure in chronic obstructive pulmonary disease. *Am Rev Respir Dis* 1985;132:42–47.
14. Stubbing DG, Pengelly LD, Morse JLC, Jones NL. Pulmonary mechanics during exercise in subjects with chronic airflow obstruction. *J Appl Physiol* 1980;49:511–515.
15. Boushy SF, Thompson HK Jr, North LB, et al. Prognosis in chronic obstructive pulmonary disease. *Am Rev Respir Dis* 1973;108:1373–1383.
16. Inkley SR, Oldenburg FC, Vignos PJ Jr. Pulmonary function in Duchenne muscular dystrophy related to stage of disease. *Am J Med* 1974;56:297–306.

17. Enson Y, Giuntini C, Lewis ML, et al. The influence of hydrogen ion concentration and hypoxia on the pulmonary circulation. *J Clin Invest* 1964;43:1146–1162.

18. Griggs RG, Donohoe KM, Utell MJ, et al. Evaluation of pulmonary function in neuromuscular disease. *Arch Neurol* 1981;38:9–12.

19. Leith DE. Lung biology in health and desease: respiratory defense mechainisms, part 2. In: Brain JD, Proctor D, Reid L, eds. *Cough.* New York: Marcel Dekker, 1977:545–592.

20. Bach JR. Mechanical insufflation-exsufflation: comparison of peak expiratory flows with manually assisted and unassisted coughing techniques. *Chest* 1993;104:1553–1562.

21. Redding GJ, Okamoto GA, Guthrie RD, Rollevson D, Milstein JM. Sleep patterns in nonambulatory boys with Duchenne muscular dystrophy. *Arch Phys Med Rehabil* 1985;66:818–821.

22. Smith PEM, Edwards RHT, Calverley PMA. Ventilation and breathing pattern during sleep in Duchenne muscular dystrophy. *Chest* 1989;96:1346–1351.

23. Soudon P. Ventilation assisteè au long cours dans les maladies neuro-musculaire: experience actuelle. *Readaptation Revalidatie* 1987;3:45–65.

24. Shneerson J. *Disorders of ventilation.* Boston: Blackwell Scientific Publications, 1988:43.

25. Ohtake S. Nocturnal blood gas disturbances and treatment of patients with Duchenne muscular dystrophy. *Kokyu To Junkan* 1990;38:463–469.

26. Begin P, Grassino A. Inspiratory muscle dysfunction and chronic hypercapnia in chronic obstructive pulmonary disease. *Am Rev Respir Dis* 1991;143:905–912.

27. Canny GJ, Szeinberg A, Koreska J, et al. Hypercapnia in relation to pulmonary function in Duchenne muscular dystrophy. *Pediatr Pulmonology* 1989;6:169–171.

28. Juan G, Calverley P, Talamo C. Effect of carbon dioxide on diaphragmatic function in human beings. *N Engl J Med* 1984;310:874–879.

29. Higgins ITT. Epidemiology of bronchitis and emphysema. In: Fishman AP, ed. *Pulmonary diseases and disorders*, 2nd ed. New York: McGraw-Hill, 1988:70–90.

30. Fishman AP. The spectrum of chronic obstructive disease of the airways. In: Fishman AP, ed. *Pulmonary diseases and disorders*, 2nd ed. New York: McGraw-Hill, 1988:1159–1171.

31. Department of Health Education and Welfare. *Smoking and health: A report of the Surgeon General.* DHEW Publication No. (PHS) 79-50066. Washington, D.C., 1979.

32. Leeder SR, Colley JRT, Corkhill R, et al. Change in respiratory symptom prevalence in adults who alter their smoking habits. *Am J Epidemiol* 1977;105:522–529.

33. Buist AS, Nagy JM, Sexton GJ. The effect of smoking cessation on pulmonary function: a 30-month follow-up of two smoking cessation clinics. *Am Rev Respir Dis* 1979;120:953–957.

34. Kark JD, Leguish M, Rannon L. Cigarette smoking as a risk factor for epidemic A (HI NI) influenza in young men. *N Engl J Med* 1982;307:1042–1046.

35. Bosse R, Sparrow D, Rose CL, et al. Longitudinal effect of age and smoking cessation on pulmonary function. *Am Rev Respir Dis* 1981;123:378–381.

36. Hillberg RE. Chronic obstructive pulmonary disease: causes and clinicopathologic considerations. In: Bach JR, ed. *Pulmonary rehabilitation: the obstructive and paralytic conditions.* Philadelphia: Hanley & Belfus, 1996:17–38.

37. Tager IB. Chronic bronchitis. In: Fishman AP, ed. *Pulmonary diseases and disorders*, 2nd ed. New York: McGraw-Hill, 1988:1543–1551.

38. Rochester DF, Braun NMT. Determinants of maximal inspiratory pressure in chronic obstructive pulmonary disease. *Am Rev Respir Dis* 1985;132:42–47.

39. Stubbing DG, Pengelly LD, Morse JLC, Jones NL. Pulmonary mechanics during exercise in subjects with chronic airflow obstruction. *J Appl Physiol* 1980;49:511–515.

40. Bach JR, Robert D, Leger P, et al. Sleep fragmentation in kyphoscoliotic individuals with alveolar hypoventilation treated by nasal IPPV. *Chest* 1995;107:1552–1558.

41. Bach JR. Amyotrophic lateral sclerosis: predictors for prolongation of life by noninvasive respiratory aids. *Arch Phys Med Rehabil* 1995;76:828–832.

42. Bach JR. Prevention of morbidity and mortality with the use of physical medicine aids. In: Bach JR, ed. *Pulmonary rehabilitation: the obstructive and paralytic conditions.* Philadelphia: Hanley & Belfus, 1996:303–329.

43. Wysocki M, Tric L, Wolff MA, Gertner J, Millet H, Herman B. Noninvasive pressure support ventilation in patients with acute respiratory failure. *Chest* 1993;103:907–913.

44. Bach JR, Alba AS. Tracheostomy ventilation: a study of efficacy with deflated cuffs and cuffless tubes. *Chest* 1990;97:679–683.

45. Bach JR, Saporito LR. Criteria for extubation and tracheostomy tube removal for patients with ventilatory failure: a different approach to weaning. *Chest* 1996;110:1566–1571.

46. Bach JR, Bach GA. Do you suffer from intubation and tracheostomy paradigm paralysis? *Respiratory Interventions* 1993;93:3,13.

47. Bach JR. A comparison of long-term ventilatory support alternatives from the perspective of the patient and care giver. *Chest* 1993;104:1702–1706.

48. Bach JR, Intintola P, Alba AS, Holland I. The ventilator-assisted individual: cost analysis of institutionalization versus rehabilitation and in-home management. *Chest* 1992;101:26–30.

49. Bach JR, Alba A, Pilkington LA, Lee M. Long-term rehabilitation in advanced stage of childhood onset, rapidly progressive muscular dystrophy. *Arch Phys Med Rehabil* 1981;62:328–331.

Glossary

air stacking—insufflations are stacked in the lungs to expand them maximally; this is done by taking a deep breath then adding consecutive volumes of air delivered via a mouthpiece or nasal interface and holding them with a closed glottis until no more air can be held and the lungs and chest wall are fully expanded

alpha1-antiprotease—an enzyme that protects lungs by inactivating neutrophil-derived elastase; capable of being destroyed by toxins such as cigarette smoke

alveolar ventilation—the passage of air into and out of the small air sacs (alveoli) of the respiratory exchange membrane of the lungs by the intermittent action of the diaphragm and other inspiratory muscles

alveolus—the microscopic air sacs of the lung from which oxygen diffuses into the blood and carbon dioxide diffuses out of the blood

amyotrophic lateral sclerosis—a disease of peripheral and spinal nerves of unknown cause that usually occurs between 50 and 70 years of age and can occur in juveniles and young adults, thereby at times creating confusion with disorders like spinal muscular atrophy

anterior horn cell diseases—disorders of the cell bodies of the peripheral nerves, the cell bodies located in the anterior (front) areas in the spinal cord that cause spinal muscular atrophy, amyotrophic lateral sclerosis, and poliomyelitis

apnea—absence of breathing for an abnormally long period of time

atelectasis—areas of collapse of lung air sacs (alveoli) due to underventilation or accumulation of airway secretions

Becker muscular dystrophy—a sex-linked recessive dystrophin deficient muscular dystrophy similar but milder than Duchenne muscular dystrophy

BiPAP—bi-level positive airway pressure, a method of ventilatory assistance

body ventilator—a device that acts on the body to assist breathing

bronchodilators—medications that open the airways of patients with asthma or bronchospasm from any cause

bronchoscopy—passage of a tube through the mouth or nose into the airways to remove airway secretions or perform a biopsy under direct vision

bulbar muscles—muscles located in the head and neck that include the oropharyngeal (mouth and throat) muscles, permitting speech, swallowing, and coughing

cannula—tubing entering the nose or mouth to deliver air or supplemental oxygen

capnograph—a device that measures the blood carbon dioxide level by analyzing the concentration of carbon dioxide in the exhaled air

carbon dioxide tension—the partial pressure of carbon dioxide in the blood; its level correlates inversely with lung ventilation, that is, blood carbon dioxide tensions increase (hypercapnia) when the lungs are under- (hypo) ventilated and decrease (hypocapnia) when the lungs are over- (hyper) ventilated

cardiomyopathy—weakness of the heart muscle caused by muscle pathology affecting the heart

chronic alveolar hypoventilation—lung underventilation that results in elevated CO_2 levels (hypercapnia)

compliance—(pulmonary compliance) essentially the elasticity of the lungs that decreases when one cannot take or does not receive deep breaths, leading to loss of lung tissue and lung stiffening

cor pulmonale—failure of the right side of the heart due to decreased blood oxygen levels (hypoxia) and increased blood carbon dioxide levels (hypercapnia) from lung underventilation

CO_2—carbon dioxide

CPAP (continuous positive airway pressure)—continuous pressure applied through a mask covering the nose, mouth, or mouth and nose that acts as a splint to keep the otherwise obstructed upper airway open and acts to expand the lungs but does not directly help one breathe; this is not a method of ventilatory or inspiratory muscle assistance

CPAP masks—nasal interfaces for the delivery of CPAP or nasal ventilation for ventilatory assistance

cystic fibrosis—the most commonly inherited disease of the lungs that causes profuse secretion of thick airway mucus that is difficult to cough out and obstucts airways

Duchenne muscular dystrophy—the most common, progressive, inherited disease of muscle

dyspnea—shortness of breath

dystrophin—the defective or absent protein of Duchenne and Becker muscular dystrophies

end-tidal carbon dioxide levels—the concentration or partial pressure of carbon dioxide in the last bit of air that one exhales that closely reflects the partial pressure of carbon dioxide in the arterial blood

Emerin—the defective protein in Emery-Dreifuss muscular dystrophy

Emery-Dreifuss muscular dystrophy—a sex-linked inherited muscular dystrophy affecting males; this condition has a high incidence of heart arrhythmias as well as the typical muscle degeneration seen with other muscular dystrophies

forced expiratory volumes—patients with obstructive airway disease have a decreased ability to forcibly expel air from their lungs because attempts to do so result in widespread collapse of airways and the trapping of air in the lungs

global alveolar hypoventilation—diffuse underventilation of all segments of the lungs

glottis—the opening between the vocal folds at the upper orifice of the larynx; the mouth of the windpipe

hypocapnia—decreased blood carbon dioxide levels due to alveolar hyperventilation

hypercapnia—increased blood carbon dioxide levels due to inability of the breathing muscles to ventilate the lungs adequately

hypoxia (hypoxemia)—decreased blood oxygen levels due to increased blood carbon dioxide levels, mucus plugging of the airways, or lung disease such as pneumonia

IPPB (intermittent positive pressure breathing)—the delivery of deep insufflations to expand the lungs more fully

IPPV (intermittent positive pressure ventilation)—a form of inspiratory muscle aid or ventilatory assistance provided by delivering air to the lungs via the mouth, nose, mouth-and-nose, or an indwelling tracheostomy tube

inspiratory capacity (predicted)—the volume of air that one should be able to inhale as a function of age, sex, and height, i.e., most adult males have predicted inspiratory capacities of over 3,000 ml

insufflation—providing greater volumes of air than one can inhale with one's own inspiratory muscles

intubation—passage of a tube via either the nose (nasotracheal tube) or the mouth (orotracheal tube) through the throat and larynx (translaryngeally) and into the trachea for ventilatory assistance and airway suctioning

larynx—the voice organ at the upper portion of the windpipe including the vocal folds

maximum insufflation capacity—the maximum volume of air that can be mechanically delivered to the patient's lungs and held by the patient in the lungs

mechanical insufflation–exsufflation—a technique whereby a device is used to provide a deep volume of air to the lungs (insufflation) immediately followed by a forced expiration (exsufflation) to create 10 L per s of expiratory flow to expel airway secretions

metabolic alkalosis—the relatively increased retention of bicarbonate and increased excretion of chloride by the kidneys that occurs most often as an attempt by the body to compensate for increased acidity of the blood that results from increased levels of CO_2 dissolved in the blood by lung hypoventilation

microatelectasis—areas of collapse of lung air sacs (alveoli) due to underventilation or accumulation of airway secretions that are too small to be documented by chest radiograph

muscular dystrophy—a myopathy in which there is ongoing muscle degeneration and regeneration

myopathy—any disorder characterized by anatomical, biochemical, or electrical abnormalities in muscle fibers and in which there is no evidence that they are due to nervous system dysfunction

myoneural junction—the junction where communication or synapse takes place between the nerves and muscle cells

neuropathy—any general anatomical, biochemical, or electrical disorder of nerves

neutrophil-derived elastase—an enzyme that makes a hole in biologic membranes thus allowing neutrophil entry

normocapnic—when blood carbon dioxide partial pressures are within normal physiological limits, approximately 34–44 mm Hg

oximeter—a device that can continuously measure the oxyhemoglobin saturation of the blood

oxygen—a gas needed by the body's metabolic processes the blood levels of which are decreased by underventilation (hypercapnia), airway mucus plugging, and lung disease

oxyhemoglobin saturation—oxyhemoglobin is the main oxygen-carrying protein in the blood, and, normally, it is 95% or more saturated with oxygen

O_2—oxygen

peak cough flows—the maximum flows that can be generated while coughing whether coughing occurs with or without assistance

PEEP (positive end-expiratory pressure)—pressure given at the end of a mechanically assisted breath

pneumonia—infection in the lungs usually caused by bacteria multiplying in airway secretions that cannot be expulsed from the lungs

pulmonary fibrosis—an infiltrative disease of the lung tissues that results in destruction of the respiratory exchange membrane and chronic respiratory failure

respirator—*See ventilator*

respiratory exchange membrane—the membrane interface between the lung's alveolar walls and the capillary membrane walls through which oxygen diffuses from the alveoli into the blood and carbon dioxide diffuses from the blood into the alveoli

scoliosis (or kyphoscoliosis)—curvature and rotation of the spinal column with resulting back and chest deformity often caused by inability of weakened muscles to hold up the spinal column

spinal muscular atrophy—an inherited disease of peripheral nerves (anterior horn cells in the spinal cord) that has been arbitrarily separated into types 1 through 5 based on severity

spirometer—a device used for measuring volumes of air such as that with vital capacity measurements

stenosis—narrowing of a passage, e.g., the narrowing of the trachea caused by complications of translaryngeal intubation or an indwelling tracheostomy tube

suctioning—the passage of a catheter into the airways to aspirate out airway secretions and other debris

thoracic—pertaining to the spine at the level of the chest

tidal volume—the volume of air one inhales during one normal breath measured in milliliters

trachea—the windpipe

tracheostomy—a surgical hole (stoma) that creates a passage through the neck to the windpipe (trachea) for placement of a tube (tracheostomy tube) through which ventilatory support and airway suctioning can be done

ventilator—a device that intermittently provides negative or positive pressure to assist or substitute for the inspiratory muscle function needed for breathing (sometimes called a *respirator*)

ventilation—*See alveolar ventilation*

ventilation-perfusion mismatching—when areas of the lung that are properly ventilated have inadequate blood supply for gas exchange or when areas of the lungs with good blood supply are inadequately ventilated

vital capacity—the maximum volume of air that one can inhale then blow through a device (spirometer), measured in milliliters

3

Evolution of Mechanical Ventilation: Its Successes and Shortcomings

Yuka Ishikawa and John R. Bach

Paracelsus has been given credit for being the first to mechanically attempt ventilatory support by using his chimney bellows in 1530. The delivery of intermittent positive pressure ventilation (IPPV) via the mouth with chimney bellows continued to be used in Europe through the 19th century (1). Despite the description of successful ventilatory support via an indwelling tracheostomy tube in 1869, until the late 1950s, the standard of care was to provide ventilatory support by only noninvasive means. This was particularly advantageous for maintaining normal oral communication and taking food by mouth because noninvasive methods rarely hamper and never eliminate oral communication or swallowing as does the delivery of IPPV via indwelling tracheostomy or translaryngeal tubes. Recently, with better understanding of complications associated with the delivery of IPPV via indwelling translaryngeal and tracheostomy tubes, there has been a trend to return to noninvasive approaches. The criteria needed for both undergoing tracheostomy as well as tracheostomy tube removal and conversion to noninvasive respiratory alternatives are presented in Chapter 2. In this chapter, we review the history of mechanical ventilation and the reasons for these trends.

Body Ventilators

The tank-style ventilator was the first device used for both acute and long-term mechanical ventilatory support; and tank-style ventilators continue to be used by many individuals and are the primary method of ventilatory support in some intensive care units around the world (2). The first tank ventilator was described

Tracheostomy and Ventilator Dependency: Management of Breathing, Speaking, and Swallowing. Edited by Donna C. Tippett, MPH, MA, CCC-SLP. Thieme Medical Publishers, Inc. New York © 2000.

by the Scottish physician, John Dalziel in 1838 (3). These ventilators consist of either a tank or chamber that contains the patient with only the head protruding. Negative pressure is created in the chamber, which in turn, cyclically creates negative intrapleural pressure that results in insufflation.

The best known and the first of the tank-style ventilators to receive widespread use was the iron lung. The iron lung was developed in 1928 by Philip Drinker and Louis Agassiz Shaw of Boston (4). It had a sliding bed with head-wall attached and a rubber collar. Pressure changes were created in the tank by an electrically powered rotary blower (the first electrically powered ventilator) and an alternating valve. In 1931, John Emerson of Cambridge, Massachusetts, built a simplified, inexpensive, and more convenient iron lung that operated quietly, permitted speed changes, and could be operated by hand if electricity failed (Fig. 3–1). Then, in 1936, Fred Snite Jr., son of Colonel Frederick Snite, a prominent Chicago financier, was stricken with poliomyelitis while traveling with his family in Beijing. A Drinker iron lung was removed from an opium den in Beijing and Snite, Jr. returned to the United States using it with much fanfare and in the company of a large entourage of Chinese and American healthcare professionals (5). The Drinker had been sent to China as a gift from New York University. It had been used in the opium den to ventilate people who had overdosed on opium. This stimulated public awareness and resulted in the mass production of Emerson iron lungs in time for the severe poliomyelitis epidemics that were to come. The first chest shell ventilator, essentially a smaller analog to the iron lung, covered only the chest and upper abdomen. It was developed by Ignez von Hauke of Austria in 1876 (6). In the new models available today, negative pressure from a negative pressure generator (ventilator) is cycled under the shell to expand the chest and abdomen. Custom-molded designs have been described subsequently for people with scoliosis (7). Chest shell ventilators were used for long-term daytime supported ventilation with the user sitting as well as for nocturnal support with the user supine; however, the use of chest shell ventilators for daytime aid has been largely supplanted by more practical and effective methods including mouthpiece IPPV, intermittent abdominal pressure ventilator (IAPV) use (8), and at times, glossopharyngeal breathing (GPB).

The prototype wrap-style ventilator was the Tunnicliffe breathing jacket. It was described in 1955 and continues to be used in England today (9). Similar models are available today in the United States. This ventilator, and the wrap ventilators that followed (Lifecare International Inc., Westminster, Colorado), consist of a

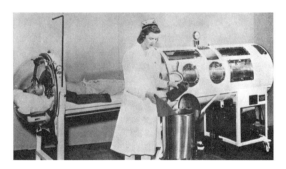

Fig. 3–1. J.H. Emerson Company's iron lung of 1932. While under nursing care patients received air via a dome which covered their heads instead of via a simple mouthpiece. Photo courtesy of J.H. Emerson Company, Cambridge, Massachusetts.

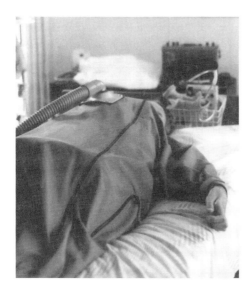

Fig. 3–2. The pneumowrap ventilator being used by a spinal cord-injured individual with late-onset ventilatory insufficiency.

firm plastic grid covering at least the thorax and upper abdomen. The grid and the body under it are covered by a wind-proof jacket that is sealed around the neck and extremities. Negative pressure is cycled under the wrap and grid and as the chest and abdomen expand, air enters the upper airway to ventilate the lungs. The only significant changes from the original design in modern wrap ventilators are the materials used to fabricate the jacket and the length and form of the extremity sleeves (Fig. 3–2).

The Rocking Bed Ventilator (J. H. Emerson Company, Cambridge, MA) has been used for ventilatory assistance since 1932 (Fig. 3–3) (10). It rocks the patient 15° to 30°, thereby using gravity to cyclically displace abdominal contents for diaphragmatic excursion. This device is generally less effective than other body ventilators, but is adequate for many patients (11).

The prototype IAPV was the Bragg-Paul Pulsator which was described by C.J. McSweeney in 1938 (12). "The apparatus consists of a distensible rubber bag applied around the patient's chest in the form of a belt, this belt being rhythmically

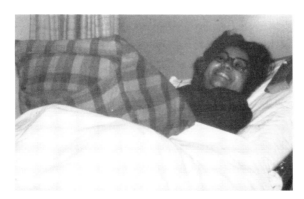

Fig. 3–3. The rocking bed ventilator used by a postpoliomyelitis individual.

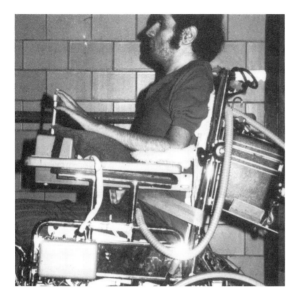

Fig. 3–4. An air sac lies within a girdle which this high-level spinal cord-injured individual is wearing beneath his clothing. The ventilator hose is connected to the air sac.

filled with, and emptied of, air" (12). The modern IAPV (Fig. 3–4) (13) consists of an elastic inflatable bladder incorporated within an abdominal corset worn beneath outer clothing. If the patient has any inspiratory capacity or is capable of GPB, he or she can add autonomous tidal volumes to the mechanically assisted inspirations. These noninvasive ventilatory support methods do not hamper oral communication and can often facilitate it by providing the deeper breaths that many need for greater vocal intensity.

The Switch to Tracheostomy IPPV

Trendelenburg was the first to describe the use of a tracheostomy tube with an inflated cuff for assisting ventilation during anesthesia of a human in 1869 (14). The use of transoral intubation for ventilatory support during anesthesia was described soon afterward (15). In 1893, a hand-powered bellows was devised for delivering IPPV. Rubber tubing connected it to the patient via either a tight-fitting oral–nasal interface or a tracheostomy tube (16,17). Tracheostomy and the use of a mechanical bellows for ventilatory support became widely used for anesthesia during World War I (18). Despite this, and the fact that tracheostomies were often placed to manage airway secretions for those ventilated by iron lungs in the 1940s, tracheostomy tubes were not used for long-term ventilatory support until an inadequate supply of body ventilators made this a necessity during the 1952 Danish poliomyelitis epidemic (19).

   Although iron lungs and other negative pressure body ventilators provided adequate ventilatory support, individuals generally had to remain stationary and recumbent when using them, and evacuation of airway secretions was very difficult for supine patients with limited access to the body for manually assisted coughing. Noninvasive IPPV had not yet been reported and mechanical forced exsufflation devices that assist in the elimination of airway secretions were not available (20–22). Thus, tracheostomy was increasingly popular for ventilatory assistance after 1952 and subsequently was the standard of care. Tracheostomy IPPV with the positive pressure ventilator rolled behind the patient's wheelchair permitted optimal mobility. Tracheostomy also provided a closed system for ventilatory support that was amenable to precise monitoring of ventilatory volumes and pressures, oxygen delivery, and the use of the high-technology respirators and alarm systems that were to come.

More recently, with the appreciation of the many complications associated with invasive means of ventilatory support, with clear patient preference for noninvasive methods (23), and decreased cost (24) and morbidity (25) associated with the latter, the need for and indications for tracheostomy IPPV for ventilatory support and airway secretion management have become more restricted.

Difficulties Associated with Invasive Approaches

With widespread use of endotracheal methods, numerous reports appeared of complications related to tracheostomy and long-term tracheostomy IPPV. In a review of the literature, 2.7% of acute mortality associated with ventilator use (range 0.5 to 3%) was due to the tracheostomy itself (26). Complications can be categorized as follows: intraoperative, early postoperative, and late postoperative (27). Intraoperatively, injury can occur to the vocal folds, recurrent laryngeal nerves, and esophagus. Pneumothorax, air embolism, and bronchial obstruction can occur. In the immediate postoperative stage, pneumothorax, pneumomediastinum, pneumoperitoneum, and hemorrhage can occur. The late operative stage can be complicated by infection, tracheomalacia, tracheoesophageal fistula, tracheal stenosis, subglottic stenosis, tracheocutaneous fistula, tracheal scarring, and possible obstruction from granulation tissue formation.

Infection is the most insidious complication of tracheostomy. The site is colonized by bacteria within only a few hours following tracheostomy. This is associated with the development of acute tracheobronchitis, pneumonia, mediastinitis, pericarditis, cellulitis, wound infection, and abscesses (27). Individuals with long-term indwelling tracheostomy tubes are often colonized with enteric gram-negative bacilli, especially that of the *Pseudomonas* species. This occurs because the presence of a foreign body, such as a tracheostomy tube, that protrudes from the patient, can form a nidus for the implantation of bacteria and hamper their elimination by antibiotic therapy or cleansing. Niederman and colleagues studied serial paired culture samples from the oropharynx and the tracheobronchial tree of 15 subjects with long-term indwelling tracheostomies (28). Thirteen had chronic pulmonary disease and two had neuromuscular disease. In 49 sets of cultures gram-negative bacilli were present in 36.7% of upper airway cultures and 75.5% of lower airway cultures. At the tracheobronchial site, seven subjects had persistent enteric gram-negative bacilli colonization, all with *Pseudomonas* species, while only one subject had this in the oropharynx. Subjects with persistent tracheobronchial colonization received antibiotics more often, and developed purulent tracheobronchitis more often (100% versus 25%) than those without persistent colonization (28). These findings suggest enhanced susceptibility for more frequent and more persistent enteric gram-negative bacilli colonization of the lower respiratory tract than of the upper respiratory tract and that these two mucosal sites become colonized independently of one another. Furthermore, persistent colonization was associated with more clinical illness and may have predisposed individuals to symptomatic infection (28), fatal mucus plugging, chronic purulent bronchitis, granulation formation, and sepsis from stomal infection or sinusitis.

The prevalence of other complications from tracheostomy varies. In a study by Conway and colleagues, patients with tracheostomies for sleep apnea were studied (29). The most significant complications reported in this study were granulation formation, bleeding, and stomal narrowing. Tracheal obstruction from mucus plugging and obstruction by partial dislodgment of the tracheostomy tube have also been reported (30). Hafez and colleagues, reported surgical repair techniques used for inominate artery erosion from prolonged endotracheal intubation or tracheostomy (31). The inominate artery comes off of the ascending aorta and passes adjacent to the trachea. Arterial erosion occurs as a result of direct pressure by the elbow of the cannula against the artery or indirectly through the tracheal wall by a high pressure cuff. Of the 12 patients studied, 10 had indwelling tracheostomy tubes for a period of eight days to three months. Although inominate erosion is uncommon, when it occurs, the ensuing hemorrhage is usually fatal. In this study, eight of the 12 patients died perioperatively or postoperatively (31).

Long-term tracheostomy can cause damage to the trachea and larynx as a result of pressure, irritation, and deformation by the cannula. The convex margin of the tracheostomy cannula pushes against, and thus may erode, the upper anterior tracheal wall (32). Tracheal stenosis is also a major potential complication of long-term tracheostomy with strictures developing in three main regions of the airway. If the tracheostomy is performed too high, then damage can occur to the cricoid cartilage, and subglottic stenosis can develop. Stenosis can also occur at the level of the cuff and the tracheal stoma (33). Infection appears to promote subglottic stenosis as the result of contamination carried from the tracheostomy site to the subglottic area by ciliary action (34). The contamination is colonized by bacteria whose activity results in the formation of granulation tissue. Granulation tissue and cicatrix formation gradually decrease airway patency (stenose).

Other potential long-term complications include sudden death from cardiac arrhythmias, mucus plugging, accidental disconnections, and other causes. Complications including tracheomalacia and tracheal perforation, hemorrhage, tracheoesophageal fistula, painful hemorrhagic tube changes, vocal fold adhesions, and psychosocial disturbances have been summarized and more completely referenced elsewhere (35,36). In particular, tracheostomy IPPV users are always in fear of ventilator failure or accidental disconnection from the ventilator. This can result in asphyxia and death, and the profuse airway secretions and need for their management in tracheostomy IPPV users can create embarrassment and self-consciousness. Noninvasive IPPV users, on the other hand, often never need fear ventilator failure because many can use glossopharyngeal breathing to ventilate the lungs. Airway secretions are only a concern for these individuals during intercurrent upper respiratory tract infections. Translaryngeal intubation and tracheostomy can also prevent autonomous breathing through the upper airway, and can preclude effective coughing, whether spontaneous or assisted (37).

The presence of a tracheostomy tube necessitates regular bronchial suctioning, tracheostomy site care, and tube changes. Supplemental humidification must be provided and attended to daily. Swallowing difficulties occur as the result of restriction of upward laryngeal movement and rotation by anchoring of the trachea to the strap muscles and skin of the neck. This results in reduced glottic closure and increased laryngeal penetration thus increasing the chances of aspiration. Interference with relaxation of the cricopharyngeal sphincter, compression of the esophagus, and changes in intratracheal pressure can add to the difficulties (38,39). When an inflated cuff is used, the appreciation of the taste of food is also virtually lost because food aromas are no longer transported to the nose. In addition, in many states a tracheostomy is considered an "open wound." This can prohibit community living for the individual without having them incur prohibitively expensive nursing care for tracheal suctioning and wound care (24).

Tracheal suctioning causes irritation, increases secretions, may be accompanied by severe hypoxia (40), and is at best effective in clearing only superficial airway secretions. Routine tracheal suctioning misses mucus plugs adherent between the tube and the tracheal wall, *and* it misses the left mainstem bronchus 54 to 92% of the time (41), accounting for the higher incidence of left lung pneumonia.

Richard and colleagues performed a retrospective study for the incidence of laryngeal stenosis in 315 neurologically impaired patients. Fifty-five percent of the patients were intubated translaryngeally for a mean of 17 days but did not subsequently undergo tracheostomy. Three percent underwent tracheostomy only, and 42% underwent tracheostomy after translaryngeal intubation for a mean of 13 days. The incidence of laryngotracheal stenosis was significantly higher after tracheostomy than after translaryngeal intubation–only [42 (29.3%) of 143 versus 22 (12.8%) of 172]. The incidence of glottic or subglottic stenosis did not appear to increase when the duration of intubation increased to a mean of 17 days. Their data, thus, suggest maintaining translaryngeal intubation for longer periods when there is any possibility of accomplishing ventilator weaning or conversion to the use of noninvasive methods of ventilatory support and thus avoiding tracheostomy (42). Likewise, in a study by Stauffer and colleagues, 150 patients with indwelling translaryngeal or tracheostomy tubes were compared. Adverse consequences occurred in 62% of all translaryngeally intubated patients and in 66% of all patients with indwelling tracheostomy tubes, whether during placement or use of mechanical ventilation. The most frequent problems associated with the translaryngeal tubes were the use of excessive cuff pressure requirements (19%), self-extubation (13%), and inability to seal the airway (11%). Patient discomfort and difficulty in suctioning tracheobronchial secretions were also ubiquitous. Problems associated with the presence of indwelling tracheostomy tubes included stomal infection (36%), stomal hemorrhage (36%), excessive cuff pressure requirements (23%), and subcutaneous emphysema or pneumomediastinum (13%). Complications of tracheostomy were judged to be more severe than those of endotracheal intubation. Follow-up studies of survivors revealed a high prevalence of tracheal stenosis after tracheostomy (65%), but significantly lower after endotracheal intubation (19%) (30). This study also noted that patients appeared to tolerate endotracheal intubation well for up to 22 days. Dunham and La Monica, too, concluded that patients can tolerate translaryngeal intubation for up to two weeks without significant complications (43).

The potentially severe complications of translaryngeal intubation and tracheostomy should be considered when faced with an individual with ventilatory failure. Although prolonging translaryngeal intubation appears to be warranted rather than resorting to tracheostomy, the best approach for avoiding both the acute and long-term complications of these invasive methods is by using noninvasive inspiratory and expiratory muscle aid alternatives (44).

Noninvasive IPPV Methods

Noninvasive IPPV methods, which can greatly facilitate the patient's ability to communicate, are more effective than body ventilators, and are preferred over body ventilator use as well as over tracheostomy IPPV (45). These were first described in 1969 (46).

IPPV can be delivered noninvasively very simply via oral (Fig. 3–5) (47,48), nasal (Fig. 3–6) (23,49–51), or oral–nasal (Fig. 3–7) interfaces (52). Ventilatory support in this manner neither interferes with speech, nor eating, nor significantly alters patient appearance, and all of the complications and difficulties associated with indwelling tubes are avoided. Mouthpiece IPPV, and when effective, IAPV use, are the preferred methods for daytime ventilatory assistance.

By 1964, a number of patients had switched from nocturnal body ventilator use, which was no longer very effective for them, to up to 24-h mouthpiece IPPV (47). With the advent of the Bennett lip seal (Nellcor–Puritan-Bennett, Pleasan-

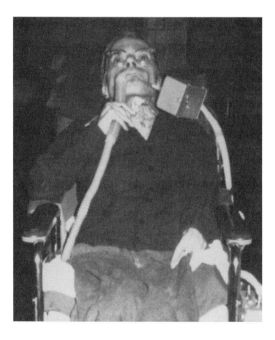

Fig. 3–5. A man with muscular dystrophy using mouthpiece ventilation for 24-h ventilatory support.

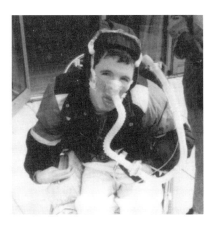

Fig. 3–6. A man with Duchenne muscular dystrophy who uses 24-h nasal ventilation here seen using a custom-molded low-profile acrylic nasal interface. Reprinted, with permission, from McDermott, Bach, Parker et al. (52).

ton, CA) in 1972, mouthpiece IPPV could be delivered during sleep with less insufflation leakage out of the mouth and little risk of the mouthpiece falling out of the mouth (Fig. 3–8). Mouthpiece IPPV with lipseal retention tends to be a more effective method of nocturnal noninvasive IPPV than nasal IPPV.

Nasal IPPV is the generally preferred method for nocturnal ventilatory support. It was first used as an alternative to tracheal intubation for 24-h ventilatory support in 1984 (53). Nasal continuous positive airway pressure (CPAP) masks are often used as the interfaces for nasal IPPV, however, nasal CPAP masks were not originally designed to be conduits for the ventilatory pressures needed for ventilatory support. Excessive nasal bridge pressure and insufflation leakage into the eyes are common complaints when using nasal IPPV via CPAP masks. There are now many commercially available nasal interfaces available for IPPV

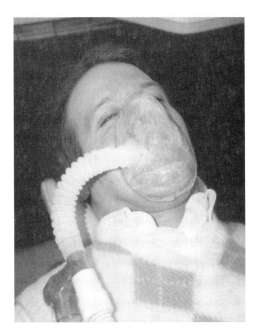

Fig. 3–7. A man with spinal cord injury using a custom-molded acrylic strapless oral–nasal interface for nocturnal ventilatory support. Reprinted, with permission, from McDermott, Bach, Parker et al. (52).

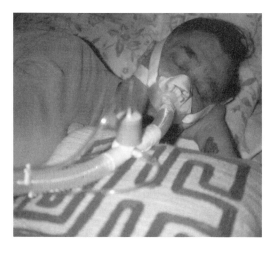

Fig. 3–8. A man using nocturnal lipseal ventilation with his nose plugged with nasal pledgets and covered to prevent ventilator delivered air from leaking out of the nose (insufflation leakage).

including the Gold Seal Gel Mask with its convenient reusable headgear retention system (Softcap), the Monarch, and the Contour Nasal Mask (Respironics Inc., Murrysville, PA); the Sullivan (ResMed Inc., Elmonte, CA); the Adam circuit (Nellcor-Puritan-Bennett, Pleasanton, CA); the Phantom (Sleep Net Inc., Manchester, N.H.); and the Health Dyne Nasal Mask (Marietta, GA). Each design applies pressure differently to the nasal area. It is impossible to predict which one will be preferred by any particular nasal IPPV user. Many people use different models on alternate nights to vary skin contact pressure. Custom-molded nasal interfaces can now also be obtained both commercially (SEFAM Company, distributed by Respironics, Inc., Murrysville, PA) and individually in New Jersey (52) and in France (54).

Oral–nasal interfaces were described for long-term supported ventilation in 1989 (55). These interfaces used strap retention systems like those used for mouthpiece and nasal IPPV, however, since effective ventilatory support could be provided by either nasal or mouthpiece IPPV, or when necessary, mouthpiece IPPV with the nose plugged by either a clip or cotton pledgets and tape (Fig. 3–8) (46), strap retained oral–nasal interfaces have not been used widely for long-term ventilatory support.

Strapless oral–nasal interfaces with bite-plate retention have been used in Europe since 1985 and were first described in the medical literature in 1989 (55). These interfaces not only provide an essentially hermetic seal for the delivery of IPPV, but simple tongue thrust is all that is necessary to expel them in the event of vomiting or other need. The bite-plate retention is also important for individuals living alone who are unable to don straps because of limited upper extremity range of motion or strength (52). Speech can also be perfectly functional during their use. All noninvasive IPPV methods can be used for daytime as well as for nocturnal ventilatory support.

Difficulties with noninvasive IPPV include the fact that about 4% of nocturnal mouthpiece IPPV users with no ventilator-free breathing ability have periods of excessive insufflation leakage through the nose that cause frequent nocturnal arousals (46). The nose can be clipped or plugged with cotton before sleep for these individuals. Generally, however, nasal insufflation leakage during lipseal IPPV is not a clinical problem because the high ventilator insufflation volumes (1,200 to, at times, 2,000 ml) used tend to compensate for nasal leakage. The use of the low pressure alarm, and conditioned reflexes also prevent excessive leak associated decreases in SaO_2 during sleep.

Orthodontic deformities can also occur for long-term mouthpiece or nasal interface users. Other potential difficulties include allergy to the plastic lipseal and aerophagia. We have never had to discontinue noninvasive IPPV for any patient because of noninvasive IPPV-associated aerophagia. Normally, the gastroesophageal spincter can withstand usual peak IPPV airway pressures without leak. Aerophagia tends to occur when ventilator-delivered volumes result in peak pressures over about 25 cm H_2O. Abdominal distention often occurs sporadically. The air passes as flatus once the patient gets up or is placed in a wheelchair in the morning. When severe, a rectal tube can usually decompress the colon.

Management of Airway Secretions

A normal cough involves the expulsion of about 2.5 L of air upon glottic opening after thoracoabdominal pressures exceeding 120 cm H_2O have been generated by the abdominal and intercostal muscles. The explosive decompression generates peak cough flows (PCF) of 6 to 16 L/s. Thus, both a deep breath and optimal airway pressures are necessary. Although quantitation of manually assisted PCF and the importance of generating them were reported in 1966 (56), the concept has been virtually ignored until recently.

Individuals with functional pharyngeal musculature can master glossopharyngeal breathing. The importance of deep GPB-assisted breaths on cough effectiveness and speech volume was described in 1956 (57). GPB involves the use of the tongue and pharyngeal muscles to add to an inspiratory effort by projecting (gulping) boluses of air past the glottis. The glottis closes with each "gulp." One breath usually consists of six to nine gulps of 60 to 100 ml each. During the training period, the efficiency of GPB can be monitored by spirometrically measuring the milliliters of air per gulp, gulps per breath, and breaths per minute (44). GPB can provide an individual with weak inspiratory muscles and little or no measurable vital capacity (VC) with normal lung ventilation without using a ventilator and with the ability to take the deep breaths needed to generate adequate PCF (37,47). GPB is, however, rarely useful in the presence of an indwelling tracheostomy tube. It cannot be used when the tube is uncapped as it is during tracheostomy IPPV, and even when capped, the gulped air tends to leak around the outer walls of the tube and out the tracheostomy site as airway volumes and pressures increase during the air stacking process of GPB. The safety and versatility afforded by effective GPB are key reasons to eliminate tracheostomy in favor of noninvasive aids.

Mechanically assisted coughing, i.e., mechanical insufflation–exsufflation (MI-E), was developed and used in 1952 to supplement manual techniques. The first widely used mechanically forced exsufflation device or insufflator–exsufflator, was known as the Cof-flator. It was extensively studied and first reported to be very effective in clearing airway secretions in 1953 and 1954 (20–22); however, it went off the market as tracheostomy and tracheal suctioning became the standards of care in the early 1960s. A new mechanical insufflator–exsufflator (In-Exsufflator, J.H. Emerson Company, Cambridge, MA) came on the market in February of 1993 as renewed efforts to use noninvasive IPPV were increasingly made since the descriptions of nasal IPPV in 1987.

MI-E delivers a deep insufflation via a mouthpiece, mask, tracheostomy, or translaryngeal tube to the lungs then, with a pressure drop from about +40 cm H_2O to –40 cm H_2O, exsufflation creates 10 L/s of expiratory flow which brings up mucus, food, or other airway debris from the airways. A manually applied abdominal thrust should be applied in conjunction with the exsufflation phase of the machine. The insufflation and exsufflation pressures are independently adjusted for comfort and efficacy. One treatment consists of about five cycles of MI-E followed by a period of normal breathing or ventilator use for 20 to 30 s to avoid hyperventilation. Five or more treatments are given in one sitting, and the treatments are repeated until no further secretions are expulsed and oxyhemoglobin saturation (SaO_2) levels, if decreased by the airway debris, have returned to either normal or baseline.

An increase in VC of 15 to 42% was noted immediately following treatment in 67 individuals with "obstructive dyspnea" and a 55% increase in VC was noted following MI-E in individuals with neuromuscular conditions (58). We have observed 15 to 400% improvement in VC and normalization of SaO_2 as MI-E eliminates mucus plugs for acutely ill ventilator-assisted neuromuscular patients (37).

MI-E use can be required as frequently as every 5 to 20 min during respiratory tract infections or when used by someone who consistently aspirates food. Although no medications are usually required for effective MI-E in neuromuscular ventilator users, liquifying sputum with heated aerosol treatments can facilitate mucus elimination when secretions are inspissated. When used to maintain SaO_2 within normal limits by quickly eliminating desaturation causing mucus plugs, and when noninvasive IPPV is provided as needed to maintain normal alveolar ventilation, episodes of respiratory failure can be prevented and long-term ventilatory support maintained without resorting to tracheostomy for the majority of patients with advanced neuromuscular disease (44). Oxygen therapy should always be avoided for these patients unless assisted ventilation has first been used to normalize alveolar ventilation (blood carbon dioxide tensions) and assisted coughing fails to normalize SaO_2. Patients with hypoxia and oxyhemoglobin desaturation, despite normal ventilation and aggressive assisted coughing, have intrinsic lung disease, most often atelectasis, and often pneumonia, and may be chronically aspirating upper airway secretions. Thus, those with severely impaired pharyngeal musculature who essentially continually aspirate their oral secretions and whose SaO_2 cannot be normalized by MI-E have a high risk of recurrent pneumonia. It is our clinical impression that the aspiration of food or airway secretions does not signal a high risk for pulmonary complications unless chronic oxyhemoglobin desaturation occurs irrespective of attempts at assisted coughing and assisted ventilation (when necessary) to reverse it.

Summary

With the reported success of nocturnal nasal IPPV in 1987 (49,53,51) and the development of other noninvasive IPPV methods to complement the IAPV, GPB, and mouthpiece IPPV for up to 24-h ventilatory support (46,52,59), there are now many noninvasive alternatives to inconvenient body ventilators and tracheostomy IPPV (23,60–64). In addition, the versatility afforded by the development of bi-level positive airway pressure and the greater sophistication of portable volume ventilators also provide impetus to explore further the use of noninvasive respiratory aids for individuals with ventilatory insufficiency due to parenchymal or obstructive lung disease in both acute care and long-term care settings (65–81).

References

1. Gordon AS. History and evolution of modern resuscitation techniques. In Gordon AS, ed. *Cardiopulmonary resuscitation conference proceedings.* Washington, DC: National Academy of Sciences, 1966:7.
2. Corrado A, Gorini M, De Paola E. Alternative techniques for managing acute neuromuscular respiratory failure. *Semin Neurol* 1995;15:84–89.
3. Woollam CHM. The development of apparatus for intermittent negative pressure respiration (1) 1832–1918. *Anaesthesia* 1976;31:537–547.
4. Drinker PA, McKhann CF. The iron lung: first practical means of respiratory support. *JAMA* 1986;255:1476–1479.
5. Gorham J. A medical triumph: the iron lung. *Respir Care* 1979;9:71–73.
6. Von Hauke I. Der Pneumatische Panzer. Beitrag zur mechanischen Behandlung der Brustkrankheiten. *Wiener Medizinische Presse* 1874;15:785, 836.
7. Newman JH, Wilkins JK. Fabrication of a customized cuirass for patients with severe thoracic asymmetry. *Am Rev Respir Dis* 1988;137:202–203.
8. Bach JR, Alba AS. Total ventilatory support by the intermittent abdominal pressure ventilator. *Chest* 1991;99:630–636.
9. Spalding JMK, Opie L. Artificial respiration with the Tunnicliffe breathing jacket. *Lancet* 1958;274:613.
10. Eve FG. Actuation of inert diaphragm by gravity method. *Lancet* 1932;2:995–998.
11. Bryce-Smith R, Davis HS. Tidal exchange in respirators. *Curr Res Anaesth Analges* 1954;33:73–77.
12. McSweeney CJ. The Bragg-Paul pulsator in treatment of respiratory paralysis. *Br Med J* 1938;1:1206–1209.
13. Adamson JP, Lewis L, Stein JD. Application of abdominal pressure for artificial respiration. *JAMA* 1959;169:153–155.
14. Trendelenburg F. Beitrage zur den Operationen an den Luftwagen 2. Tamponnade der Trachea. *Arch Klin Chir* 1871;12:121–233.
15. MacEwen W. Clinical observations on the introduction of tracheal tubes by the mouth instead of performing tracheotomy or laryngotomy. *Br Med J* 1880;2:122–126.
16. Fell GE. Forced respiration. *JAMA* 1891;16:325–328.
17. Hochberg LA. *Thoracic surgery before the 20th century.* New York: Vantage Press, 1960:684.
18. Magill IW. Development of endotracheal anesthesia. *Proc R Soc Med* 1928;22:83–84.
19. Lassen HCA. The epidemic of poliomyelitis in Copenhagen, 1952. *Proc R Soc Med* 1954;47:67–71.
20. Barach AL, Beck GJ, Bickerman HA, et al. Physical methods simulating cough mechanisms. *JAMA* 1952;5:85–91.
21. Bickerman HA, Itkin S. Exsufflation with negative pressure: elimination of radiopaque material and foreign bodies from bronchi of anesthetized dogs. *Arch Int Med* 1954;93:698–704.
22. The OEM Cof-flator Portable Cough Machine. St. Louis, MO: Shampaine Industries Inc.
23. Bach JR, Alba AS. Management of chronic alveolar hypoventilation by nasal ventilation. *Chest* 1990;97:52–57.

24. Bach JR, Intintola P, Alba AS, Holland I. The ventilator-assisted individual: cost analysis of institutionalization versus rehabilitation and in-home management. *Chest* 1992;101:26–30.

25. Bach JR, Rajaraman R, Ballanger F, Tzang A, et al. Neuromuscular ventilatory insufficiency: the effect of home mechanical ventilator use vs. oxygen therapy on pneumonia and hospitalization rates. *Am J Phys Med Rehabil* 1998;77:8–19.

26. Salmon LFW. Tracheostomy procedure. *Social Medical* 1968;347:1975.

27. Blair PA. Complications of tracheostomy. *J Louisana St Med Soc* 1987;139:15–18.

28. Niederman M, Ferranti R, Zeigler A, et al. Respiratory infection complicating long-term tracheostomy: the implication of persistent gram-negative tracheobronchial colonization. *Chest* 1984;85:39–44.

29. Conway W, Victor L, Magilligan D, Fujita S, Zorick F, Roth T. Adverse effects of tracheostomy for sleep apnea. *JAMA* 1981;246:349–353.

30. Stauffer J, Olson D, Petty T. Complications and consequences of endotracheal intubation and tracheotomy: a prospective study of 150 critically ill adult patients. *Am J Med* 1981;70:65–71.

31. Hafez A, Couraud L, Velly JF, Bruneteau A. Late cataclysmic hemorrhage from the inominate artery after tracheostomy. *Thorac Cardiovasc Surg* 1984;32:315–316.

32. Eliachar I, Stegmoyer R, Levine H, Sivak E, Mehta A, Tucker H. Planning and management of long-standing tracheostomy. *Otolaryngo Head Neck Surg* 1987;97:385–391.

33. Heffner J, Miller S, Sahn S. Tracheostomy in the intensive care unit: part 2: complications. *Chest* 1986;90:430–436.

34. Kirchner J. Tracheotomy and its problems. *Surg Clin North Am* 1980;60:1093–1098.

35. Bach JR, O'Connor K. Electrophrenic ventilation: a different perspective. *J Am Paraplegia Soc* 1991;14:9–17.

36. Bellamy R, Pitts FW, Stauffer S. Respiratory complications in traumatic quadriplegia. *J Neurosurg* 1973;39:596–600.

37. Bach JR. Mechanical insufflation-exsufflation: comparison of peak expiratory flows with manually assisted and unassisted coughing techniques. *Chest* 1993;104:1553–1562.

38. Bonanno P. Swallowing dysfunction after tracheostomy. *Ann Surg* 1971;174:29–33.

39. Logemann JA. *Evaluation and treatment of swallowing disorders*. San Diego: College-Hill Press Inc, 1983:119.

40. Bach JR, Sortor S, Sipski M. Sleep blood gas monitoring of high cervical quadriplegic patients with respiratory insufficiency by non-invasive techniques [abstract]. *Abstracts Digest*, 1988:102. 14th Annual Scientific Meeting of the American Spinal Cord Injury Association, Available from L.H. Johnson, 2020 Peachtree Road, NW, Atlanta, GA.

41. Fishburn MJ, Marino RJ, Ditunno JF. Atelectasis and pneumonia in acute spinal cord injury. *Arch Phys Med Rehabil* 1990;71:197–200.

42. Richard I, Giraud M, Perrouin-Verbe B, Hiance D, Mauduyt de la Greve I, Mathe J. Laryngotracheal stenosis after intubation or tracheostomy in patients with neurological disease. *Arch Phys Med Rehabil* 1996;77:493–497.

43. Dunham M, La Monica C. Prolonged tracheal intubation in the trauma patient. *J Trauma* 1984;24:120–124.

44. Bach JR. Prevention of morbidity and mortality with the use of physical medicine aids. In: Bach JR, ed. *Pulmonary rehabilitation: the obstructive and paralytic conditions*. Philadelphia: Hanley & Belfus, 1996:303–329.

45. Bach JR. A comparison of long-term ventilatory support alternatives from the perspective of the patient and care giver. *Chest* 1993;104:1702–1706.

46. Bach JR, Alba AS, Saporito LR: Intermittent positive pressure ventilation via the mouth as an alternative to tracheostomy for 257 ventilator users. *Chest* 1993;103:174–182.

47. Bach JR, Alba AS, Bodofsky E, et al. Glossopharyngeal breathing and non-invasive aids in the management of post-polio respiratory insufficiency. *Birth Defects* 1987;123:99–113.

48. Curran FJ, Colbert AP: Ventilator management in Duchenne muscular dystrophy and postpoliomyelitis syndrome: twelve years' experience. *Arch Phys Med Rehabil* 1989;70:180–185.

49. Ellis ER, Bye PTP, Bruderer JW, et al. Treatment of respiratory failure during sleep in patients with neuromuscular disease, positive-pressure ventilation through a nose mask. *Am Rev Respir Dis* 1987;135:148–152.

50. Hill NS, Eveloff SE, Carlisle CC, et al.: Efficacy of nocturnal nasal ventilation in patients with restrictive thoracic disease. *Am Rev Respir Dis* 1992;145:365–367.

51. Kerby GR, Mayer LS, Pingleton SK. Nocturnal positive pressure ventilation via nasal mask. *Am Rev Respir Dis* 1987;135:738–740.

52. McDermott I, Bach JR, Parker C, et al. Custom-fabricated interfaces for intermittent positive pressure ventilation. *Int J Prosthodont* 1989;2:224–233.

53. Bach JF, Alba A, Mosher R, et al. Intermittent positive pressure ventilation via nasal access in the management of respiratory insufficiency. *Chest* 1987;92:168–170.

54. Leger P, Jennequin J, Gerard M, et al. Home positive pressure ventilation via nasal mask for patients with neuromuscular weakness or restrictive lung or chest-wall disease. *Respir Care* 1989;34:73–79.

55. Ratzka A. Uberdruckbeatmung durch Mundstuck. In Frehse U, ed. *Spatfolgen nach Poliomyelitis: Chronische Unterbeatmung und Möglichkeiten selbstbestimmter Lebensführung Schwerbehinderter.* München, West Germany: Pfennigparade eV, 1989;5:149.

56. Kirby NA, Barnerias MJ, Siebens AA. An evaluation of assisted cough in quadriplegic patients. *Arch Phys Med Rehabil* 1966;47:705–707.

57. Feigelson CI, Dickinson DG, Talner NS, et al. Glossopharyngeal breathing as an aid to the coughing mechanism in the patient with chronic poliomyelitis in a respirator. *N Engl J Med* 1956;254:611–613.

58. Barach AL, Beck GJ. Exsufflation with negative pressure: physiologic and clinical studies in poliomyelitis, bronchial asthma, pulmonary emphysema and bronchiectasis. *Arch Int Med* 1954;93:825–841.

59. Viroslav J, Sortor S, Rosenblatt R. Alternatives to tracheostomy ventilation in high level SCI [abstract]. *J Am Paraplegia Soc* 1991;14:87.

60. Carrey Z, Gottfried SB, Levy RD. Ventilatory muscle support in respiratory failure with nasal positive pressure ventilation. *Chest* 1990;97:150.

61. Carroll N, Branthwaite MA. Control of nocturnal hypoventilation by nasal intermittent positive pressure ventilation. *Thorax* 1988;43:349–352.

62. Gay PC, Patel AM, Viggiano RW, et al. Nocturnal nasal ventilation for treatment of patients with hypercapnic respiratory failure. *Mayo Clin Proc* 1991;66:695–698.

63. Heckmatt JZ, Loh L, Dubowitz V. Night-time nasal ventilation in neuromuscular disease. *Lancet* 1990;335:579–581.

64. Vianello A, Bevilacqua M, Salvador V, et al. Long-term nasal intermittent positive pressure ventilation in advanced Duchenne's muscular dystrophy. *Chest* 1994;105:445–448.

65. Ambrosino N, Foglio K, Rubini F, et al. Noninvasive mechanical ventilation in acute respiratory failure due to chronic obstructive pulmonary disease: correlates for success. *Thorax* 1995;50:755–759.

66. Benhamou D, Girault C, Faure C, et al. Nasal mask ventilation in acute respiratory failure: experience in elderly patients. *Chest* 1992;102:912–917.

67. Brochard L, Isbey D, Piquet J, et al. Reversal of acute exacerbations of chronic obstructive pulmonary disease by inspiratory assistance with a face mask. *N Engl J Med* 1990;323:1523–1525.

68. Foglio C, Vitacca M, Quadri A, et al. Acute exacerbations in severe COLD patients: treatment using positive pressure ventilation by nasal mask. *Chest* 1992;101:1533–1536.

69. Fortenberry JD, Del Toro J, Jefferson LS, et al. Management of pediatric acute hypoxemic respiratory insufficiency with bi-level positive pressure (BiPAP) nasal mask ventilation. *Chest* 1995;108:1059–1061.

70. Hodson ME, Madden BP, Steven, MH, et al. Noninvasive mechanical ventilation for cystic fibrosis patients—a potential bridge to transplantation. *Eur Respir J* 1991;4:524–529.

71. Lapinsky SE, Mount DB, Mackey D, et al. Management of acute respiratory failure due to pulmonary edema with nasal positive pressure support. *Chest* 1994;105:229–232.

72. Leger P, Bedicam JM, Cornette A, et al. Nasal intermittent positive pressure ventilation: long-term follow-up in patients with severe chronic respiratory insufficiency. *Chest* 1944;105:100–103.

73. Marino W. Intermittent volume cycled mechanical ventilation via nasal mask in patients with respiratory failure due to COPD. *Chest* 1991;99:681–684.

74. Meduri GU, Abou-Shala N, Fox RC, et al. Noninvasive face mask mechanical ventilation in patients with acute hypercapnic respiratory failure. *Chest* 1991;100:445–447.

75. Meecham Jones DJ, Paul EA, Jones PW, et al. Nasal pressure support ventilation plus oxygen compared with oxygen therapy alone in hypercapnic COPD. *Am J Respir Crit Care Med* 1995;152:538–541.

76. Pennock BE, Crawshaw L, Kaplan PD. Noninvasive nasal mask ventilation for acute respiratory failure: institution of a new therapeutic technology for routine use. *Chest* 1994;105:441–444.

77. Piper AM, Parker S, Torzillo PJ, et al. Nocturnal nasal IPPV stabilizes patients with cystic fibrosis and hypercapnic respiratory failure. *Chest* 1992;102:846–850.

78. Renston JP, DiMarco AF, Supinski GS. Respiratory muscle rest using nasal BiPAP ventilation in patients with stable severe COPD. *Chest* 1994;105:1053–1057.

79. Strumpf DA, Millman RP, Carlisle CC, et al. Nocturnal positive-pressure ventilation via nasal mask in patients with severe chronic obstructive pulmonary disease. *Am Rev Respir Dis* 1991;144:1234–1236.

80. Waldhorn RE. Nocturnal nasal intermittent positive pressure ventilation with bi-level positive airway pressure (BiPAP) in respiratory failure. *Chest* 1992;101:516–519.

81. Wysocki M, Tric L, Wolff MA, et al. Noninvasive pressure support ventilation in patients with acute respiratory failure. *Chest* 1993;103:907–911.

Glossary

air embolism—air enters the vascular system and is carried to a smaller blood vessel where it lodges and blocks blood flow

air stacking—insufflations are stacked in the lungs to expand them maximally; this is done by taking a deep breath, then adding consecutive volumes of air delivered via a mouthpiece or nasal interface and holding them with a closed glottis until no more air can be held and the lungs and chest wall are fully expanded

alveolar ventilation—the passage of air into and out of the small air sacs (alveoli) of the respiratory exchange membrane of the lungs by the intermittent action of the diaphragm and other inspiratory muscles

atelectasis—areas of collapse of lung air sacs (alveoli) due to underventilation or accumulation of airway secretions

BiPAP—bi-level positive airway pressure, a method of ventilatory assistance

body ventilator—a device that acts on the body to assist breathing

carbon dioxide tension—the partial pressure of carbon dioxide in the blood; its level correlates inversely with lung ventilation, that is, blood carbon dioxide tensions increase (hypercapnia) when the lungs are under (hypo) ventilated and decrease (hypocapnia) when the lungs are over (hyper) ventilated

cellulitis—inflammation of the soft connective tissues

CPAP (continuous positive airway pressure)—continuous pressure applied through a mask covering the nose, mouth, or mouth and nose that acts as a splint to keep the otherwise obstructed upper airway open and acts to expand the lungs but does not directly help one breathe; this is not a method of ventilatory or inspiratory muscle assistance

CPAP masks—nasal interfaces for the delivery of CPAP or nasal ventilation for ventilatory assistance

glossopharyngeal breathing (GPB)—the "gulping" of air into the lungs to permit ventilator-free breathing or provide maximal insufflations (deep lung volumes) without need for a ventilator or other air delivery system

glottis—the opening between the vocal folds at the upper orifice of the larynx; the mouth of the windpipe

hypercapnia—increased blood carbon dioxide levels due to inability of the breathing muscles to ventilate the lungs adequately

hypoxia (hypoxemia)—decreased blood oxygen levels due to increased blood carbon dioxide levels, mucus plugging of the airways, or lung diseases such as pneumonia

IPPB (intermittent positive pressure breathing)—the delivery of deep insufflations to expand the lungs more fully

IPPV (intermittent positive pressure ventilation)—a form of inspiratory muscle aid or ventilatory assistance provided by delivering air to the lungs via the mouth, nose, mouth-and-nose, or an indwelling tracheostomy tube

insufflation—providing greater volumes of air than one can inhale with one's own inspiratory muscles

intubation—passage of a tube via either the nose (nasotracheal tube) or mouth (orotracheal tube) through the throat and larynx (translaryngeally) and into the trachea for ventilatory assistance and airway suctioning

larynx—the voice organ at the upper portion of the windpipe including the vocal folds

mechanical insufflation–exsufflation—a technique whereby a device is used to provide a deep volume of air to the lungs (insufflation) immediately followed by a forced expiration (exsufflation) to create 10 L/s of expiratory flow to expel airway secretions

mediastinitis—inflammation in the space between the folds of the lining of the lungs (pleura) and the intervening space that separates the right from the left lungs

negative pressure body ventilators—body ventilators that work by creating negative pressure around the chest and abdomen to cause air to enter the nose and mouth to ventilate the lungs

oxyhemoglobin saturation—oxyhemoglobin is the main oxygen-carrying protein in the blood, and, normally, it is 95% or more saturated with oxygen

peak cough flows—the maximum flows that can be generated while coughing whether coughing occurs with or without assistance

pericarditis—inflammation of the lining of the heart

PEEP (positive end-expiratory pressure)—pressure given at the end of a mechanically assisted breath

pneumomediastinum—air entering between the folds of the lining of the lungs (pleura) and the intervening space that separates the right from the left lungs

pneumonia—infection in the lungs usually caused by bacteria multiplying in airway secretions that cannot be expulsed from the lungs

pneumoperitoneum—air entering the abdominal cavity

pneumothorax—a tear in the lining of the lung that permits air to escape from the lung and enter the space between the lining of the lung and the lining of the rib cage

respirator—*See ventilator*

subcutaneous emphysema—the pathological presence of air under the skin

stenosis—narrowing of a passage, e.g., the trachea, caused by complications of translaryngeal intubation or an indwelling tracheostomy tube

suctioning—the passage of a catheter into the airways to aspirate airway secretions and other debris

thoracic—pertaining to the spine at the level of the chest

tidal volume—the volume of air one inhales during one normal breath measured in milliliters

trachea—the windpipe

tracheocutaneous fistula—a pathological tract between the trachea and the skin

tracheoesophageal fistula—a pathological tract between the trachea and the esophagus

tracheomalacia—the softening and thinning out of the trachea

tracheostomy—a surgical hole (stoma) that creates a passage through the neck to the windpipe (trachea) for placement of a tube (tracheostomy tube) through which ventilatory support and airway suctioning can be performed

ventilator—a device that intermittently provides negative or positive pressure to assist or substitute for the inspiratory muscle function needed for breathing (sometimes called a *respirator*)

ventilation—See *alveolar ventilation*

vital capacity—the maximum volume of air that one can inhale then blow through a device (spirometer), measured in milliliters

4

Tracheotomy, Tracheostomy Tubes, and Mechanical Ventilation

ALICE K. SILBERGLEIT, GLENDON M. GARDNER AND MICHAEL C. IANNUZZI

Speech–language pathologists working with individuals with tracheostomy and/or ventilator dependency come across a myriad of terminology by medical, nursing, and respiratory care staff regarding tracheostomy tubes and ventilator settings. The purpose of this chapter is to familiarize the practicing clinician with basic information regarding the history and indications of tracheotomy, components of tracheostomy tubes, specialty tracheostomy tubes, and speaking valves which can be used to enable voicing in this patient population. In addition, commonly used forms of ventilatory support, available options for adjustments of a ventilator, and indications for changing ventilator settings are addressed.

Tracheotomy

Tracheotomy is the surgical opening of the trachea to the outside environment through the tissues of the anterior neck. Trache**ot**omy signifies a temporary opening, whereas *trache**ost**omy* is a permanent opening which must be reversed surgically if it is to be closed. Commonly, the two terms are used interchangeably. Tracheotomy is one of the oldest described surgical procedures. Several authors refer to the *Ebers Papyrus* of Egypt, dated approximately 1550 BC, and the Indian sacred Hindu book *Rigveda*, 2000 BC as the earliest descriptions of tracheotomy (1–3). Throughout the ensuing years, the surgical procedure was favored by some physicians and completely condemned by others. Antyllus, in 117 AD, wrote of

Tracheostomy and Ventilator Dependency: Management of Breathing, Speaking, and Swallowing. Edited by Donna C. Tippett, MPH, MA, CCC-SLP. Thieme Medical Publishers, Inc. New York © 2000.

"a transverse incision between two of the rings," which continues to be used today (2). In ancient times, the indication for tracheotomy was to relieve airway obstruction. At the beginning of the 19th century, the most common reason for performing tracheotomy was the treatment of diphtheric croup which often killed its victims (4).

Procedure

The procedure can be performed as either an open surgical procedure or percutaneously with trocars (sharpened tubes) with essentially the same result. The open procedure begins with an incision through the skin of the anterior lower neck. The dissection continues down to the strap muscles which are then separated in the midline, exposing the thyroid gland. Depending on the patient's anatomy, the thyroid isthmus is either ligated and divided or retracted superiorly or, less commonly, inferiorly. This exposes the anterior wall of the trachea. The trachea can be entered in a variety of ways including a simple vertical or horizontal incision, excision of a portion of the anterior wall, or creation of a flap of the wall. If a permanent tracheostomy is being created, flaps are designed at the skin and the tracheal wall which when sutured together provide a smooth epithelium-lined tract between the trachea and the outside environment. A temporary tracheotomy tract is generally not epithelium-lined and, without a tube in place to keep it open, closes, and heals within days to weeks. A temporary tracheotomy may be kept open indefinitely with the use of a tube and sometimes forms a mature tract on its own.

Indications

Tracheotomy is performed for basically two reasons: to bypass airway obstruction at or above the trachea or manage the airway for long-term ventilatory support. Airway obstruction may be due to a variety of conditions. Examples include benign or malignant tumors of the pharynx, larynx, trachea, thyroid gland, or other structures in the neck. Surgery or radiation therapy to treat these tumors may cause enough edema to block an already limited airway. Infection, such as deep neck abscesses or inflammatory conditions such as Wegener's granulomatosis, may also necessitate tracheotomy. Stenosis of the airway at the level of the larynx or trachea may be congenital or due to trauma such as long-term endotracheal intubation. Bilateral vocal fold immobility, usually due to paralysis, causes obstruction at the level of the glottis. Tracheotomy may also be used to treat severe obstructive sleep apnea or facilitate pulmonary toilet in a patient who chronically aspirates. Tracheotomy, however, does not prevent aspiration. In fact, it is well documented that the presence of a tracheostomy tube contributes to the risk of aspiration, particularly if a cuffed tracheostomy tube is present (5).

For individuals with acute critical illnesses who recover rapidly, the airway can be managed with a transnasal or transoral endotracheal tube. Many patients, however, may require long-term support and the best modality to manage the airway in these situations has been debated. Long-term use of transoral or transnasal endotracheal tubes potentially creates complications (6,7). The tube must pass between the vocal folds and through the cricoid ring to reach the trachea and it is at these locations that a firm plastic tube may do damage (8). A very thin epithelium overlies the hard vocal processes of the arytenoid and the inner aspect of the cricoid cartilages. Erosion of this epithelium by the endotracheal tube can lead to ulceration, granulation tissue formation, and scarring (9). Cricoarytenoid joint motion may be severely impaired causing airway obstruction or dysphonia (10–12). Scarring at the level of the cricoid cartilage can cause clinically significant subglottic stenosis.

The likelihood of a significant laryngeal injury due to endotracheal intubation increases with gastroesophageal reflux disease, infection, motion of the tube or the patient, use of too large a tube, prolonged intubation, and chronic disease such as diabetes mellitus. Estimates of how often these complications occur vary, but most studies that include endoscopic inspection of the larynx during the course of translaryngeal intubation or immediately after extubation demonstrate that as many as 65% of patients have various degrees of injury (13–15). Because of these potential complications, if more than seven days of ventilatory support are anticipated, tracheotomy should be considered.

A tracheostomy tube may be preferred for other reasons. The tracheostomy tube is more secure and less likely to be inadvertently displaced than a transoral endotracheal tube. It may provide for easier nursing care. Due to its lower position in the airway and shorter length, it eliminates dead space and decreases the work of breathing and occasionally facilitates weaning from mechanical ventilation. The decision to perform a temporary trache**ot**omy versus a permanent trache**ost**omy is based on the underlying problem and the prognosis for recovery. If recovery is expected within a reasonable amount of time, e.g., a formerly healthy trauma patient requiring long-term ventilatory support, trache**ot**omy should be performed. A tracheotomy stoma will usually heal spontaneously within days to weeks after the tube has been removed. On the other hand, an extremely obese elderly patient with Pickwickian syndrome and severe obstructive sleep apnea who has failed to benefit from other interventions and is unlikely to recover, would benefit from a trache**ost**omy. The stoma in this case is smooth and epithelium-lined and will not completely close even without a tube.

Complications

The potential complications of tracheotomy include those common to all surgical procedures such as infection and bleeding but also include pneumothorax or pneumomediastinum. A complication shared by tracheotomy and standard endotracheal intubation is trauma to the trachea caused by the cuff located near the end of the tube. Erosion of the tracheal wall at the cuff site may lead to injury to the brachiocephalic artery and vein with resultant, usually fatal hemorrhage. Fortunately this rarely occurs. Tracheal stenosis and/or tracheomalacia may also result from excessive cuff pressure. A false passage, usually anterior to the trachea, can be created during routine tube changing. If this is not recognized immediately, pneumomediastinum or pneumothorax and possibly respiratory arrest and death may occur. (See Chapter 3 for additional information regarding complications.)

Tracheostomy Tubes

There are three basic parts of a tracheostomy tube: the outer cannula, inner cannula, and obturator (Fig. 4–1). The obturator is used to place the outer cannula of the tracheostomy tube into the tracheotomy stoma site. It is immediately removed after insertion and replaced with an inner cannula. The inner cannula functions to collect secretions that could potentially obstruct the airway (16). Inner cannulas may be disposable or nondisposable. Disposable inner cannulas are usually replaced at least daily. Nondisposable ones are cleaned and replaced daily or several times per day depending upon the amount of secretions. Inner cannulas serve to keep the airway free of thick or incrusted secretions. There are some tracheostomy tubes available that do not have inner cannulas. These tubes are made of silicone which is intended to reduce the risk of secretion buildup (17).

Tracheostomy tubes are made from a variety of material. Portex tracheostomy tubes are made from polyvinyl chloride (PVC). The advantage of this material is that it is flexibile yet maintains the shape of the tube. The Portex tube is thermosensitive which allows the tube to soften at body temperature conforming to

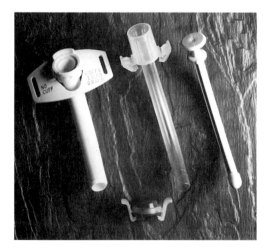

Fig. 4–1. Shiley outer cannula, inner cannula, and obturator (left to right). Photo courtesy of Mallinckrodt Medical, Inc., Hazelwood, Missouri.

the patient's anatomy (18). As reported by Dikeman and Kazandjian (17), tubes made from PVC are more porous and tend to retain bacteria. For this reason, PVC tubes may not be sterilized and reused. Silicone or a combination of silicone and PVC is also used in tracheostomy tubes. Silicone is durable but softer than PVC and contains fewer chemical additives, possibly reducing the risk of chemicals leaking into the tissues of the trachea. Silicone tends to reduce the risk of secretion incrustation and bacteria buildup on the tracheostomy tube and may be reused after sterilization. Silicone and PVC can be combined to produce a softer material than PVC alone; this type of tube is considered disposable and cannot be reused. Although metal tracheostomy tubes have been available for years and are considered more sanitary than PVC tubes, they are rigid and heavy and may cause increased irritation at the stoma site.

Tracheostomy tubes are available in a variety of sizes and lengths which vary among manufacturers. For example, a number 4 tracheostomy tube made by one manufacturer may not have the same inner and outer cannula dimensions as a number 4 tube made by another (Table 4–1). Thus when changing a tracheostomy tube, if different manufactured tubes are used it is important to note the inner and outer cannula dimensions rather than simply the size.

The design of the angle of tracheostomy tubes also varies between manufacturers, and specialty tubes are available for individuals with extra long tracheas, or short or thick necks. The following section reviews some of the specialty tracheostomy tubes currently available.

Specialty Tracheostomy Tubes

Single and Multiple Fenestrated Tracheostomy Tubes (Figs. 4–2 and 4–3) have openings on the superior surface of the outer cannula to allow airflow from the trachea through the fenestration and up through the vocal folds. Fenestrated tubes are available on both cuffed and cuffless tracheostomy tubes. Fenestrated inner cannulas are also available.

The Bivona Tight to the Shaft Tracheostomy Tube (Figs. 4–4 and 4–5) was designed to minimize the amount of cuff material which remains loose around the shaft of the outer cannula when the cuff is deflated. When the cuff of this tube is completely deflated, it retracts tight to the shaft of the tracheostomy tube and adds no distinguishable dimension to the outer diameter of the tube's shaft (19).

The Bivona Adjustable Neck Flange Hyperflex Tracheostomy Tube (Fig. 4–6) was designed for trauma patients and patients with thick necks. Distinguishing features of this tube are the flexible wire reinforced silicone shaft which limits kinking of the tube and a longer shaft to conform to unusual tracheal anatomy or pathology. In addition, this tube has an adjustable neck flange so that cuff position and shaft length may be altered without the need for a tracheostomy tube change (20).

The Moore Tracheostomy Tube (Fig. 4–7) is a flexible tube designed to conform to the individual's anatomy. It is made of radiopaque medical grade silicone which reduces the risk of secretion incrustation. In addition, the standard long length of the tube can be trimmed for individual use (21).

Table 4–1. Cross-reference chart of tracheostomy tube sizes.

NEONATAL AND PEDIATRIC

Bivona®

Neonatal

Product Code(s) Aire-Cuf®	Cuffed TTS™ Cuff	Fome-Cuf®	I.D. mm	O.D. mm	Length mm
65N025	67N025	85N025	2.5	4.0	30
65N030	67N030	85N030	3.0	4.7	32
65N035	67N035	85N035	3.5	5.3	34
65N040	67N040	85N040	4.0	6.0	36

Cuffless: 60N025, 60N030, 60N035, 60N040

Pediatric

Product Code(s) Aire-Cuf®	Cuffed TTS™ Cuff	Fome-Cuf®	I.D. mm	O.D. mm	Length mm
65P025	67P025	85P025	2.5	4.0	38
65P030	67P030	85P030	3.0	4.7	39
65P035	67P035	85P035	3.5	5.3	40
65P040	67P040	85P040	4.0	6.0	41
65P045	67P045	85P045	4.5	6.7	42
65P050	67P050	85P050	5.0	7.3	44
65P055	67P055	85P055	5.5	8.0	46

Cuffless: 60P025, 60P030, 60P035, 60P040, 60P045, 60P050, 60P055

Flextend™

Cuffless	I.D. mm	O.D. mm	Shaft (mm)	FlexTend (mm)
60PF25	2.5	4.0	38	10.0
60PF30	3.0	4.7	39	10.0
60PF35	3.5	5.3	40	15.0
60PF40	4.0	6.0	41	15.0
60PF45	4.5	6.7	42	17.5
60PF50	5.0	7.3	44	20.0
60PF55	5.5	8.0	46	20.0

Shiley

Neonatal

Product Code	I.D. mm	O.D. mm	Length mm
Cuffless			
3.0 NEO	3.0	4.5	30
3.5 NEO	3.5	5.2	32
4.0 NEO	4.0	5.9	34
4.5 NEO	4.5	6.5	36

Pediatric

Product Code	I.D. mm	O.D. mm	Length mm
Cuffless			
3.0 PED	3.0	4.5	39
3.5 PED	3.5	5.2	40
4.0 PED	4.0	5.9	41
4.5 PED	4.5	6.5	42
5.0 PED	5.0	7.1	44
5.5 PED	5.5	7.7	46

Portex

Neonatal

Product Code	I.D. mm	O.D. mm	Length mm
Cuffless			
553025	2.5	4.8	30
553030	3.0	5.2	32
553035	3.5	5.8	34

Pediatric

Product Code	I.D. mm	O.D. mm	Length mm
Cuffless			
555025	2.5	4.8	30
555030	3.0	5.2	36
555035	3.5	5.8	40
555040	4.0	6.6	44
555045	4.5	7.1	48
555050	5.0	7.7	50
555055	5.5	8.3	52

Adjustable Hyperflex™

Cuffless

Product Code(s)	I.D. mm	O.D. mm	Maximum Usable Length (mm)
60HA25	2.5	4.0	55
60HA30	3.0	4.7	60
60HA35	3.5	5.3	65
60HA40	4.0	6.0	70
60HA45	4.5	6.7	75
60HA50	5.0	7.3	80
60HA55	5.5	8.0	85

ADULT

Bivona®

Low Pressure Cuffed Tubes

MR Aire-Cuf® Fome-Cuf® — Single Cannula

Product Code(s)	I.D. mm	O.D. mm	Length mm
750150	5.0	7.3	60
750160	6.0	8.7	70
750170	7.0	10.0	80
750180	8.0	11.0	88
750190	9.0	12.3	98
750195	9.5	13.3	98

Cuffed Weaning or Fenestrated Tubes

TTS™ Cuff — Single Cannula

Product Code(s)	I.D. mm	O.D. mm	Length mm
670150	5.0	7.3	60
670160	6.0	8.7	70
670170	7.0	10.0	80
670180	8.0	11.0	88
670190	9.0	12.3	98
670195	9.5	13.3	98

Shiley

Inner Cannula

Product Code	I.D. mm	O.D. mm	Length mm
4DCT	5.0	8.5	67
6DCT	7.0	10.0	78
8DCT	8.5	12.0	84
10DCT	9.0	13.0	84

Inner Cannula Low Pressure Cuff

Product Code	I.D. mm	O.D. mm	Length mm
4DFEN	5.0	8.5	67
6DFEN	7.0	10.0	78
8DFEN	8.5	12.0	84
10DFEN	9.0	13.0	84

Portex

Inner Cannula

Product Code	I.D. mm	O.D. mm	Length mm
503060	5.0	8.5	67
503070	6.0	9.9	73
503080	7.0	11.3	78
503090	8.0	12.6	84
503100	9.0	14.0	84

Inner Cannula Low Pressure Cuff

Product Code	I.D. mm	O.D. mm	Length mm
513060	5.0	8.5	67
513070	6.0	9.9	73
513080	7.0	11.3	78
513090	8.0	12.6	84
513100	9.0	14.0	84

(continued)

Table 4-1. (continued)

ADULT

Cuffed Single Cannula Tubes

Bivona®

Product Code(s)		I.D. mm	O.D. mm	Length mm
MR Aire-Cuf®	Fome-Cuf®			
750150	850150	5.0	7.3	60
750160	850160	6.0	8.7	70
750170	850170	7.0	10.0	80
750180	850180	8.0	11.0	88
750190	850190	9.0	12.3	98
750195	850195	9.5	13.3	98

Shiley — Low Pressure Cuff

Product Code	I.D. mm	O.D. mm	Length mm
5SCT	5.0	7.0	58
6SCT	6.0	8.3	67
7SCT	7.0	9.6	80
8SCT	8.0	10.9	89
9SCT	9.0	12.1	99
10SCT	10.0	13.3	105

Portex — Single Cannula

Product Code	I.D. mm	O.D. mm	Length mm
530060	6.0	8.3	55
530070[1]	7.0	9.7	75
530080[1]	8.0	11.0	82
530090[1]	9.0	12.4	87
530100	10.0	13.8	98

[1] Available Inner Cannula reduces lumen by 2 mm

Cuffless Profile Tubes

Bivona® — Single Cannula

TTS™ Cuff	Cuffless	I.D. mm	O.D. mm	Length mm
670150	60A150	5.0	7.3	60
670160	60A160	6.0	8.7	70
670170	60A170	7.0	10.0	80
670180	60A180	8.0	11.0	88
670190	60A190	9.0	12.3	98
670195	60A195	9.5	13.3	98

Shiley — Inner Cannula

Product Code	I.D. mm	O.D. mm	Length mm
4CFS	5.0	8.5	67
6CFS	7.0	10.0	78
8CFS	8.5	12.0	84
10CFS	9.0	13.0	84

Portex — Single Cannula

Product Code	I.D. mm	O.D. mm	Length mm
550060	6.0	8.3	55
550070	7.0	9.7	75
550080	8.0	11.0	82
550090	9.0	12.4	87
530100	10.0	13.8	98

Adjustable Hyperflex™

Bivona®

TTS™ Cuff	MR Aire-Cuf®	I.D. mm	O.D. mm	Maximum Usable Length (mm)
67HA60	75HA60	6.0	8.7	110
67HA70	75HA70	7.0	10.0	120
67HA80	75HA80	8.0	11.0	130
67HA90	75HA90	9.0	12.3	140

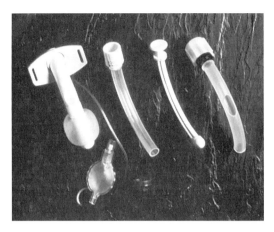

Fig. 4–2. Single fenestrated outer cannula (far left) with fenestrated inner cannula (far right). Photo courtesy of Mallinckrodt Medical, Inc., Hazelwood, Missouri.

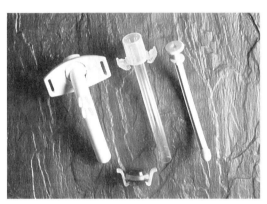

Fig. 4–3. Multiple fenestrated outer cannula (far left). Photo courtesy of Mallinckrodt Medical, Inc., Hazelwood, Missouri.

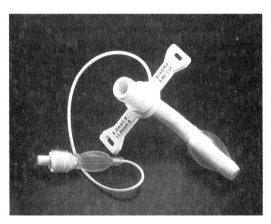

Fig. 4–4. Bivona Tight to the Shaft Tracheostomy Tube with Inflated Cuff. Photo courtesy of Bivona Medical Technologies, Inc., Gary, Indiana.

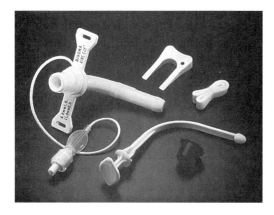

Fig. 4–5. Bivona Tight to the Shaft Tracheostomy Tube with Deflated Cuff. Photo courtesy of Bivona Medical Technologies, Inc., Gary, Indiana.

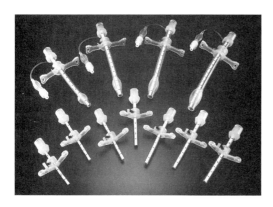

Fig. 4–6. Bivona Adjustable Neck Flange Hyperflex Tracheostomy Tubes. Photo courtesy of Bivona Medical Technologies, Inc., Gary, Indiana.

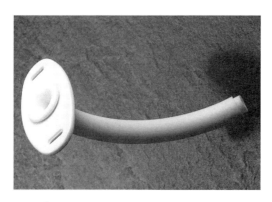

Fig. 4–7. Moore Tracheostomy Tube. Photo courtesy of Boston Medical Products, Westborough, Massachusetts.

The Tracoe Comfort Tracheostomy Tube (Fig. 4–8) is flexible at room temperature and becomes more pliable at body temperature. It also has a featherlight weight to improve patient comfort (21).

The Tracoe Flex Tracheostomy Tube (Fig. 4–9) is also flexible at room temperature and becomes more pliable at body temperature to improve patient comfort. An additional feature of this tube is a swivel neck plate which can move horizontally or vertically to allow greater range of movement (21).

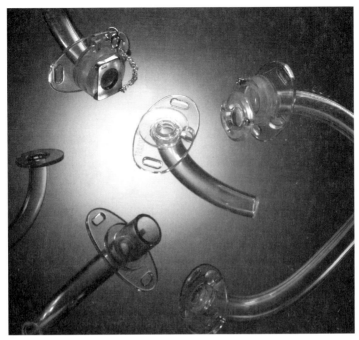

Fig. 4–8.   Tracoe Comfort Tracheostomy Tube. Photo courtesy of Boston Medical Products, Westborough, Massachusetts.

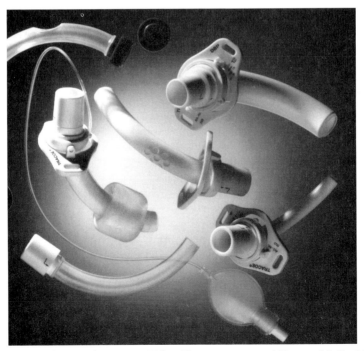

Fig. 4–9.   Tracoe Flex Tracheostomy Tube. Photo courtesy of Boston Medical Products, Westborough, Massachusetts.

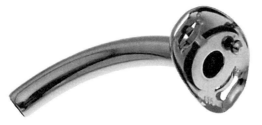

Fig. 4–10. Stainless Steel Jackson Tracheostomy Tube. Photo courtesy of Pilling Weck, Fort Washington, Pennsylvania.

Metal or Sterling Silver Jackson Tracheostomy Tubes (Fig. 4–10) are available in stainless steel or sterling silver. A fenestrated model may be special ordered to facilitate speech (22).

Double Cuffed Tracheostomy Tubes (Figs. 4–11 and 4–12) are typically used to alternate inflation of the cuffs and therefore, potentially reduce the risk of granulation formation within the trachea (18). In cases of tracheomalachia a longer shaft length with a double cuff may be necessary.

Cuffs of Tracheostomy Tubes

Tracheostomy tubes may be cuffless or cuffed as seen in Figures 4–1 and 4–2, respectively. Metal tracheostomy tubes do not have cuffs (Fig. 4–10). Using a syringe into the pilot balloon, the cuff of a tracheostomy tube is inflated to create a seal against the trachea thus allowing airflow directly into the lungs while bypassing the upper airway (Fig. 4–13). Potential complications of an inflated cuff

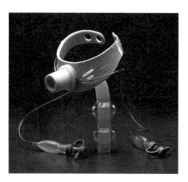

Fig. 4–11. Portex Double Cuffed Tracheostomy Tube. Photo courtesy of SIMS Portex, Inc., Keene, New Hampshire.

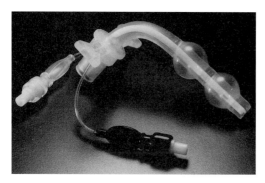

Fig. 4–12. Bivona Double Cuffed Tracheostomy Tube with Extended Shaft. Photo courtesy of Bivona Medical Technologies, Inc., Gary, Indiana.

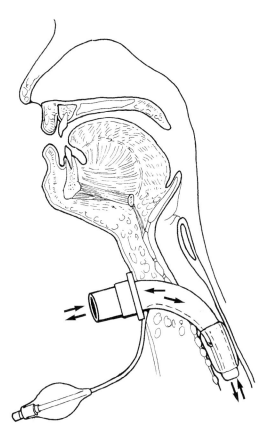

Fig. 4–13. Arrows show route of air-flow to and from the lower airway with an inflated tracheostomy tube cuff.

include irritation of the posterior tracheal wall as the tracheostomy tube and cuff move up and down during swallowing, breathing, or changes in body positioning; the formation of granulation tissue on the trachea at the site of the cuff due to irritation over a period of time to the posterior tracheal wall; an overinflated cuff delivering excess pressure on the anterior esophageal wall thus limiting the diameter of the esophagus, causing dysphagia; and limitation of laryngeal elevation during swallowing which may lead to aspiration (5).

Cuffs, like tracheostomy tubes, come in a variety of shapes and materials. There are barrel-shaped cuffs (Fig. 4–2), spherical-shaped cuffs (Fig. 4–11), and oval-shaped cuffs (Fig. 4–14). Barrel-shaped cuffs provide an even distribution of cuff pressures within the trachea, and spherically shaped cuffs provide a smaller area of contact along the tracheal wall when inflated. The oval or egg-shaped cuff is a foam cuff which has a sponge-like consistency. This particular type of cuff is filled with air at rest and reinflates spontaneously after deflation. The foam cuff conforms to a patient's trachea and is useful in reducing the risk of collapsing the tracheal walls in cases of tracheomalacia or trauma to the trachea (17). It should be noted that due to the foam cuff's spontaneous reinflation properties, airflow to the upper airway for voicing purposes is not possible. Patients with foam cuffs

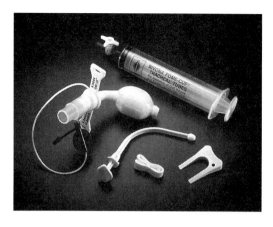

Fig. 4–14. Oval-Shaped Foam Cuff. Photo courtesy of Bivona Medical Technologies, Inc., Gary, Indiana.

are not candidates for voicing with one-way speaking valves or via capping of the outer cannula as a deflated cuff is required for these situations.

As a patient's medical status improves, the cuff is usually deflated to prepare for weaning from the tracheostomy tube, relieve pressure from the posterior tracheal wall at the site of the cuff to begin swallowing therapy, or facilitate upper airway airflow through the vocal folds to allow the patient to phonate (Fig. 4–15).

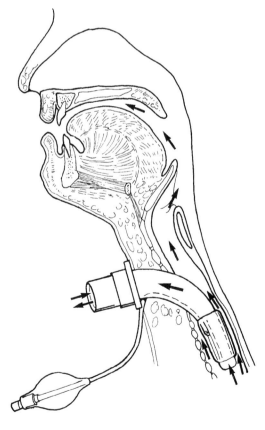

Fig. 4–15. Arrows show the route of airflow to the upper airway as well as the lower airway when a tracheostomy tube cuff is deflated.

Voicing Options for Patients with Deflated Cuffs or Cuffless Tracheostomy Tubes

A cuffed tracheostomy tube creates a seal against the tracheal wall preventing airflow from the lungs and trachea from entering the upper airway, i.e., larynx, mouth, and nasopharynx. When the cuff is inflated, inhalation and exhalation occur directly via the trachea to and from the atmosphere. To allow airflow between the trachea and the upper airway the cuff of the tracheostomy tube must be deflated. If voicing with a deflated or cuffless tracheostomy tube is being considered, cuff manipulation should be done only by a trained healthcare professional. In addition, an otolaryngologic examination is necessary to assess laryngeal status and identify vocal fold pathology which may affect the voice. There are basically three different variations of voicing with a deflated cuff or cuffless tracheostomy tube:

1. The inner cannula remains in place using digital occlusion over the proximal opening of the tracheostomy tube. The patient inhales, the outer hub of the inner cannula is digitally occluded and the patient voices upon exhalation.
2. The inner cannula is removed allowing the patient to voice via digital occlusion of the proximal end of the outer cannula as above. If the patient is nearing the process of decannulation, capping of the outer cannula may be tolerated so that both inhalation and exhalation occur through the mouth and nose.
3. In cases where a fenestrated outer cannula tracheostomy tube is used, voicing may occur by removing the inner cannula and digitally occluding or capping the proximal end of the outer cannula. Air flows both around the distal end of the tracheostomy tube and up through the fenestration to allow for greater airflow through the vocal folds and a stronger voice. If a fenestrated inner cannula is in place, removing the inner cannula is not necessary. In some cases the fenestration of the outer cannula may be situated too close to the posterior tracheal wall or may actually touch the trachea. If this occurs, air will not be able to flow through the fenestration to reach the vocal folds, and the patient will not be able to voice. Changing the size or type of the tracheostomy tube so that the fenestrated portion of the tracheostomy tube is situated freely within the trachea may improve voicing in such situations.

    Since air flows along the path of least resistance, occlusion of the outer cannula is necessary for more efficient use of breath support and for a stronger sounding voice. If the proximal end of the outer cannula remains open in any of the above scenarios, some air will flow out of the patient's nose and mouth as well as out the trachea and a breathy, low volume, weak sounding voice will occur.

ONE-WAY SPEAKING VALVES

An additional method of voicing with a deflated or cuffless tracheostomy tube involves the use of a one-way speaking valve. Speaking valves are placed on the outer hub of the inner cannula of the tracheostomy tube and open during inhalation and close during exhalation so that air is directed up through the vocal folds (Fig. 4–16). Speaking valves are frequently used as a transition step prior to full decannulation of the tracheostomy tube. Speaking valves eliminate the need

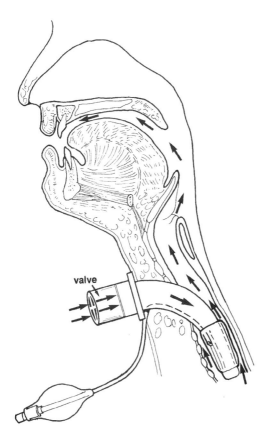

valve

Fig. 4–16. Arrows show the route of inhalation through a speaking valve and exhalation via the upper airway with a speaking valve in place and the tracheostomy tube cuff fully deflated.

for digital occlusion of the tracheostomy tube and so reduce the risk of infection from unclean hands occluding the tracheostomy tube opening. Speaking valves also allow patients to phonate who have upper extremity weakness and are unable to digitally occlude a tracheostomy tube. A cuffless tracheostomy tube or a tracheostomy tube with a deflated cuff must be in place when using a speaking valve. If a cuff is inflated (Fig. 4–17) while a speaking valve is in place, the patient will not be able to exhale. Air will not be able to exit the upper airway due to the obstruction of the inflated cuff, and air will not be able to exit the tracheostomy tube because of the seal the speaking valve provides at the proximal end of the tracheostomy tube upon exhalation. Some common speaking valves currently available are described briefly; for further information see Chapter 5.

The Passy-Muir Tracheostomy and Ventilator Speaking Valves (Passy-Muir Inc., Irvine, California) attach to the standard 15-mm hub of an inner cannula. It is unique from other valves due to its biased closed position. In other words, the valve is closed at rest and opens during inhalation. The valve then begins to close prior to the end of inhalation. This design enables a small column of air to be trapped between the valve and the tracheostomy tube thus acting as a buffer against secretion buildup which could potentially occlude the function of the valve. It has been reported that the biased closed position requires less effort to

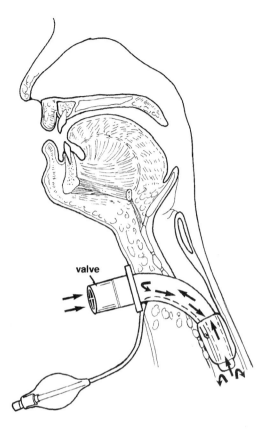

valve

Fig. 4–17. Arrows show inhalation through the speaking valve and trapping of air within the trachea during attempts to exhale when a speaking valve is in place and the tracheostomy tube cuff is inflated.

close than do valves that have an open bias (23). Some studies have shown that the Passy-Muir valve improves oxygen saturation, reduces the risk of aspirating if wearing the valve during eating, and helps facilitate patient tolerance of the ventilatory weaning process (24–26). There are four models of the Passy-Muir valve (Fig. 4–18). The aqua valve is designed for in-line use with ventilators as it has a tapered end to easily accommodate ventilator tubing, however, all of the valves are interchangeable and can be used with tracheostomy patients who are either on or off of a ventilator. Additional options to the 2000 series Passy-Muir speaking valves include an adapter for supplemental oxygen and an attachment to secure the valve to the tracheostomy tube collar so that it remains near the patient should it become dislodged, i.e., during a cough.

The Montgomery Tracheostomy Speaking Valve (Boston Medical Products, Westborough, Massachusetts) (Fig. 4–19) fits onto the standard 15-mm hub of an inner cannula. It has a unique cough release feature designed to prevent the valve from popping off of the tracheostomy tube during a cough. When a cough occurs, the silicone diaphragm partially dislodges, but may be easily tucked back into its housing at the end of the cough (27). The Montgomery Speaking Valve is also available in a model specifically designed for in-line ventilator use called the VENTRACH speaking valve.

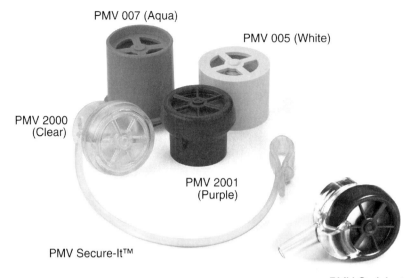

PMV 007 (Aqua)

PMV 005 (White)

PMV 2000
(Clear)

PMV 2001
(Purple)

PMV Secure-It™

PMV O₂ Adapter
with PMV 2001

Fig. 4–18. Passy-Muir Tracheostomy and Ventilator Speaking Valves. Photo courtesy of Passy-Muir, Inc., Irvine, California.

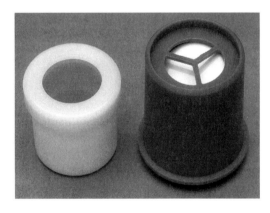

Fig. 4–19. Montgomery Speaking Valve (left) and Montgomery VEN-TRACH Speaking Valve (right). Photo courtesy of Boston Medical Products, Westborough, Massachusetts.

The Shiley Phonate Speaking Valve (Mallinckrodt Medical Inc., Hazelwood, Missouri) (Fig. 4–20) attaches to the standard 15-mm hub of an inner cannula. It also has a cough release design (28). This valve is available with or without a supplemental oxygen port.

The Hood Speaking Valve (Hood Laboratories, Pembroke, Massachusetts) (Fig. 4–21) attaches to all 15-mm connectors of tracheostomy tubes (29). It is also available in a model which attaches to the Hood Stoma Stent thus eliminating the need for finger occlusion to voice in patients wearing the stent.

The Tucker Valve (Pilling Weck, Fort Washington, Pennsylvania) (Fig. 4–22) is designed for the Jackson Sterling Silver Tracheostomy Tube. It is built into the silver inner cannula. It is a hinged flap which lifts up to allow air into the trachea

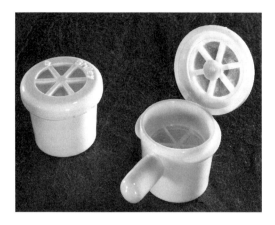

Fig. 4–20. Shiley Phonate Speaking Valve with (right) and without (left) oxygen port. Photo courtesy of Mallinckrodt Medical, Inc., Hazelwood, Missouri.

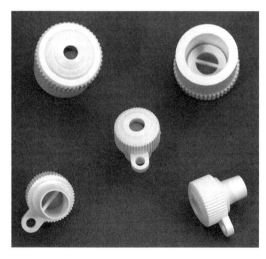

Fig. 4–21. Hood Speaking Valves for tracheostomy tubes (top row); Hood Speaking Valves that attach to the Hood Stoma Stents (middle and bottom rows). Photo courtesy of Hood Laboratories, Pembroke, Massachusetts.

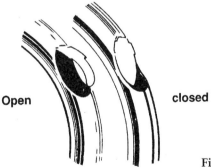

Open   closed

Tucker Valve

Fig. 4–22. Tucker Valve. Photo courtesy of Pilling Weck, Fort Washington, Pennsylvania.

upon inhalation and then drops down to seal the inner cannula during exhalation thus redirecting air around the tube and out the upper airway. The Tucker Valve may be used with a fenestrated or nonfenestrated sterling silver outer cannula (22).

Intubation and Mechanical Ventilation

Tracheal intubation and mechanical ventilation are indicated to support an individual during a life-threatening illness and correct respiratory failure. Respiratory failure is classified into three categories: *hypoxic, hypercapnic* or a combination of the two. Hypoxic respiratory failure occurs when there is failure of gas exchange and hypercapnic respiratory failure occurs when there is failure of the ventilatory pump. Tracheal intubation without mechanical ventilation is indicated to protect the compromised upper airway in a patient who can maintain adequate respiratory function.

Mechanical Ventilation: General Principles

For ventilation to occur, the lungs and the chest wall must expand and then return to their resting volumes. Expansion occurs by the development of a transpulmonary pressure gradient (Ptp). *Ptp* is the difference between intrapulmonary pressure (Ppul) and intrapleural pressure [Ptp = Ppul − Ppl]. During spontaneous unassisted breathing, contraction of the diaphragm and other accessory muscles of inspiration result in a more negative Ppl, generating a pressure gradient and the movement of tidal volume (Vt) into the lungs. Relaxation of the ventilatory muscles returns these pressures and volumes to their resting levels, thus the elastic recoil of the thoracic cage and the lung increases intrathoracic pressure, causing an increase in alveolar and airway pressure, allowing exhalation of the tidal volume.

All forms of ventilatory support function by developing a transpulmonary pressure gradient. A transpulmonary pressure gradient can be created either by increasing Ppul or lowering Ppl. Positive pressure ventilation creates Ptp by increasing Ppul with the application of above atmospheric pressure. Negative pressure ventilation creates a Ptp by causing a more negative Ppl with the application of subatmospheric or negative extrathoracic pressure. Other forms of ventilatory support, namely such gravity-assisted devices as the pneumobelt and rocking bed, also act by creating Ptp and do so by assisting diaphragmatic movement.

Types of Ventilatory Support

Invasive ventilatory support refers to mechanical ventilation via an endotracheal or tracheostomy tube. Noninvasive ventilation refers to ventilation without an endotracheal tube and includes negative pressure ventilation, gravity-assist devices, and positive pressure ventilation administered through a mask. (Also see Chapter 3.)

Negative pressure ventilation (NPV) is any type of ventilation in which the surface of the thorax is exposed to subatmospheric or negative pressure during inspiration. A negative pressure ventilator consists of two components: a "chamber" surrounding the patient's chest and abdomen, and a negative pressure generator. The chamber may cover only the anterior surface of the thorax and abdomen such as a cuirass, or chest shell, or cover all or nearly all extracranial portions of the body, such as with the iron lung and body suit. The main mode for delivering NPV is with cyclical negative pressure. Inspiration is initiated with the application of negative pressure and expiration is passive. The advantage of NPV is that it avoids endotracheal intubation. NPV can be used for nighttime respiratory muscle rest for patients with chronic obstructive pulmonary disease (COPD) or neuromuscular disorders. The main disadvantage of NPV is that it limits nursing care access to the patient. In addition, some patients complain of difficulty with sleep and some develop obstructive sleep apnea (30).

Gravity-assist devices, namely, the rocking bed and pneumobelt, are means of noninvasive ventilatory support. Both rely on the effect of gravity to assist diaphragmatic motion and are particularly suited to patients with severe diaphragmatic weakness or paralysis, most notably for patients with polio. The rocking bed induces a rocking motion of the abdominal viscera within the thorax to assist inspiration. This action has been likened to a piston within a (thoracic) cylinder (31). The pneumobelt (32) or intermittent abdominal pressure respirator consists of an inflatable bladder inside a corset. The corset is fitted around the abdomen with the bladder connected to a positive pressure generator. As the bladder is inflated, the abdominal wall is compressed, the diaphragm is elevated, and exhalation occurs. As the bladder deflates, abdominal pressure is relieved and inspiration occurs passively with gravity pulling the viscera and diaphragm back to their original positions. Because this action depends on gravity, the pneumobelt must be used in the sitting position.

To use the rocking bed, the rocking rate is set between 12 and 16 cycles per minute, and the patient is coached to exhale during head down rocking and to inhale while the head moves up (33). After synchronization has been achieved, the rate is adjusted to optimize minute ventilation. To use the pneumobelt, the rate is set to approximate the spontaneous respiratory rate and an inspiratory: expiratory (I:E) ratio at 1:1.5 (34). Bladder peak inflation pressures are begun at 20–25 cm H_2O. Inflation pressure is gradually increased until the patient's assisted tidal volume is in the desired range. Maximum peak pressures used are 30–50 cm H_2O. Since both the rocking bed and pneumobelt assist ventilation by augmenting diaphragmatic motion, their indication is for patients with diaphragmatic weakness or paralysis. The rocking bed is suited for nocturnal use and pneumobelt for daytime use, and the two may be used in complementary fashion. The effectiveness of both the rocking bed and pneumobelt are variable and depend on the patient's body habitus, therefore, these modes of ventilation are not suited to treat acute respiratory failure. Furthermore, the rocking bed and pneumobelt are not considered for first-line intervention since noninvasive positive pressure ventilation administered via a nasal or face mask is generally more convenient.

Positive pressure ventilation (PPV) is the ventilatory support most commonly used to treat respiratory failure. As noted, positive pressure ventilation creates a Ptp by increasing Ppul with the application of above atmospheric pressure. There are two main modes of positive pressure ventilation: volume-targeted and pressure-targeted. With volume-targeted ventilation, a specific tidal volume is delivered, although the peak airway pressure may vary. In pressure-targeted ventilation, the peak inspiratory plateau pressure is established during inspiration, but the tidal volume may vary depending on the patient's lung compliance and airway resistance.

Modes of Volume-Targeted PPV

Volume-targeted ventilation can be delivered as controlled-mode ventilation (CMV), assist-control ventilation (ACV), intermittent mandatory ventilation

(IMV), and synchronous intermittent mandatory ventilation (SIMV). With controlled-mode ventilation, spontaneous breathing must be abolished so this mode is primarily used in the operating room where the patient is paralyzed. Because long periods of CMV can cause disuse atrophy and uncoordination of respiratory muscles (35), assisted modes of ventilation are preferred. Assisted modes allow for greater patient comfort and help minimize respiratory muscle atrophy since breaths provided are triggered by the patient's inspiratory efforts.

With assist-control ventilation, all breaths are mechanical positive pressure breaths. A backup rate of mechanical breaths is set and starts if no patient effort occurs within a preselected time. To illustrate, if a patient is breathing 12 times per minute with the assist-control backup rate set at 10 breaths and the tidal volume set at 500 cc, the patient receives a minute ventilation of 6 L (500 cc × 12). Each of the 12 breaths is initiated by the patient, and the ventilator delivers 500-cc tidal volumes with each breath. If the patient does not breathe at a rate above the backup rate, the patient's minute ventilation would be 5 L resulting from 10 breaths at a 500-cc tidal volume.

With the assist-control mode, all breaths are machine assisted. Intermittent mandatory ventilation (IMV) differs from assist-control in that IMV allows spontaneous breathing through the ventilator circuit without any ventilatory support. Spontaneous breathing occurs in between the volume-targeted breaths delivered by the ventilator at the IMV rate. In another words, patients can breathe spontaneously, and, in addition to their own spontaneous minute ventilation, receive a number of mechanical breaths (IMV rate) with a preset tidal volume. As the IMV rate is lowered the patient assumes a greater proportion of their minute ventilation. To illustrate, consider a patient on an IMV mode with the ventilator set at an IMV rate of 7 and a tidal volume at 500 cc. If the patient is breathing at a rate of 12 with their own spontaneous tidal volume through the ventilator circuit of 300 cc, their minute volume would be 7 breaths × 500 cc plus 5 breaths at 300 cc or a total of 5 L. This patient would be contributing 1.5 L to the 5-L minute ventilation.

Synchronized intermittent mandatory ventilation (SIMV) is essentially the same as IMV but incorporates a demand valve that must be patient activated so that each spontaneous breath allows the mechanical breaths to be delivered in concert with the patient's effort. At present, all IMV circuits are synchronized so IMV and SIMV are used interchangeably.

CMV, as noted above, has been replaced by the AC mode on today's modern ventilators since CMV does not allow spontaneous breaths. If controlled ventilatory support is desired, the assist control mode is used and the patient given appropriate sedation and neuromuscular blockade to minimize or eliminate respiratory effort.

Assist control mode is generally favored for nearly all patients because of patient synchrony. If the patient feels uncomfortable with the sensation of "air hunger," the response generally should be to sedate with morphine sulfate which decreases the sensation of dyspnea and administer therapy directed at the underlying problem. It is unlikely that changing the mode of mechanical ventilation will improve the situation.

SIMV may be more comfortable for some patients. How to predict which patients would do better with SIMV is simply not known. As noted above, SIMV is usually associated with greater work of breathing compared to AC ventilation, and thus is less frequently used as an initial ventilator mode. It is controversial whether SIMV or AC with T-piece weaning allows for faster liberation from mechanical ventilation during the weaning process.

Pressure-Targeted PPV

With pressure-targeted ventilation, the pressure delivered is set but the tidal volume varies with the time available for inspiration, and the patient's respiratory compliance and airway resistance. Pressure-targeted PPV is not generally used as a mode of mechanical ventilation in patients whose respiratory compliance or airway resistance is changing. Changes in respiratory compliance may occur, for example, with cardiogenic pulmonary edema or from worsening lung injury such as in the acute respiratory distress syndrome (ARDS). Changes in airway resistance may occur from tracheobronchial secretions and bronchospasm.

Pressure-targeted ventilation has the advantage that it addresses the risk for ventilator-induced lung injury due to large inflation volumes. Peak airway pressures are lower in pressure-cycled than in volume-cycled machine breaths. The major disadvantage is the tendency for inflation volumes to vary with changes in the mechanical properties of the lung.

Modes of Pressure-Targeted PPV

The main modes of pressure-targeted PPV are pressure-controlled (PCV) and pressure-support ventilation (PSV). Pressure-controlled ventilation is similar to the volume-targeted CMV in that the cycled breathing is completely controlled by the ventilator with no participation by the patient. Pressure-support ventilation is similar to assist-control mode in that the patient initiates the breaths. At the onset of each spontaneous breath, the negative pressure generated by the patient opens a valve that delivers the inspired gas at a preselected pressure (usually 5–10 cm H_2O).

Each of these modes of mechanical ventilation has advantages and disadvantages (See Table 4–2). The primary consideration in choosing a mode of ventilation is to consider two specific goals: (1) a reduction of the work of breathing; and (2) the assurance of patient comfort and synchrony with the ventilator. There is currently no consensus on the optimum mode of ventilatory support. While each of the modes have been reviewed, nearly all patients should be placed on assist-control mode. In the majority of cases in which there is a problem with mechanical ventilation, the reason is not that the assist-control mode is the wrong choice. The reason for difficulties with mechanical ventilation generally relates to the underlying critical condition of the patient. It is generally more fruitful to pay attention to the patient's medical condition than in choosing one of the other modes of mechanical ventilation. Choosing a mode other than assist control should only be done after thoughtful evaluation by a critical care specialist.

Noninvasive Pressure Support

Spontaneous breathing in which a positive pressure is maintained throughout the respiratory cycle is called *continuous positive airway pressure* (CPAP). The major

Table 4–2. Advantages and disadvantages of selected modes of mechanical ventilation.

Mode	Advantages	Disadvantages
CMV	Rests respiratory muscles	No patient-ventilator interaction. Must use sedation/ neuromuscular blockade
ACV	Reduced work of breathing. Patient determines amount of ventilatory support	May lead to inappropriate hyperventilation
SIMV	Improved patient-ventilator interaction	May increase work of breathing
PCV	Limits peak inspiratory pressure and may minimize baurotrauma	Potential hypoventilation or hyperventilation with changes in lung resistance or compliance
PSV	Decreased work of breathing. May offer greater comfort to some patients	Same as (PCV)

use of CPAP is in nonintubated patients. CPAP can be delivered through specialized face or nasal masks equipped with adjustable pressurized valves. A further development of CPAP is BiPAP (Bi-level Positive Airway Pressure, Respironics, Inc., Murrysville, PA). BiPAP is a variable flow generator that permits independent control of inspiratory (IPAP) and expiratory (EPAP) pressures. The option of varying EPAP may have an advantage in that positive expiratory pressure may recruit collapsed alveoli increasing FRC (36).

Setting the Ventilator

The ventilator should be set so that the patient's ventilatory rquirements are met and the patient appears comfortable. Patients should not be breathing out of phase with the ventilator nor should they be at the same level of distress noted before initiation of ventilation. Ventilator settings are based on the patient's size and condition and require frequent reassessment. The settings include fractional inspired oxygen (FIO_2), tidal volume, respiratory rate, flow rate, sensitivity, and positive end expiratory pressure (PEEP).

FIO$_2$

In general, the lowest acceptable FIO_2 should be selected to obtain the target arterial oxygen saturation (PaO_2), namely, an oxygen saturation of greater than 90%. When the patient's supplemental oxygen requirement is not known, the FIO_2 is first set at 100% and dialed down under pulse oximetry or arterial blood gas monitoring.

TIDAL VOLUME

For volume-targeted ventilation such as with assist-control or IMV mode, the tidal volume selected in adults usually varies from 5 to 15 ml/kg of ideal body weight. Factors such as risk for barotrauma, lung/thorax compliance, and ventilatory needs are considered when choosing the tidal volume. To minimize risk of ventilator-induced lung injury, peak alveolar pressure as estimated from the plateau pressure is monitored.

The incidence of injury increases as the plateau pressure rises. It had been customary to use tidal volumes of 10–15 ml/kg of body weight which is two to three times higher than normal tidal volume. Patients with normal lungs typically feel more comfortable when they are ventilated at these higher tidal volumes, however, in patients with lung injury whose total lung capacity is reduced, the higher tidal volumes may overdistend lung units and cause lung injury. Although data are incomplete, there is a growing tendency to lower the tidal volumes delivered to 5–7 ml/kg or less in order to achieve a plateau pressure no higher than 35 cm of water (37,38). Using smaller tidal volumes may lead to increased arterial carbon dioxide tension. To avoid high peak airway pressure, carbon dioxide tension is allowed to rise while maintaining a pH around 7.2 with the administration of bicarbonate. This strategy is called *permissive hypercapnia* or *controlled hypoventilation* (39). The strategy is that hypercapnia is permitted provided that the hazards of alveolar overdistention are judged more deleterious to survival than the potential hazards of allowing the arterial pH to be decreased.

RESPIRATORY RATE

The setting of respiratory rate depends on the mode of mechanical ventilation, desired minute ventilation, target $PaCO_2$ level, and the level of spontaneous ventilation. The IMV rate, or for assist-control mode, the backup rate, should be about four breaths per minute less than the patient's spontaneous rate. This ensures that the ventilator continues to supply an adequate minute ventilation should the patient suddenly become apneic or have a decrease in respiratory drive. With pressure-support ventilation the rate is not set.

FLOW RATE

Peak inspiratory flow rate should match patient peak inspiratory demands, which is usually between 40 and 100 L/min. To avoid barotrauma, consideration must also be given to the peak alveolar pressure. For a given airway resistance and lung compliance, higher peak flow rates result in higher peak alveolar pressure. In patients with COPD, better gas exchange is often achieved at higher flow rates probably because the resulting increase in expiratory time allows more complete emptying of gas-trapped regions (40). With pressure-targeted ventilation, the peak inspiratory flow is not set but rather determined by the set pressure, respiratory resistance, and patient effort.

SIGH BREATHS

During normal spontaneous breathing an individual normally inspires deeply a number of times per hour. These breaths help to reestablish lung volume that has diminished because of shallow breathing and to reverse any alveolar collapse. Since most ventilators use large tidal volumes (greater than physiology) to ventilate patients, sighs are normally not administered. In fact, few ventilators now incorporate the sigh option.

SENSITIVITY

Most ventilators are triggered by a drop in airway pressure, and their sensitivity is usually set at -1 to -2 cm water. If the amount of pressure drop necessary is decreased, the system becomes more sensitive thus requiring less patient effort to trigger the ventilator.

PEEP

PEEP refers to positive end expiratory pressure applied during mechanical ventilation. PEEP, by maintaining lung volume above the critical closing level, improves ventilation–perfusion matching thus lowering oxygen requirements. PEEP is not a specific therapy but best thought of as a means to help reduce iatrogenic lung injury by allowing ventilation with low inflation volume and allowing the FIO_2 to be reduced to less toxic levels. A potential deleterious effect of PEEP is that PEEP also increases intrathoracic pressure and may limit venous return and right heart filling leading to a decreased cardiac output and decreased oxygen delivery (41). PEEP is mostly used in patients with acute respiratory failure due to acute lung injury. Recently, low levels of PEEP can be beneficial in patients with COPD with the main goal to counterbalance instrinsic PEEP (42).

ALARMS

Alarms may be adjusted to indicate high or low minute ventilation and high or low tidal volumes. When a selected threshold is not maintained, an audible alarm and visual indicator activate, which indicate that hypoventilation exists and warrants immediate attention. Airway pressure is also monitored with alarms for high peak airway pressure, a low inspiratory pressure and a loss of PEEP/CPAP. An abrupt decrease in peak airway pressure of greater than 5 to 10 cm H_2O may indicate a circuit leak which could predispose to hypoventilation. An acute peak airway pressure elevation of greater than 5 to 10 cm H_2O may indicate potential problems including mucus plugging, increased secretions, water condensate in hoses of the delivery circuit, bronchospasm, kinked tracheal tube, tension pneumothorax or patient asynchrony with the ventilator.

Summary

In summary, the above information provides the reader with a foundation of knowledge regarding tracheostomy and mechanical ventilation. This chapter focuses upon a review of the procedure and indications for tracheotomy and its potential complications as well as detailed information regarding the current availability of tracheostomy tubes, the advantages and disadvantages of the styles and types of tubes presently manufactured, and speaking valve options which are used with tracheostomy tubes. The indications, general principles, and modes of mechanical ventilation along with ventilator settings were also presented.

References

1. Brandt L, Goerig M. Die Geschichte der Tracheotomie. *Anaesthetist* 1986;35:279–283.
2. Stock CR. What is past is prologue: a short history of the development of tracheostomy. *ENT Journal* 1987;66:166–169.

3. Frost EAM. Tracing the tracheostomy. *Ann Otol* 1976;85:618–624.
4. Quiroga VA. Diphtheria and medical therapy. *New York St J Med* 1990;90:256–262.
5. Logemann J. Evaluation of swallowing disorders. In: Logemann J, ed. *Evaluation and treatment of swallowing disorders*. Boston: Little Brown, 1983:87–125.
6. Benninger MS, Alessi D, Archer S, et al. Vocal fold scarring: current concepts and management. *Oto-H&N Surg* 1996;115:474–482.
7. Leonard R, Senders C, Charpied G. Effects of long-term intubation on vocal fold mucosa in dogs. *J Voice* 1992;6:86–93.
8. Weymuller EA. Laryngeal injury from prolonged endotracheal intubation. *Laryngoscope* 1988;98 (Supp No. 45): 1–15.
9. Lusk RP, Wooley AL, Holinger LD. Laryngeal stenosis in pediatric laryngology. In: Holinger LD, Lusk RP, Green CG, eds. *Pediatric laryngology and bronchoesophagology*. Philadelphia: Lippincott-Raven Publishers, 1997:165–186.
10. Goodwin WJ, Isaacson G, Kirchner JC, Sasaki CT. Vocal cord mobilization by posterior laryngo-plasty. *Laryngoscope* 1988;98:846–848.
11. Hoasjoe DK, Franlin SW, Aarstad RF, et al. Posterior glottic stenosis mechanism and surgical management. *Laryngoscope* 1997;107:765–679.
12. Zalzal GH. Posterior glottic fixation in children. *Ann Otol Rhin Layngol* 1993;102:680–686.
13. Colice GL, Stukel TA, Dain B. Laryngeal complications of prolonged intubation. *Chest* 1989; 96:877–884.
14. Kastanos N, Miro RE, Perez AM, et al. Laryngotracheal injury due to endotracheal intubation: incidence, evolution, and predisposing factors. A propsective long term study. *Crit Care Med* 1983;362–367.
15. Whited RE. Laryngeal dysfunction following prolonged intubation. *Ann Otolo* 1979;88:474–478.
16. Silbergleit AK, Basha MA. Speech-language pathology in the intensive care unit. In: Johnson AF, Jacobson BJ, eds. *Medical speech-language pathology. A practitioner's guide*. New York: Thieme, 1998:65–95.
17. Dikeman KJ, Kazandjian MS. Endotracheal tubes and tracheostomy tubes. In: Dikeman KJ, Kazandjian MS, eds. *Communication and swallowing management of tracheostomized and ventilator-dependent adults*. San Diego: Singular Publishing Group, 1995:61–96.
18. SIMS, Inc. Product Information Brochure, Keene, New Hampshire, 1996:8.
19. Bivona Medical Technologies Product Information, Gary, Indiana, December, 1994.
20. Bivona Medical Technologies Product Information, Gary, Indiana, April, 1994.
21. Boston Medical Products Product Catalog, Westborough, Massachusetts, 1998.
22. Pilling Weck Product Brochure, Research Triangle Park, North Carolina, 1996.
23. Mason M, Watkins C. Protocol for use of the Passy-Muir tracheostomy speaking valves. *Eur Resp J* 1992;5(Suppl. 15):148s–153s.
24. Frey JA, Wood S. Weaning from mechanical ventilation augmented by the Passy-Muir speaking valve. Presented at the International Conference of the American Lung Association and the American Thoracic Society, Anaheim, California, 1991.
25. Eibling DE, Gross RD. Subglottic air pressure: a key component of swallowing efficiency. *Ann Otol Rhinol Laryngol* 1996;105:253–258.
26. Stachler, RJ, Hamlet SL, Choi J, Fleming S. Scintigraphic quantification of aspiration reduction with the Passy-Muir Valve. *Laryngoscope* 1996;106:231–234.
27. Montgomery Speaking Valve, Boston Medical Products 1996 Product Catalog, Westborough, Massachusetts, 1996:18.
28. Shiley Phonate Speaking Valve: Product Information Pamphlet. Mallinckrodt Medical, Inc., Irvine, California, 1994.
29. Hood Speaking Valve Product Information. Hood Laboratories, Pembroke, Massachusetts, 1997.
30. Levy, RD, Bradley TD, Newman SL, Macklem PT, Martin JG. Negative pressure ventilation: effects on ventilation during sleep in normal subjects. *Chest* 1989;95:95–9.
31. Eve FC. Acutation of the inert diaphram. *Lancet* 1932;2:995–997.
32. Adamson JP, Lewis L, Stein JD. Application of abdominal pressure for artificial respiration. *JAMA* 1959;169:1613–1617.
33. Hill NS. Use of the rocking bed, pneumobelt, and other noninvasive aids to ventilation. In: Tobin MJ, ed. *Principles and practice of mechanical ventilation*. New York: McGraw-Hill Inc, 1994.

34. Hill NS. Clinical application of body ventilators. *Chest* 1986;90:897–905.
35. Pontoppiadan H, Geffin B, Lowenstein E. Acute respiratory failure in the adult. *N Engl J Med* 1972;287:743.
36. Katz JA. PEEP and CPAP in perioperative respiratory care. *Respir Care* 1984;29:614–629.
37. Amato MB, Barbas CSV, Medeiros DM, et al. Effect of a protective ventilation strategy on mortality in the acute respiratory distress syndrome. *N Engl J Med* 1998;338:347–354.
38. Stewart TE, Meade MO, Cook DJ, Granton JT, et al. Evaluation of a ventilation strategy to prevent barotrauma in patients at high risk for acute respiratoyr distress syndrome. *N Engl J Med* 1998;338:355–361.
39. Darioli R, Perret C. Mechanical controlled hypoventilation in status asthmaticus. *Am Rev Respir Dis* 1984;129:385–387.
40. Gottfried SB, Rossi A, Milic-Emili J. Dynamic hyperinflation, intrinsic PEEP, and the mechanically ventilated patient. *Crit Care Digest* 1986;5:30–36.
41. Dorinsky PM, Whitcomb ME. The effect of PEEP on cardiac output. *Chest* 1984; 210–216.
42. Pinsky MR. Through the past darkly: ventilatory management of patients with chronic obstructive pulmonary disease. *Crit Care Med* 1994;22:1714–1717.

Appendix

RESOURCES

1. Bivona Medical Technologies, Inc.
   5700 West 23rd Avenue
   Gary, Indiana 46406
   1-800-348-6064
2. Boston Medical Products
   117 Flanders Road
   Westborough, Massachusetts 01581
   1-800-433-2674
3. Hood Laboratories
   575 Washington Street
   Pembroke, Massachusetts 02359
4. Mallinckrodt Medical, Inc.
   675 McDonnell Blvd.
   P.O. Box 5840
   Hazelwood, Missouri 63134
   1-888-744-1414
5. Passy-Muir, Inc.
   4521 Campus Drive, Suite 273
   Irvine, California 92612
   1-714-833-8255 (California)
   1-800-634-5397 (Outside California)
6. Pilling Weck
   420 Delaware Drive
   Fort Washington, Pennsylvania 19034
   1-800-523-6507
7. SIMS Portex, Inc.
   10 Bowman Drive
   Keene, New Hampshire 03431
   1-800-258-5361

5

Communication, Tracheostomy and Ventilator Dependency

DONNA C. TIPPETT AND LURA VOGELMAN

Current concepts of health recognize not only prevention of disease but also restoration of function. The World Health Organization defines health as "a complete state of physical, mental, and social well-being, and not merely the absence of disease or infirmity" (1). This concept implies a continuum of health which includes the stages of optimum health, suboptimum health, overt illness or disability, and approaching death (2). Attempts to maintain optimum health are preventive, and efforts to address overt illness or disability are rehabilitative. Rehabilitation addresses a variety of disabilities that affect physical, emotional, and vocational well-being. Impaired communication ability is a disability that can diminish well-being profoundly.

Impaired ability to communicate orally can result when tracheotomy is performed for severely impaired respiratory function of the pharynx and larynx as well as for ventilating patients who cannot breathe independently. Inability to communicate orally is a catastrophe for anyone. This is especially true for those who are quadriplegic or quadriparetic and, therefore, unable to write. Such individuals are unable to express concerns or ask questions including those that bear on their medical status. In addition to being frightening and frustrating, their experience is dangerous to the extent that they cannot convey vital information to caregivers. Many people who have ventilatory insufficiency live for several years if they opt for life-sustaining therapy. Many of these individuals face a lack of oral communication as a condition of life unless special measures are taken toward its preservation.

Preserving oral communication in patients with tracheostomies is the primary focus of this chapter. Approaches applicable to those patients who breathe inde-

Tracheostomy and Ventilator Dependency: Management of Breathing, Speaking, and Swallowing. Edited by Donna C. Tippett, MPH, MA, CCC-SLP. Thieme Medical Publishers, Inc. New York © 2000.

pendently and to those who depend on coupling to a ventilator are reviewed. For the former, valving the tracheostomy cannula to provide inspiration through the cannula and expiration through the larynx is often practical and effective. For the latter, deflating the cuff, which is often inflated to seal the cannula in the trachea, may preserve oral communication without sacrificing alveolar ventilation. Although the literature includes references to these practices, it also suggests that their recognition is restricted. Our experiences justify confidence in the effectiveness of these compensations for the communication impairments which result from tracheostomy with or without ventilator dependency. These efforts to facilitate oral communication in ventilator-dependent and nonventilator-dependent individuals with tracheostomies can improve the quality and safety of life for thousands of people and their families.

Scope of the Problem

Tracheostomy is frequently performed for patients who have neuromuscular diseases, some of which render the patient incapable of independent breathing. Lesions may be in the central nervous system (e.g., brain stem infarction, trauma to the spinal cord) (3); peripheral nervous system (e.g., amyotrophic lateral sclerosis, Guillain–Barré syndrome) (4–9); neuromuscular junction (e.g., botulism, myasthenia gravis) (10); or muscle (e.g., muscular dystrophy) (11) (Fig. 5–1). Pathology which is not primarily neuromuscular may also lead to tracheostomy as in the instance of obstructive airway disease, surgery of the head and neck, adult respiratory distress syndrome, and injuries that result in instability of the chest wall.

NEUROMUSCULAR ETIOLOGIES ASSOCIATED WITH
TRACHEOSTOMY AND VENTILATOR DEPENDENCY

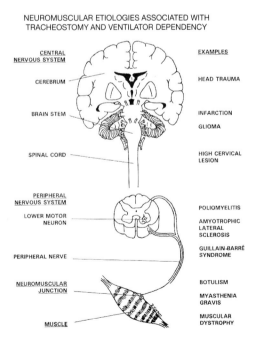

Fig. 5–1. Sites of neuromuscular pathology identified with tracheostomy with or without ventilator dependency. Reprinted, with permission, from Tippett and Siebens (67).

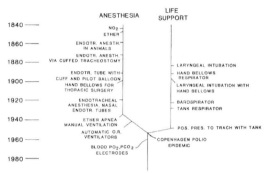

Fig. 5–2. Diagram depicting the landmarks in the development of mechanical intermittent positive pressure ventilation in anesthesia and surgery on the left and for life support of compromised patients on the right. The two paths did not fully merge until after the poliomyelitis epidemic of 1952 in Copenhagen. Reprinted, with permission, from Snider (12).

In the 1940s and 1950s, poliomyelitis caused severe respiratory muscle weakness in large numbers of young people worldwide. In response to this epidemic, devices for upper airway care and mechanical support of respiration were developed. The use of mechanical ventilator support in surgery and anesthesia and as a life support system progressed separately until 1952 (Fig. 5–2). It was in Denmark where the scarcity of tank respirators first prompted interest in positive pressure breathing as it was being used in anesthesia. Positive pressure ventilation via tracheostomy quickly became the preferred method of managing the respiratory paralysis of poliomyelitis (12). Regional systems of health care evolved and the polio respiratory centers came into being (13,14). After the introduction of effective vaccines, poliomyelitis was virtually eradicated, and the need for the respiratory care centers specifically for "polio survivors" diminished. Nevertheless, survivors of various diseases and traumas today continue to require tracheostomy and mechanical ventilator support. Exponential advances in the technology of mechanical ventilation occurred in the 1960s. By the end of the 1970s, intensive care capability was available in most American hospitals, including the advanced life support techniques of mechanical ventilation, dialysis, and IV alimentation (15).

In 1985, there were 48,000 temporary tracheostomies (ICD-9 31.1) and 6,000 permanent tracheostomies (ICD-9 31.21, ICD-9 31.29) (16). In 1986, Make and colleagues (17) surveyed 121 acute and chronic inpatient healthcare facilities and nine home care vendors in Massachusetts. They found that neuromuscular ventilatory insufficiency was the most common diagnosis, and that the prevalence of ventilator-dependent individuals was 2.8 per 100,000 in the United States (approximately 7,000 persons). More recently, the American Association for Respiratory Care (AARC) commissioned the Gallup Organization of Princeton, New Jersey to conduct a survey documenting the number of chronic ventilator-dependent individuals in the United States. In December 1990, 300 respiratory care department managers and 100 pulmonary physicians were interviewed by telephone. Based upon these interviews, it was estimated that there are 11,419 chronic ventilator-dependent patients being treated in hospitals in the continental United States at any given time (18).

In addition to information regarding incidence and prevalence, there are data showing that utilization of mechanical ventilation is increasing. For example, the number of patients mechanically ventilated for 24 h or more at Massachusetts General Hospital increased from 66 in 1958 to 2,000 in 1982 (12). At Rochester General Hospital the number of patients who received more than 3 h of mechanical ventilation was 98 in 1974 and 251 in 1983 (19). At Rush-Presbyterian-St. Luke's Medical Center in Chicago, ventilation use increased from approximately 8,000 days in 1979 to more than 12,000 days in 1989 (20).

Ventilator dependency can be prolonged even for patients who are weaned eventually. For example, in patients with Guillain–Barré syndrome, mean duration of ventilator dependency ranged from 37 to 63 days (4–7); in patients with myasthenia gravis, duration of ventilator dependency ranged from one to 32 days (10).

Thus, the tracheostomy populations are sizable, their etiologies are diverse, and the durations of ventilator dependency are substantial. Given the size and diversity of this population, it is not surprising that speech–language pathologists have become involved increasingly over the last 10 years in the evaluation and treatment of speaking and swallowing in individuals with tracheostomies and ventilator dependency. Evidence of our new role includes the increasing number of seminars on tracheostomy and ventilator dependency, the appearance of articles and books on this topic, and the publication of the *Position Statement and Guidelines for the Use of Voice Protheses in Tracheotomized Persons With or Without Ventilatory Dependence* by the American Speech-Language-Hearing Association (21) which defines the requisite knowledge and scope of practice of speech–language pathologists working with these individuals.

Effect of Tracheostomy on Speaking

Independent Breathing

The presence of a tracheostomy tube alters the normal flow of air through the upper airway for the production of speech. When the tracheostomy cannula has a cuff which is inflated, a circumstance under which the airway is protected from the aspiration of some secretions and foodway contents, phonation is sacrificed. The exchange of air during inspiration and expiration occurs at the level of the cannula, permitting delivery of air to the lungs. As the cuff is inferior to the larynx, vocal folds, mouth and nasal passages, cuff inflation precludes airflow through these structures (Fig. 5–3). When the cuff is deflated, or with a cuffless tube, air exchange occurs through the mouth and nose as well as through the open tracheostomy cannula. Phonation is impossible or effortful because subglottic pressure is not sufficient for speech production. The goal in the rehabilitation of speech production in individuals with tracheostomy is the restoration of airflow through the larynx during expiration. Achieving this goal is dependent on the presence of a deflated cuff or a cuffless tracheostomy cannula as well as occlusion of the tube during expiration (Fig. 5–4).

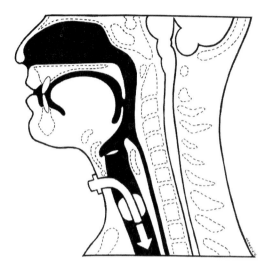

Fig. 5–3. Tracheostomy cannula with cuff inflated. Reprinted, with permission, from Tippett and Siebens (67).

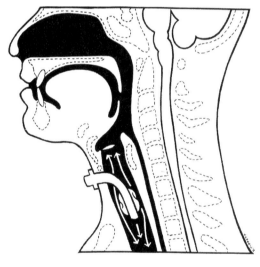

Fig. 5–4. When the tracheostomy cannula is occluded, air flows around the deflated cuff and through the larynx during both inspiration and expiration. Reprinted, with permission, from Tippett and Siebens (67).

Evaluation of Candidacy for Communication Options

Tracheostomy and Independent Breathing

The evaluation of communication options begins with the examination of oral motor components in nonspeech tasks. The respiratory mechanism, larynx, velum/pharynx, tongue, lips/face/teeth, and jaw are tested using traditional oral peripheral measures (see Chapter 6 for the Dysarthria/Dysphagia Battery). Individuals who are successfully "mouthing" words to communication partners have a better prognosis for the restoration of oral communication than those individuals who do not demonstrate this skill (22).

The history of the individual's respiratory function and airway status begins with information related to the diagnosis necessitating the tracheostomy, e.g., neuromuscular diseases, obstructive airway disease, surgery of the head and neck, adult respiratory distress syndrome, injury to the chest wall. Tracheal stenosis, tracheomalacia, and vocal fold paralysis are conditions that may occur prior to, or as a result of, the tracheostomy. The presence of any of these conditions is confirmed by an otolaryngologist during a flexible fiberoptic examination. Positive findings complicate, or may preclude, oral communication. Granulation tissue may form in reaction to the presence of the tracheostomy. Depending on the size and location of the granulomas, communication may be adversely affected. Additional history of mechanical ventilation, weaning complications, and recency of tracheostomy is beneficial in the planning of speech–language pathology intervention.

The size and type of tracheostomy cannula may influence oral communication. Ideally, the cannula should not be greater than ⅔ to ¾ of the diameter of the tracheal lumen, thus allowing ample airflow around the cannula (23). Smaller individuals typically have smaller tracheas and benefit from downsizing to cannulas of lesser diameters if speech cannot be produced during a trial of finger occlusion (and other factors have been excluded). A Shiley no. 6 cannula, or its equivalent, is usually compatible with achieving phonation in most patients.

Evaluation also includes a screening of manual dexterity. Fine motor skills must be sufficient to perform finger occlusion or to apply and remove a speaking valve if these are to be considered viable options for independent communication. Alternatively, for those individuals who are not candidates for digital occlusion or speaking valves, motor skills must be adequate to produce gestures, access alternative/augmentative communication systems, or operate electrolarynges.

Observation of the presence and management of oral and pharyngeal secretions through spontaneous swallowing suggests how well the individual will be able to tolerate cuff deflation and predict the "wetness" in voice quality. It is common for secretions to accumulate superiorly to an inflated cuff as these secretions cannot be eliminated by coughing and throat-clearing. A trial of cuff deflation is advantageous in determining the individual's ability to cough, expectorate, or swallow these secretions. Copious secretions account for a wet-hoarse voice quality that diminishes overall speech intelligibility. In extreme cases, there exists an inability to tolerate cuff deflation even for brief trials. The normal protection of the airway is provided by vocal fold adduction and an effective cough. The absence of these may result in aspiration of secretions that can compromise the individual's medical status. For those individuals, alternatives to cuff deflation must be considered.

The presence of language and/or cognitive impairments may interfere with the ability to produce meaningful communication after airflow is restored for speech production. Deficits in language and/or cognition also dictate the level of instruction necessary to teach communication options. Evaluation of these skills presents a challenge when working with patients who are without oral communication and motor skills necessary to generate written responses. For these individuals, testing is frequently limited to responses in the form of nonoral signals of affirmation or negation to yes/no questions. Inquiries may include orientation, recall of biographical information, and recall of general knowledge items. For those individuals who possess functional motor skills to respond by writing, selected portions, or an entire, formal aphasia or cognitive/language battery can be a useful means of measurement.

Alternatives to Cuff Deflation for Communication

Tracheostomy and Independent Breathing

Short-term solutions to communication problems, as well as long-term options for individuals who are not candidates for cuff deflation, include writing, "mouthing," gestures, electrolarynges, alternative/augmentative communication systems, and fenestrated tracheostomy cannulas. Writing allows the generation of novel messages to untrained partners. Limitations to the effectiveness of written communication include the experiential and educational levels of the communication partners and the necessity of close physical proximity to read the message. Functional language abilities, fine motor skills, positioning, and endurance are additional factors that need to be considered when exploring written language as an option.

"Mouthing" can be an effective method of communication, and is preferred by many individuals with tracheostomies because of its naturalness. Drawbacks include the variability among partners in reading "mouthed" words and the articulatory precision of the "speaker."

Gestures are another natural means of communication and seldom require extensive training. Amerind, a formal gestural system, is highly predictable and easy to acquire (24). Resourceful individuals may use a combination of modalities. Success is predicated on the flexibility of the person with tracheostomy and the communication partner.

Electrolarynges are designed to provide a vibratory source for those who do not have functioning vocal folds, usually after a laryngectomy. These devices can also be considered as communication options for individuals with tracheostomies who have intact articulatory skills. Electrolarynges are a short-term solution for communication for those who have potential for oral communication or a long-term solution for those with vocal fold or upper airway compromise. The two types of electrolarynges are intraoral and neck placement devices. Intraoral systems have thin plastic tubes attached to a battery operated sound source. The tubing is placed 1.5–2 inches behind the teeth and activated by depressing a hand-held button in synchrony with speech onset (Fig. 5–5). Neck placement devices are operated by placing the flat surface of the device against the cheek, lateral aspect of the neck, or under the chin (Fig. 5–6). Placement is highly individualized and requires thorough experimentation on the part of the speech–language pathologist. Training is necessary for the timing of speech onset and precise articulation. Independent communication is limited by the user's manual ability to operate the on/off button and by the ability of communication partners to understand the mechanical sound produced by the electrolarynx. Sunners (25) reported that four of five patients with temporary tracheostomies were able to use electrolarynges to communicate with staff and family. Success depended on the individual's cognitive, language, and emotional status. Instruction times ranging from

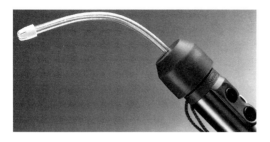

Fig. 5–5. Intraoral electrolarynx. Photo courtesy of Siemens Hearing Instruments, Inc., Prospect Heights, Illinois.

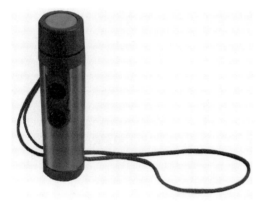

Fig. 5–6. Neck type electrolarynx. Photo courtesy of Siemens Hearing Instruments, Inc., Prospect Heights, Illinois.

15 min to 2 h duration were sufficient for initiation of functional communication. Godwin and Heffner (26) estimated that more than 90% of patients with tracheostomies who have normal cognitive and language skills are able to use electrolarynges for communication.

Alternative/augmentative communication systems can be simple or complex. The alternative/augmentative communication system may contain letters, words, pictures, or symbols. The type of device is dictated by individual needs and abilities. A communication needs assessment is the first step in developing an alternative/augmentative communication system. Beukelman and colleagues (27) suggested identifying communication partners, environments in which patients will need to communicate, types of messages which patients will need to convey, and positions in which patients will operate alternative/augmentative communication systems (e.g., bed, wheelchair). Hearing, vision, and cognitive/language abilities of the alternative/augmentative communication user must be considered as well. Postural modifications and mounting devices require input from occupational and physical therapy in order to guarantee the successful use of the device. Means of indicating communicative intentions may be via direct selection, scanning, or encoding. Table 5–1 summarizes some communication options when cuff deflation is not viable (28).

The traditional fenestrated tracheostomy tube is designed to allow airflow through the upper airway via single or multiple ports on the convex surface of the cannula. Air flows through the port or ports and passes into the upper airway for speech production during exhalation. The cuff does not need to be deflated to allow speech (Figs. 5–7 and 5–8). The advantage of the fenestration is commonly thought to be prevention of aspiration of secretions into the airway by maintaining the inflated cuff as a barrier, however, secretions may be readily aspirated through the fenestration, and the fenestration itself may become plugged with secretions, thereby interfering with oral communication. Other problems include the formation of granulation tissue around the port site (26), and occlusion of the port by positioning of the tube against the posterior tracheal wall. Furthermore, individuals are exposed to the drawbacks associated with inflated cuffs when fenestrated tubes are used. An unfenestrated inner cannula must be used when suctioning to prevent the catheter tip from catching on the port. Newer designs have fenestrations on the inner as well as outer cannulas, thus eliminating the necessity to remove the inner tube before initiating speech.

An adaptation of the traditional fenestrated tracheostomy tube is the Tucker tube. This fenestrated design uses a specialized inner cannula that fits a metal Jackson or Tucker tube. A metal flap is hinged to an opening in the inner cannula in such a manner that airflow causes the flap to open during inspiration and close during expiration. Thus, exhalation occurs through the larynx, and speech production is possible. The inner cannula can be removed for cleaning of the secretions that accumulate around the hinged flap (29, 30) (Fig. 5–9).

As individual anatomy varies greatly, it is logical that precut fenestrations may not be functional for every patient. Cane and colleagues (31) described a method for adapting the size and position of ports to accommodate these variations. The proper positioning of the fenestrations reduces the risk of the ports being obstructed by the pharyngeal wall.

Oral Communication Options with Cuff Deflation

Tracheostomy and Independent Breathing

Oral communication options with cuff deflation in individuals who have tracheostomies and ability to breathe independently include plugs, buttons, digital occlusion of the tracheostomy cannula, and application of unidirectional tracheostomy speaking valves to cannulas.

For those individuals who are able to tolerate continuous occlusion of the cannula, plugging the tracheostomy tube is possible for restoring oral communication. With the plug in place, inspiration and expiration occur through the trachea, larynx, pharynx, and oral and nasal cavities. Typically, candidates for decannulation are appropriate for plugging as part of the weaning process. Plugs can be used when it is important to have airway access, although the individual may not need to breathe through the cannula at all times. Most weaning protocols dictate a downsizing of the tracheostomy cannula in conjunction with plugging. Trials of total occlusion via plugging should be carefully monitored for changes in oxygen saturation, heart rate, respiratory rate, and patient comfort. The work of breathing may increase markedly with plugging in patients with reduced ventilatory capacity. Clearance of secretions by coughing may be made more difficult by the presence of the plugged tracheostomy cannula. Airway obstruction may result if congealed secretions accumulate in the trachea around the cannula (26).

Table 5-1. Communication options for persons dependent on a tracheostomy or ventilator[a].

	Method	Brief Description	Equipment	Some Benefits	Potential Problems
Larynx as a sound source for speech	Continuous or intermittent occlusion of trach. Must not occlude airway	1. Caregiver or patient put finger or chin over trach during exhalation to cause air to move through vocal cords. 2. Caregiver or patient put finger over trach during exhalation to allow speech. 3. Plug the trach. Often used prior to weaning from trach.	Nonfenestrated trach (cuffless or deflated) Fenestrated trach (trach can be inflated) Tracheostomy button	Speech. "Cough" for clearing upper airway. Make noise to get attention.	Hygiene/infection. Someone must occlude trach. Must synchronize occlusion with exhalation. May require close monitoring.
	One-way speaking valve. Trach must not occlude airway	Valve attached to trach allows air to flow in, but instead of going out trach during expiration, the air goes through the patient's nose and mouth making speech possible. Contraindicated for patients with laryngeal or tracheal stenosis.	Examples are Olympic Trach-Talk, Montgomery Speaking Valve, Hood, Kistner, Passy–Muir Trach Valve (available in pediatric size)	Speech. Upper airway clearance. Useful when patient a) is not ready for plugging and may require oxygen; b) cannot use fingers; c) wants to use both hands and talk; d) is ventilator dependent.	Patient may not be able to apply/remove valve independently. Valves can pop off with cough. Valve may not be easily cleaned and may require replacement every 3 months.
	Talking trachs	*Primarily for patients on ventilators.* A conduit is attached to a source of compressed air which is separate from the ventilator. Patient/caregiver occludes the conduit to direct airflow through larynx.	Examples are Portex Talking Tubes, Bivona Talking Trach Tube, Communi-trach	Speech. Useful because it a) allows speech throughout respiratory cycle; b) permits maintenance and monitoring of ventilator and tidal volumes; and c) allows cuff inflation.	Interference by secretions. Difficulty positioning tube. Altered voice quality. Airflow can be uncomfortable.
External sound sources for speech	Neck type electrolarynx	For patients unable to use vocal cords because of laryngeal injury or cuff inflation but who can articulate well. Need hand function, upper extremity strength.	Examples are Western Electric, Romet, Jedcom, Servox	Speech, portability and ready accessibility. Can personalize sound to some extent.	Requires learning new skills. Placement problems.
	Oral type electrolarynx	Tone generator with a plastic tube which is placed in mouth. For patients who cannot use neck type.	Example is Copper Rand	Speech. Has pitch and volume controls.	Requires learning new skills. Placement problems.
	Remote switch electrolarynx	A modification of oral type. Has remote switch so person with quadriplegia can operate. Tube mounted on headband.	Example is Copper Rand	Speech. For patients who cannot hold electrolarynx.	Placement is a problem. Requires learning new skills.

When speech is not an option				
Handwriting	For patients who can print or write. Allows them to respond, initiate, etc., and prepare messages in advance.	Magic Slate; Notepad and pen/pencil	Natural and familiar form of communication. Unlimited access to language.	Cognitive/linguistic requirements; lack of privacy.
Signs and gestures	Natural gestures for everyone. Signs used with children learning language who have good upper extremity skills.	None, but need upper extremity strength and function	Natural gestures easily understood. Signs provide access to language. Portable.	Sign language-new learning for user and partners.
Direct selection	For patients, even those with no literacy skill who can point using finger, eyes, hand, head stick, etc. to select desired messages from a display.	Alphabet boards, symbol boards, ETRANs, charts, communication devices	Access to language (words, symbols). Use of encoding to expand access to vocabulary. Provide options for speech output, rate enhancement.	Limited access to vocabulary. Requires new learning for user and partners.
Scanning (auditory and visual)	For patients unable to use direct selection because of visual and/or motor problems. Either a person or a device scans vocabulary/letters. When the desired message is reached, the user indicates, stopping the scan.	Alphabet boards, symbol boards, listener-assisted scanning charts, communication devices	Access to language. Listener-assisted scanning can be very efficient. Can use encoding to expand access to vocabulary. Options for speech output, rate enhancement.	Limited access to vocabulary. Slow. Requires new learning for user and partners.

[a]This chart was developed by Sarah Blackstone, Donna Tippett, and Carolyn Watkins.

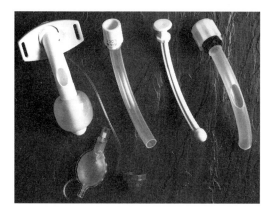

Fig. 5–7. Fenestrated cuffed tracheostomy cannula with a single port. Inner cannula is also fenestrated. Photo courtesy of Mallinckrodt Medical TPI, Inc., Irvine, California.

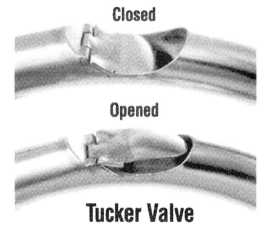

Fig. 5–8. Fenestrated cuffed tracheostomy cannula with multiple ports. Photo courtesy of Mallinckrodt Medical TPI, Inc., Irvine, California.

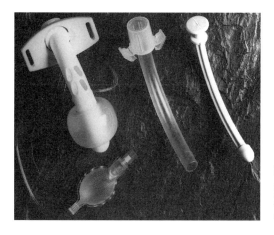

Fig. 5–9. Tucker tracheostomy tube. Leaflet on inner cannula opens on inhalation and closes on exhalation, forcing air up through the upper airway. Photo courtesy of Pilling Weck, Research Triangle Park, North Carolina.

Some patients no longer require the presence of a tracheostomy tube for ventilation or frequent pulmonary toileting, but it may be desirable to maintain the patency of the stoma. Under these circumstances, a tracheostomy button can be

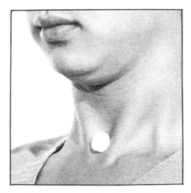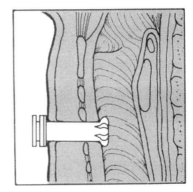

Fig. 5–10. Olympic trach button. Photo courtesy of Olympic Medical, Seattle, Washington.

used which occludes the stoma without protruding into the tracheal lumen. Buttons are plastic cylinders that are secured by a flange to the anterior tracheal wall and pose no resistance to the clearance of secretions through the tracheal lumen (Fig. 5–10). Oral communication is achieved if all other speech mechanisms are functional. In the event that an individual requires a subsequent tracheostomy tube, the stomal tract is preserved.

In those who are not candidates for plugs or buttons, preliminary attempts at oral communication are usually confined to finger occlusion. If the tracheostomy tube is cuffless, or if the cuff is deflated, the patient or communication partner can intermittently place a finger over the open cannula on expiration, thus diverting the flow of air through the upper airway and vocal folds. When the finger is released, air exchange resumes through the cannula. Assessment by the speech–language pathologist includes the individual's ability to exhale air through the mouth when the cannula is occluded. This can be facilitated by asking the individual to blow or cough while the cannula is occluded digitally. Difficulty performing this task suggests obstruction above the level of the tracheostomy. The quality of phonation provides information about the status of the vocal folds, breath support for speech production, and the effect of secretions on speech intelligibility. If prolonged intubation has occurred prior to the initiation of speech trials and the patient has become accustomed to "mouthing" words, vibration of the vocal folds may be difficult to initiate. Retraining of voice production may be necessary. Advantages of finger occlusion are that it is easy to learn and restores oral communication without the need to acquire equipment. Disadvantages include the possibility of introducing bacteria into the airway with finger occlusion, the inability to perform bimanual tasks while engaged in conversation, the need for sufficient fine motor skills to locate and occlude the cannula consistently, and, in some circumstances, dependency on a partner to occlude the cannula digitally at appropriate intervals. Successful use of finger occlusion may be an endpoint or an initial step in the process of assessment for other communication options, such as unidirectional tracheostomy speaking valves.

A unidirectional tracheostomy speaking valve coupled to the hub of a cannula can accomplish the results of finger occlusion without its drawbacks. Such valves are open during inspiration and closed during expiration forcing air through the

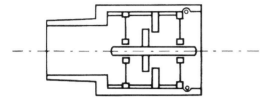

Fig. 5–11. Cross sectional illustration of the function of the one-way inspiratory tracheotomy valve. Reprinted, with permission, from Toremalm (32).

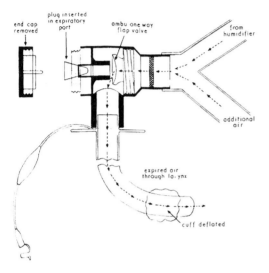

Fig. 5–12. Speaking valve for attachment to a tracheostomy tube. Reprinted, with permission, from Emery (33).

larynx. A variety of these valves are described in the literature and are summarized below.

In 1968, Toremalm (32) constructed a plunger-type, one-way valve with a moving membrane on a piston. The membrane was encased in a Teflon cylinder, attached easily, and was lightweight (Fig. 5–11). Toremalm (32) reported that 22 patients, most with transient bilateral vocal fold paralysis, successfully used his device.

Speaking valves were also developed to meet the unique needs of particular patients. In 1972, Emery (33) adapted a flap valve from an Ambu bag to make a speaking valve for an individual with polyneuritis who was able to tolerate periods without ventilator support. The end cap of the expiratory port was removed and the open port was occluded by a spigot (Fig. 5–12). Cowan in 1975 (34) adapted an Improved Jackson speaking aid tracheostomy tube to prevent complete closure of the valve during expiration and still allow phonation for a patient with a post-diphtheritic laryngeal and tracheal stenosis. When the inner cannula of the Jackson tube was in place for the attachment of the valve, the patient could not produce adequate expiratory airflow. The solution was to insert a small screw through the side of the tube, preventing complete closure of the valve and allowing a portion of the expired air to escape past the valve and out of the cannula. The remainder of the airflow traveled through the stenotic larynx and was available for speech.

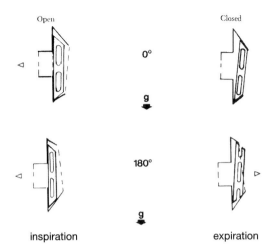

Open   Closed

0°

180°

inspiration   expiration

Fig. 5–13. Two-way valve. With the valve house in position "0" the valve body closes the valve at expiration, and the air stream is forced through the larynx, and the patient can speak and cough. If the valve house is turned to position "180," the valve body will not close the valve completely and both inspiration and expiration will occur through the valve which then functions as a humidifier. Reprinted, with permission, from Saul and Bergstrom (35).

Saul and Bergstrom (35) described a straight tracheal cannula with a two-way valve which could be rotated to allow inspiration only or inspiration/expiration. A short straight tube was placed directly in the stoma and attached by outer flanges and inner flaps. Thus, the need for suturing or securing the tube by neck bands was eliminated. A two-way adjustable valve was attached to the tube by a housing that could be rotated for speech purposes. As this tube did not extend into the tracheal lumen, there was no contact with or irritation to the tracheal mucosa (Fig. 5–13). Candidates for this type of device included individuals status post irradiation who had laryngeal stenosis, individuals with bilateral vocal fold paresis, or those with chronic respiratory disease.

French and colleagues (36) developed a simple ball valve. Its operation is shown schematically in Figure 5–14. Figure 5–14A shows the valve at rest. When the patient inhales (Fig. 5–14B), the inspiratory stream blows the ball back, allowing air to enter freely through the port. The ball is stopped from entering the cannula by a wire stop. On expiration (Fig. 5–14C), the ball seals the port, forcing airflow through the larynx. Adaptations of French's and colleagues' (36) Hopkins valve are designed to fit either an Improved Jackson metal or Shiley plastic tracheostomy cannula.

The Passy–Muir valve (37) (Passy-Muir, Inc., Irvine, California) was invented by David Muir, a 23-year-old man with quadriplegia secondary to muscular dystrophy. It consists of a centrally supported membranous flap mounted in a plastic housing. Its resting position is closed, and the flap is opened during inspiration. The positive closure system returns the silastic membrane to the biased-closed position at the end of an expiratory cycle. This valve attaches to cannulas which incorporate a universal 15 mm fitting, including pediatric sizes. Models are available that are compatible with ventilator use and in low-profile designs (Fig. 5–15).

French and colleagues (38) compared the advantages and disadvantages of the Hopkins ball valve with the Passy–Muir flap valve. Inspiratory resistance was less with the ball valve. Closing pressure was slightly lower with the flap valve inasmuch as this valve is closed in its resting position. Additionally, the ball valve is smaller, more easily concealed, more durable, and easier to clean. Both valves

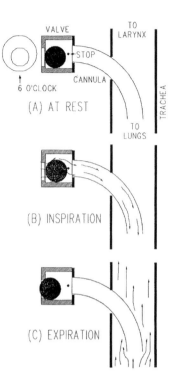

Fig. 5–14. Ball valve at rest (A), during inspiration (B), and during expiration (C). Reprinted, with permission, from Tippett and Siebens (67).

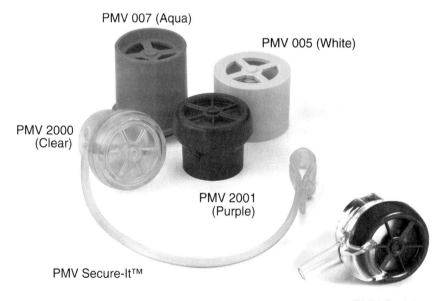

Fig. 5–15. Passy–Muir valves. Photo courtesy of Passy-Muir, Inc., Irvine, California.

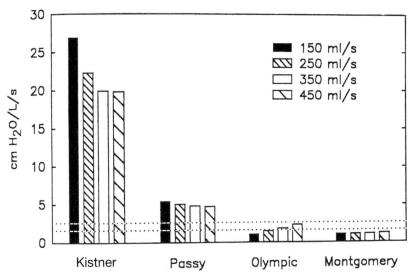

Fig. 5–16. Mean resistance of the one-way speaking valves as a function of flow rate. These results were obtained when the valves were not attached to a tracheostomy tube. The dotted lines indicate the range of nasal resistance for adults without tracheostomy. Reprinted, with permission, from Fornataro-Clerici and Zajac (39).

can be applied by the patient, the flap valve more easily than some of the adaptations of the ball valve. If one removes the inner cannula from a Shiley no. 6 tube (inner diameter = 7.0 mm; outer diameter = 10.0 mm) and attaches a ball valve to the outer cannula, resistance to inspiratory flow is comparable to the resistance when the tube is used without a valve and the inner cannula is in place.

Additional references in which technical information is cited are Toremalm (32) and Fornataro-Clerici and Zajac (39). The closing pressure of Toremalm's plunger-type valve is 2 cm H_2O (32), a disadvantageous characteristic inasmuch as this value is four times that of the Hopkins ball valve. Fornataro-Clerici and Zajac (39) compared pressure-flow characteristics of four commercially available valves. They found that there were significant differences in resistance among the valves, and that the resistance of the Kistner valve was substantially greater than that of the other valves tested and the normal upper airways (Fig. 5–16).

The variety of valve designs speaks to the ingenuity of clinicians and scientists in developing ways for individuals with tracheostomies to communicate orally. Valves obviate the need for finger occlusion, thus restoring the ability to perform bimanual tasks while speaking and reducing the introduction of bacteria through the stoma. Valving is appropriate for patients who are not able to tolerate continuous plugging. Despite the different designs of speaking valves, they share a basic function: to allow inspiration at the level of the cannula and expiration through the larynx.

The restoration of phonation is the primary benefit in the use of a unidirectional tracheostomy speaking valve. Subjective claims have been made of nonspeaking benefits, including effects on secretions, olfaction, and arterial oxygenation (37,40). Lichtman and colleagues (41) studied eight patients with tracheostomies and reported an overall 40% decrease in secretion accumulation and improvement in patients' subjective impressions of sense of smell when valves were worn. No significant differences were demonstrated in arterial oxygenation. It is unclear if the changes in secretion accumulation were a result of the resumption of a productive cough and swallowing/expectoration of secretions propelled into hypopharynx or the evaporation of secretions as a result of restored airflow to the oral and nasal cavities. Under either circumstance, the need for tracheal suctioning was reduced, in turn reducing the irritation to the airway. The improvement in olfaction was believed to be caused by the return of airflow through the nasal passages during exhalation in individuals with tracheostomy. In nontracheostomized individuals, the detection of odors occurs as air flows into the airway through the nose during inspiration. It is possible, therefore, that the odor threshold may be diminished in patients with tracheostomies as compared to those without tracheostomies because of this alteration in airflow.

Individual circumstances may require modification of conventional valving approaches. Wee (42) addressed the problem of delivering humidification to the airway when the patient is off the ventilator. The author found that some patients objected to the use of a face mask as it made them feel claustrophobic. The solution proposed was the modification of a T-piece that acted as a speaking adaptor. A light spring loaded valve was attached to a plunger mechanism. The patient or communication partner depressed the plunger to occlude the tracheostomy tube and allow speech. The release of the plunger allowed the humidified air to return (Fig. 5–17). Wee (42) proposed that this device is of benefit in the weaning process, produces minimum resistance to breathing, and is appropriate for patients who no longer need oxygen.

A design similar to Wee's (42) is incorporated in the Olympic Trach-talk valve (Olympic Medical, Seattle, Washington) (Fig. 5–18). A spring mechanism holds the valve in an open position except during exhalation. During exhalation, the force of the patient's breath closes the valve, restoring airflow through the larynx. At the end of the expiratory cycle, the spring mechanism returns to the open position for breathing. Oxygen and humidification can be delivered through the open ends of the T-piece. For suctioning purposes, a cap is removed from the distal end of the valve and the suction catheter can be inserted directly into the tracheostomy tube.

The Montgomery speaking valve (Boston Medical Products, Westborough, Massachusetts) incorporates a silastic membrane which opens on inhalation and closes on expiration (Fig. 5–19). A unique design feature of the Montgomery valve is the ability to retain the valve on the tracheostomy cannula under bursts of pressure during coughing. Rather than the valve being blown off, the "cough release" feature activates by "unhinging" a portion of the membrane to allow pressure to be released. The membrane is easily put back into place.

A special rendition of the Hopkins valve was designed to accommodate an individual who could neither reach her cannula for elective finger occlusion nor tolerate valving with every breath (43). The patient was a 25-year-old woman who presented with bilateral paresis of the shoulder and elbow flexor muscles, and bilateral vocal fold abductor paralysis (vocal folds were fixed at midline) second-

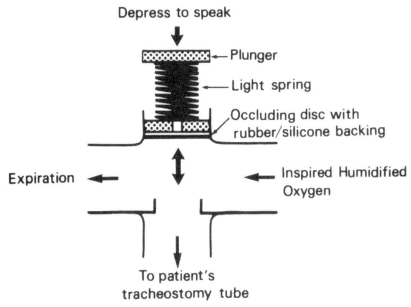

Depress to speak

Plunger

Light spring

Occluding disc with rubber/silicone backing

Expiration

Inspired Humidified Oxygen

To patient's tracheostomy tube

Fig. 5–17. Modification of a standard T-piece to form a speaking adaptor. Reprinted, with permission, from Wee (42).

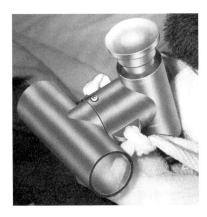

Fig. 5–18. Olympic Trach-talk valve. Photo courtesy of Olympic Medical, Seattle, Washington.

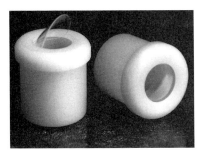

Fig. 5–19. Montgomery valve. Photo courtesy of Boston Medical Products, Westborough, Massachusetts.

ary to acute intermittent porphyria (a metabolic defect in the liver which is inherited as an autosomal dominant trait and is marked by increased production and urinary excretion of porphobilinogen and porphyrin precursor). The modified Hopkins valve was controlled by a camera shutter release mechanism which the patient manipulated with her thumb and forefinger. The shutter release was attached to a wire in the valve. The wire prevented occlusion of the cannula at rest so respiration could occur at the level of the cannula. When phonation was desired, the shutter release mechanism was depressed, the wire moved up, and the ball fell forward to occlude the cannula. Phonation was produced during expiration. The shutter mechanism was then released and inspiration could occur at the level of the cannula (Fig. 5–20).

Speaking valves are considered communication options for individuals who are medically stable and are not expected to have the tracheostomy plugged imminently. This includes patients with an ongoing need for pulmonary toileting or the delivery of oxygen through the cannula. It is not necessary for the patient to have intact speech and language skills as the valve affords benefits besides oral communication, such as the restoration of airflow to the upper airway for swallowing and secretion management (41,44).

The evaluation of an individual's candidacy for valving is conducted collaboratively with the physician, nurse, speech–language pathologist, and respiratory therapist. Initially, speech components are assessed with particular attention to the respiratory and laryngeal mechanisms. The cannula is downsized if necessary to ensure that airflow can pass around the cannula through the tracheal lumen. History of airway obstruction including granuloma tissue, tracheomalacia or stenosis is a contraindication to proceeding with valve trials. For the initial valve trial, the patient is seated upright and suctioned thoroughly for oral and tracheal secretions. Baseline measurements with pulse oximetry are made prior to applying the valve. The tracheostomy cuff is then deflated. The patient is observed for increased respiratory rate, shortness of breath, inspiratory stridor, or effortful exhalation. If the patient is without change in respiratory status and he or she appears comfortable, the cannula is occluded with a gloved finger during expiration only. Changes in respiration are noted as well as the patient's ability to cough and clear secretions while occluded. If there are no adverse changes, the patient is then asked to phonate when the cannula is occluded during exhalation. Phonation is assessed. Next the valve is applied, and the patient is asked to phonate. Initial speaking valve tasks include repetition of words and phrases, proceeding to answering simple questions, and finally to conversational speech. If

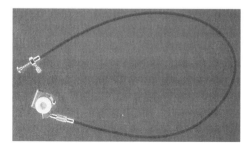

Fig. 5–20. Customized Hopkins valve.

the session is judged to be successful, then use of the valve is approved. Tolerance is determined by monitoring respiration, voice quality, and the patient's subjective assessment of comfort. Alternatively, contraindications to valving are identified, for example, obstructions to expiratory airflow resulting from either narrowing of the trachea or full or partial occlusion of the glottis (e.g., bilateral vocal fold paralysis in the medial position).

Patient and caregiver education help to ensure the successful use of the speaking valve. Repeated practice in the application of the valve may alleviate anxiety about becoming short of breath. The anatomy of the upper airway and the relationship of the tracheostomy to the vocal folds should be reviewed. Anatomical models are useful in showing these relationships. Patients should not be unsupervised with valves in place until their medical tolerance and subjective comfort are established, and education is completed. Only in this way can patients be assured that their breathing is not compromised with the valve in place and that the valve can be removed easily, if necessary.

When the patient has been able to produce voice and wear the valve without discomfort, a wearing schedule is established with the patient and caregivers. If there are no complications, then it is usual for the patient to progress quickly to wearing the valve during all waking hours within several days. If this is not possible, then timing the valve use around therapy and visitor schedules is recommended. As anxiety can increase when any changes are introduced to the medically complex patient, proceeding at the patient's comfort level is important. The use of pulse oximetry to measure the adequacy of oxygenation can be a reassurance to the patient as well as a safety monitoring device for the staff. Without the patient's agreement in the wearing schedule, any attempt to progress in the use of the valve is certain to meet with resistance. Cases 1 and 2 in Appendix A are patients who learn to use speaking valves.

There are patients who cannot tolerate a valve for more than a brief trial or who are unable to produce phonation. In the first instance, obstruction of the airway is the first consideration. If the cuff has not been fully deflated prior to the donning of the valve, the patient will experience immediate discomfort. A tracheostomy cannula that is too large for the trachea is another common cause for failure to tolerate a valve or produce adequate voice with a speaking valve. Other possible causes include vocal fold paralysis in the midline position, edema of the soft tissue in the trachea, tracheal stenosis, or tracheomalacia. Direct examination by an otolaryngologist is necessary to make the diagnosis of these conditions. Vocal fold pathology may also be present if the patient is able to tolerate the speaking valve but remains aphonic. Often prolonged intubation or the presence of a cuffed tube results in a patient becoming accustomed to "mouthing" words. Practice in relearning voicing is indicated in this instance.

Policies and procedures pertaining to tracheostomy cuff deflation and application of speaking valves vary from setting to setting. In many settings, competencies are being developed to identify a set of skills required to perform a task in a specific environment. Competencies are behavioral objectives related to a professional's scope of practice. Appendices B and C include samples of competencies for speech–language pathologists to perform tracheostomy cuff deflation and apply tracheostomy speaking valves.

Effect of Mechanical Ventilation on Speaking

In the instance of the ventilator-dependent individual, the inflated cuff affords leak-free coupling of the ventilator to the lungs (Fig. 5–21). During the inspiratory cycle, air is delivered by the ventilator and flows through the cannula to the lungs. Lung pressure increases. During the expiratory cycle, air flows out of the lungs and back to the ventilator through the cannula. Breathing in this "closed" system is controlled by adjusting ventilator settings to preserve normal concentrations and partial pressures of oxygen and carbon dioxide in arterial blood. Phonation cannot occur because air does not flow through the glottis as the tracheal lumen is sealed by the inflated cuff.

When the cuff is deflated or the tube is cuffless, the pattern of airflow is altered. During the inspiratory phase, air is delivered from the ventilator, flows through the cannula to the lungs, but also through the glottis. Phonation occurs during inspiration (Fig. 5–22). During the expiratory phase, air flows out through the cannula and back to the ventilator as well as through the nose and mouth. Phonation during expiration usually is not possible because of minimal airflow and insufficient subglottic pressure.

Evaluation of Candidacy for Communication Options

Mechanical Ventilator Dependency

When a patient is medically stable and able to be considered as a candidate for cuff deflation, brief trials are initiated with the consent of the physician and in cooperation with the respiratory therapist. The return of sensation of airflow through the upper airway may be bothersome to some patients, and it is important to proceed at a cautious rate. If the patient is unable to tolerate even brief

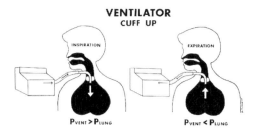

Fig. 5–21. Inspiration and expiration when a patient is coupled to a mechanical ventilator with an inflated tracheostomy cuff; air enters the lungs when air pressure in the ventilator exceeds pressure in the lungs and escapes from the lungs when lung pressure exceeds pressure in the ventilator or room. Reprinted, with permission, from Tippett and Siebens (67).

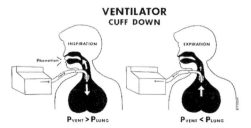

Fig. 5–22. Inspiration and expiration when a patient is coupled to a mechanical ventilator with a deflated cuff. Reprinted, with permission, from Tippett and Siebens (67).

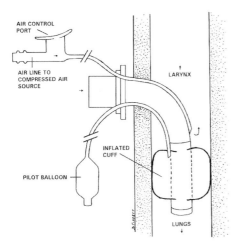

Fig. 5–23. Speaking tracheostomy cannula. Reprinted, with permission, from Tippett and Siebens (67).

periods of cuff deflation due to discomfort, inability to handle secretions, or failure to maintain adequate oxygenation, further evaluation is deferred.

Successful restoration of communication in the ventilator-dependent population is largely a factor of the individual's cognitive, language, and speech abilities (27). When cognitive, language, and oral/speech mechanisms are intact, the short-term solution of an electrolarynx and the long-term solution of cuff deflation are successful. For those with intact cognitive/language abilities, but impaired oral/speech mechanisms, various alternative/augmentative communication systems are appropriate. Attempts to restore oral communication are largely unsuccessful when there are significant cognitive/language and speech deficits.

Alternatives to Cuff Deflation for Communication

Mechanical Ventilator Dependency

Alternatives to oral communication via cuff deflation for individuals with ventilator dependency include external sound sources, augmentative/alternative communication systems, and speaking tracheostomy cannulas.

One type of external sound source specifically for ventilator-dependent individuals is the S.E.T. tube (45). This device has an extra lumen which conducts a tone to the posterior oral pharynx as part of an endotracheal tube. The tube is connected to a tone generator which the patient activates by a switch.

A speaking tracheostomy cannula restores oral communication despite dependence on mechanical ventilation through a cuffed cannula (Fig. 5–23). Air for speech is supplied independently of ventilation by a compressed air source such as an oxygen supply. Air is delivered via a narrow gauge tube that is attached to the outside of the cannula and ends in an open vent above the cuff. When the air control port is occluded, air from the source escapes through small openings above the inflated cuff and flows through the larynx, enabling the individual to speak. These tubes rely on an individual's own oropharyngeal mechanism (46), allow speech throughout the whole of the respiratory cycle (47,48) and do not

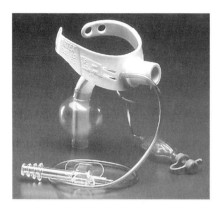

Fig. 5–24. SIMS Concord-Portex "Trach-Talk" tracheostomy tube. Photo courtesy of SIMS Portex, Inc., Keene, New Hampshire.

require adjusting ventilator output settings (47). Speaking tracheostomy tubes are viable communication options for patients who are not candidates for cuff deflation because of aspiration or compromised respiratory status. Such cannulas were first developed in England by R.J.L. Whitlock in 1967 (48) to facilitate communication for those patients who were unable to write due to paralysis or limb injuries.

In 1975, the first U.S. trials were reported by Safar and Grenvik (47) and were conducted on 25 intensive care unit patients. The Pitt speaking tracheostomy tube was used and became commercially available in the United States. Safar and Grenvik (47) concluded that "conscious patients with cuffed tracheostomy tubes can and should be given the opportunity to communicate by talking. One of several methods is the use of the Pitt speaking tracheostomy tube which meets many of the national and international specifications for tube and cuff designs" (p. 26).

Current commercially available speaking tracheostomy tubes are the Trach-Talk (SIMS Portex, Inc., Keene, New Hampshire) (Fig. 5–24) and the COMMUNI-trach I (Spectrum of California, Irvine, California) (Fig. 5–25).

Gordan (49) examined the effectiveness of the Pitt speaking tracheostomy tubes on different patient populations. He studied two groups of five patients who were ventilator-dependent, one group with neuromuscular disease and one group with respiratory failure but no history of neuromuscular disease. No members of group 1 (with neuromuscular involvement) were able to achieve intelligible, whispered speech regardless of airflow rates. All patients in group 2 were successful in producing intelligible speech at airflow rates of 4–6 L/min. At rates greater than 8 L/min, discomfort was reported by most patients. Gordan (49) concluded that the presence or absence of neuromuscular disease predicted the success or failure of the speaking tracheostomy tube to restore oral communication. Alternate communication means were recommended for patients whose ventilator dependency was attributable to a neuromuscular etiology.

Kluin and colleagues (50) studied the Portex speaking tracheostomy tube with 19 patients. Fourteen of 19 reportedly achieved intelligible speech; three of 19 were described as having "fluctuating success" secondary to mental status or build up of secretions; two of 19 did not achieve intelligible speech, one because of vocal fold paralysis and the other due to the presence of copious secretions.

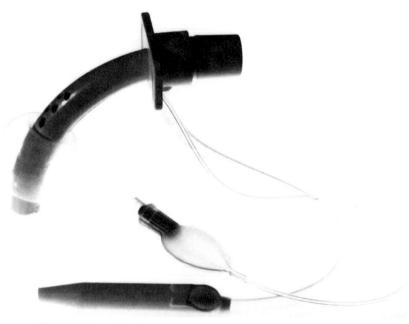

Fig. 5–25. COMMUNItrach I. Photo courtesy of Spectrum of California, Irvine, California.

Sparker and colleagues (46) compared the Portex and the COMMUNItrach speaking tracheostomy tubes. They found that 15 of 19 patients were able to achieve intelligible speech with a speaking tracheostomy tube. The authors preferred the COMMUNItrach to the Portex tubes because the former has more rigid tubing which is less susceptible to kinking. Leder and Astrachan (51) found that the multiple air ports in the COMMUNItrach results in less occlusion by secretions than is evidenced in the single port of the Portex.

In order to determine candidacy for a speaking tracheostomy tube, a review of the patient's medical history is conducted to determine any oral, laryngeal, and/or pharyngeal pathology. Examination by the speech–language pathologist and otolaryngologist reveals the anatomic or physiologic status of the components necessary for speech production (46). The recommended waiting period between the insertion of the speaking tube and the initiation of its use is three to five days. Unless the tracheostoma is adequately healed, air can leak from the stoma site or result in subcutaneous or mediastinal emphysema (47,48,52).

The adjustment of airflow rates is a delicate balance between patient comfort and clarity of speech production. Rates from 2 L/min to 15 L/min have been reported as compatible with speech. For most adults, a flow rate of 5 L/min is necessary to produce a whispered voice, and 8 to 10 L/min is necessary for normal conversational speech. Discomfort is frequently reported by patients as airflow rates increase above 10 L/min (47,48,50,52,53). It is recommended that the air delivered from the separate supply source be warmed and humidified to reduce the drying effect on the mucosa (47–49).

Before speaking trials begin, low-pressure suctioning via the speaking connector tube may be necessary to remove secretions from the area superior to the cuff (48). Sparker and colleagues (46) reported successful suctioning through the rigid tubing of the COMMUNItrach. Because the buildup of secretions is a persistent complication with the speaking tracheostomy tubes, installation of 1 to 2 mm of 10% acetylcysteine or saline solution through the speaking connector tube one or two times daily may reduce the tenacity of the secretions (54).

The ability to achieve functional speech production with the speaking tracheostomy tubes requires training of the patient and the caregiver. From one to five days of practice are common before intelligible speech is produced (50,53). In theory, voice is achievable during both the inspiratory and expiratory cycles of the ventilator, allowing for continuous speech. Leder and Traquina (53) observed that their patients could not produce intelligible speech during the inspiratory cycle, perhaps due to the "unnaturalness" of speaking out of synchrony with the normal breathing-speaking pattern. They recommended that tube occlusion be coordinated with the expiratory phase of the ventilator.

For the individual who cannot manually occlude the speaking connector tube, the communication partner needs to be signaled when to initiate and when to interrupt the airflow for speech. This requires the recognition of cues from the speaker that he or she wants to initiate speech. Electromechanical systems have been devised for independent activation of airflow by quadriplegic patients (55). Extra tubing (e.g., 50 cm) is preferable to the usual tube line length of 17 cm as it permits more convenient and varied locations of the partner providing occlusion of the line (53). A period of desensitization may be required to accommodate the adjustment to the feeling of airflow through the upper airway. Therapy using the speaking tracheostomy tube may begin with 15 min sessions, gradually increasing use of the speaking tracheostomy tube to all waking hours.

Speaking tracheostomy cannulas can present numerous problems (46,49–51,53,56). Loudness levels and voice qualities are variable across patients and across sessions. Voice quality has been described as hoarse, harsh, and with inconsistent or low volume. In part, these problems can be attributed to faulty synchronization of the onset of talking and occlusion of the speaking connector tube. However, even when this coordination has been mastered, perceptual deviations may persist.

As noted previously, secretions may occlude air vents, especially in models with a single vent. Secretions that accumulate above the cuff or in the speaking connector tube can be propelled into the larynx and pharynx when the tube is occluded for speech purposes. Positioning is an essential factor and is affected by the ventilator tubing which can pull the cannula down and away from the stoma, resulting in an inadequate air seal. Rotation of the tube, also resulting from pulling by the ventilator hosing, may cause air vents to be blocked by the tracheal wall. Neck straps which are too loose can cause anterior protrusion of the tube (53). Stomal complications can affect the tissue adjacent to the tube insertion site (51). Cleaning is difficult, and with patients who produce copious secretions, frequent changing of the tubes is necessary. Ultimately, for any communication option to be successful, the patient must be comfortable with its use. Airflow has been shown to produce annoying sensations in many patients (47,48,50,52,57). Unless modifications are made (55), the quadriplegic, ventilator-dependent patient must rely on a partner to control access to communication. For these reasons, the successful use of speaking tracheostomy cannulas is limited in the rehabilitation population. Although these tubes can serve a useful purpose (58), their inherent disadvantages often preclude their use over the long term.

Oral Communication Options with Cuff Deflation

Mechanical Ventilator Dependency

Patients with neuromuscular failure who are ventilator-dependent typically have an inflated cuff to preserve "leak-free" coupling with the ventilator. Nonoral communication (e.g., alternative/augmentative communication, writing) has been the dominant treatment alternative. However, there are precedents for using cuff deflation with patients who have a neurogenic basis for their ventilatory insufficiency.

Safar and Grenvik (47) used this technique in 1960 during the Maryland poliomyelitis epidemic. In 1973, Auchingloss and Gilbert (59) described the use of "leaking connections" between tracheostomy tubes and fixed-cycle, volume-limited ventilators with five patients. Metal tracheostomy cannulas with large slip-on cuffs were coupled to volume-set, time-cycled, piston-driven ventilators. A mini-leak technique allowed voice to be produced during lung inflation. Serious tracheal wall damage was avoided using this technique, given the continuous use of a partially inflated cuff. Successful cuff deflation was also reported with a 37-year-old man who had amyotrophic lateral sclerosis (60) and with 16 ventilator-dependent patients, one of whom had poliomyelitis (61). The latter patient's speech was considered "excellent and allowed him to carry on his business over the telephone from his home" (p. 364). Make and colleagues (61) used an increased tidal volume and partial cuff deflation to allow speech during the ventilator-delivered inspiratory cycle. In a study of Bach and Alba (62), 91 of 104 patients were adequately ventilated with deflated cuffs or cuffless tubes 24 h per day; 10 were converted to noninvasive alternatives of ventilatory support and three continued with cuff inflation. Respiration parameters were within normal limits (i.e., arterial blood gas, daytime oxygen saturation, end-tidal PCO^2). Tippett and Siebens (63) studied five ventilator-dependent, cognitively intact individuals with glottic control. They documented that cuff deflation is compatible with safe ventilation, preserves oral communication, and, additionally, can be used to restore oral alimentation. There are multiple other citations in the literature in which references are made to the use of cuff deflation and cuffless tubes to facilitate oral communication (3,8,11,52,58,64–66).

Given the drawbacks and undesirable side effects associated with cuff inflation as well as the disadvantages associated with speaking tracheostomy cannulas, cuff deflation is advocated to restore oral communication for the ventilator-dependent individual with a tracheostomy (63). During the inspiratory phase, air delivered from the ventilator flows through the cannula both into the lungs and through the glottis (Fig. 5–22). Phonation occurs during inflation of the lungs (inspiration), a paradox when compared to the usual circumstance in which phonation

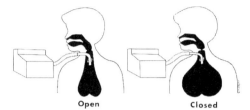

Open   Closed

Fig. 5–26. Relationship between glottic aperture and inflation of the lungs during the inspiratory cycle in a patient coupled to a ventilator; glottis is open on the left and closed or narrowed on the right. Reprinted, with permission, from Tippett and Siebens (67).

occurs during deflation (expiration). The proportions of tidal volume used for speech and for ventilation vary with glottic resistance which is under volitional control by the patient. When the glottis is narrowed, more of the tidal volume is delivered to the lungs. When there is little laryngeal resistance, inflation of the lungs diminishes (Fig. 5–26).

Tippett and Siebens (67) reported experiences with 16 ventilator-dependent patients ranging in age from 18–80 years (Table 5–2). Their group included five women and 11 men. Diagnoses were amyotrophic lateral sclerosis, spinal cord injury, Duchenne muscular dystrophy, Guillain–Barré syndrome, Arnold–Chiari malformation, acid maltase deficiency, progressive supranuclear palsy, Becker's muscular dystrophy, spinal cord stenosis, bilateral diaphragmatic paralysis and cervical hemangioblastoma.

At admission, 10 patients were not communicating orally, and six communicated using speaking tracheostomy cannulas. At discharge, 10 of the 16 patients

Table 5–2. Characteristics of ventilator-dependent patients regarding oral communication and cuff deflation at hospital admission and discharge.

Pt. no.	Age (yrs.)	Sex	Diagnosis	Oral communication Adm	Oral communication D/C	Cuff deflation Adm	Cuff deflation D/C
1	40	F	ALS	Y[a]	Y	N	Y
2	59	M	SCI	Y[a]	Y[b]	N	Y
3	21	M	DMD	N	Y	N	Y
4	70	M	GBS	N	Y[b]	N	Cuffless
5	34	M	ACM	N	Y[b]	N	Y
6	57	F	AMD	N	Y[b]	N	Y
7	74	F	PSP	N	N	Y	Y
8	18	F	SCI	N	Y	N	Y
9	24	M	BMD	N	Y	N	Y
10	80	F	SCS	Y[a]	Y[b]	N	Y
11	23	M	SCI	N	Y	Y	Y
12	29	M	SCI	Y[a]	Y	N	Y
13	66	M	SCI	Y[a]	Y	N	Y
14	75	M	BDP	N	Y	N	No tube
15	24	M	SCI	Y[a]	Y	N	Cuffless
16	42	M	CHB	N	Y	N	Y

[a] Speaking tracheostomy tube
[b] Hopkins speaking valve.

remained ventilator-dependent. Of these 10, eight were communicating orally via cuff deflation and one tolerated a cuffless tube (patient 15). Another did not achieve successful oral communication because of cognitive/language deficits and severe dysarthria. Six patients progressed to be independent of the ventilator. Hopkins ball valves were applied to the cannulas of five of the six. In summary, only two of the 16 patients used cuff deflation when admitted. At discharge, 13 practiced cuff deflation when awake, two used cuffless tubes, and one had been decannulated. The three criteria essential to success were cognition compatible with learning; laryngeal control sufficient for varying glottic resistance volitionally; and most importantly acceptance of the premise that cuff inflation may be unnecessary.

These ventilator-dependent patients were taught to use cuff deflation using strategies published previously (63). Patient, staff, and family education is a key element in the success of cuff deflation as a communication option. Anatomy and physiology of respiration, the position of the cannula, and the relationship between airway and foodway should be reviewed. A three-dimensional model showing anatomic structures in a sagittal exposure is helpful. Consideration is given to the size of the cannula. Cannulas are usually downsized to a no. 6 (Jackson or Shiley) to assure low resistance flow around the cannula in the tracheal lumen. The trachea is suctioned immediately on cuff deflation to remove the secretions which usually pool above the cuff. Ventilator adjustments are made. The tidal volume is increased to compensate for the glottic leak created by cuff deflation. Some ventilators allow adjustments of the inspiratory-to-expiratory cycles. In order to optimize phrase length, the inspiratory phase of ventilation is prolonged. Background noise is minimized to capitalize on auditory cues provided to the patient by ventilator functions. The patient is taught to speak during the output phase of the ventilator cycle by using such cues as listening, observing outward displacement of the chest, and sensing inflation of the lungs. The patient is taught by the speech–language pathologist to use these auditory and visual cues to "time" the onset of speech with the output phase of the ventilator. Some patients are bothered by the ventilator-driven air that flows through the upper airway, particularly those who have not experienced this sensation in months. Initially feelings of anxiety or discomfort may be experienced. These feelings usually are resolved with practice in timing voicing with the onset of the inspiratory cycle. In order to facilitate maximum inflation of the lungs, the patient is taught to adduct the vocal folds voluntarily. Adduction of the vocal folds is facilitated by instructions to "tighten your throat," "hold your breath," or "push down." This technique and the adjustment of ventilator settings explain the ability to maintain adequate ventilation in the presence of cuff deflation. Case 3 in Appendix A is a patient who is ventilator-dependent and learns to communicate orally.

Hoit and colleagues (68) described speech production during mechanical ventilation in seven individuals with tracheostomies. They found that individuals spoke during inspiratory flow, end-inspiratory pause, and early expiration. Subjects did not initiate speech production at the onset of the ventilator's inspiratory flow and did not utilize the full speaking time available to them. Tracheal pressures fluctuated substantially in the ventilator-dependent subjects, resulting in variations in loudness and phonatory quality. Hoit and colleagues (68) found that phonation duration was increased and vocal intensity and quality were better regulated during samples of sustained phonation when inspiratory flow was slowed and positive end-expiratory pressure (PEEP) was added. These ventilator adjustments lengthened the time tracheal pressure was above zero and flattened the tracheal pressure waveforms. Hoit and colleagues (68) also recommended that ventilator-dependent individuals be encouraged to speak as far into the expiratory cycle as possible until voicing fades. This practice results in linguistically inappropriate breaks in discourse, alerting listeners that a speaker intends to continue with a thought with the next inspiratory cycle of the ventilator. In this way, speakers are able to hold their positions in conversational exchanges. Hoit and Banzett (69) studied how the aforementioned adjustments of ventilator settings influence the quality of speech production in running speech. By decreasing the inspiratory flow time and adding PEEP, the duration of speaking time per ventilator cycle was increased, the number of syllables produced per cycle was increased, and peak tracheal pressures were decreased.

Over the past 20 years, an increasing number of patients have been managed successfully outside the hospital environment on positive pressure ventilation. Patients maintained at home developed fewer medical complications, required fewer repeat hospitalizations, and were cared for at a lower cost as compared to hospitalized patients (13,70). The use of a cuffless tracheostomy tube for home care of ventilator-dependent patients is adopted whenever feasible because of the restoration of oral communication. The care of a patient at home is described by Glover (71). Pulmonary function tests revealed no decline in status over three years, despite the presence of an uncuffed tube.

The only speaking valve compatible with ventilator use that is registered with the Food and Drug Administration is the Passy–Muir in-line valve (Passy–Muir, Inc., Irvine, California). The aqua colored valve fits the 15 mm universal hub of most tracheostomy tubes and connects to the Y-shaped piece of the ventilator circuit. Airflow from the ventilator is delivered to the lungs, but on expiration, the silastic membrane housed in the valve closes and air passes around the tracheostomy tube to the vocal folds, mouth, and nose. Candidates for these speaking valves must be able to tolerate cuff deflation and have relatively intact laryngeal and oral motor function (40).

Prentice and colleagues (72) proposed that communication and airway clearance of ventilator-dependent patients be synchronized primarily with expiration rather than inspiration. This is achieved by the use of the in-line valve. Tippett and Siebens (63) demonstrated that cuff deflation alone is sufficient for effective oral communication, upper airway clearance, and prevention of aspiration. The decision to use cuff deflation alone or with a valve should be based on individual patient performance and preference.

Influence of Cross Sectional Pharyngeal Area on Cuff Deflation

Although cuff deflation has a long history and is increasingly used at present, some resistance to this concept persists, especially with respect to the use of cuff deflation during sleep. Advances in knowledge are occurring with respect to cuff deflation which is advocated to restore oral communication for ventilator-

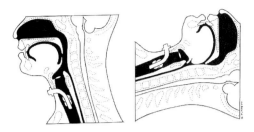

Fig. 5–27. Velum and tongue "fall" against the posterior pharyngeal wall in the supine position (right figure) narrowing the pharyngeal opening and increasing resistance to airflow. Reprinted, with permission, from Tippett and Siebens (67).

dependent individuals with tracheostomy (63,67,73). When the cuff of the tracheostomy tube is deflated, the proportions of tidal volume used for speech and ventilation vary with glottic resistance; this is under volitional control by the patient during wakefulness (Fig. 5–26). Patients can be taught to narrow or widen the glottic aperture to increase or decrease the inflation volume of the lungs, respectively, thereby becoming participants in the regulation of inspiration by varying the glottic aperture.

During sleep, resistance to airflow is not modulated by volitional control of the larynx. However, individuals with ventilator dependency remain adequately ventilated while asleep despite cuff deflation. It is hypothesized that resistance to airflow is modulated by four valve-like apertures: the lips, the tongue–palate appositions, the velopharyngeal wall, and the glottis of the relaxed larynx. In the supine position (the usual position for the ventilator-dependent individual during sleep), the pharynx offers greater resistance to flow than in the sitting position because the velum and tongue "fall" toward the posterior pharyngeal wall (Fig. 5–27).

Weller and colleagues (74) compared MRI images of craniocervical relationships of four subjects in prone and supine positions. The purpose of this study was to examine how pharyngeal cross sectional area might change in the supine position, thereby allowing a ventilator-dependent individual to have the cuff deflated during sleep and still be adequately ventilated. The narrowest retrolingual cross-sections measured 89, 232, 381, and 327 mm^2 prone as contrasted to 51, 145, 116, and 163 mm^2 supine, representing attenuations of 43, 37, 70, and 50% respectively, consequent to position. The conclusions of this study are that the pharynx has a different shape in the supine and prone positions; narrowing of the airway corresponds to higher airway resistance; and upper airway resistance is likely to be higher in the supine than prone positions. This finding supports the use of cuff deflation in individuals with ventilator dependency, permitting speech–language pathologists to present more persuasive evidence about an approach that continues to be considered nontraditional in many settings.

Quality of Life

Mechanical Ventilator Dependency and Oral Communication

Speech–language pathologists must address managed care's mandate to document treatment outcomes. Assessment of quality of life and the effect of oral communication is one approach to meet this objective. Restoration of oral communication via cuff deflation in ventilator-dependent individuals requires the collaboration of the patient, family, physician, nurse, respiratory therapist, and speech–language pathologist over several weeks. The investment of time and the costs of hospitalization and therapy are considered worthwhile because it is believed that the patient's quality of life is improved after restoration of such a basic human function. This assumption is validated by the following comment from a 32-year-old man who became a ventilator-dependent quadriplegic secondary to a gunshot wound: "Conveying messages one-to-one is very important. All my nurses prefer it much better when I can speak . . . It makes me feel much better. I feel more normal, less trapped in my body because I can take part—project my personality out of my body with my voice. So communication is important. It's certainly primary in my life and with my family" (75).

Defining quality of life is difficult. When the experts are consulted to define quality of life, there is general agreement that the evaluation of quality of life should include biomedical indicators (i.e., mortality, morbidity) and sociomedical indicators. The National Heart-Lung-Blood Institute (NHLBI) identifies three major components of quality of life, specifically: functional capacity (activities of daily living), perceptions (patient's beliefs, values, perspectives), and symptoms (what patients experience as a reflection of disease severity) (76).

There are numerous measures to assess quality of life. None are universally accepted. Many tools were first developed in the 1930s and 1940s. Some of the tools are population specific (e.g., individuals with cancer, arthritis). Some tools may be appropriate for assessing quality of life in ventilator-dependent individuals. These include the Life Domain Satisfaction Measures (77), the Semantic Differential Scale of General Affect (77), the Nottingham Health Profile (78), the Sickness Impact Profile (79), and the QL-Index (80)

The Life Domain Satisfaction Measures and the Semantic Differential Scale of General Affect were used with ventilator-dependent individuals by John Bach and colleagues (81,82). The Life Domain Satisfaction Measures are designed to explore respondents' feelings about nine domains in life. These are housing, transportation, education, job, health, family life, social life, sexual life, and life, in general. Respondents summarize their feelings by selecting a number on a scale of 1 through 7, with 1 being "completely dissatisfied" and 7 being "completely satisfied." The Semantic Differential Scale of General affect includes eight heuristic dimensions which consist of opposite or polar adjectives placed at extremes of a seven-point scale (e.g., 1 = boring/7 = interesting; 1 = miserable/7 = enjoyable; 1 = hard/7 = easy; 1 = useless/7 = worthwhile). Respondents check a number on the scale which best represents their perception. The Life Domain and Semantic Differential instruments measure two of the components of quality of life as defined by the NHLBI: functional capacity and patients' perceptions.

Studies of overall quality of life in ventilator-dependent individuals tend to fall into two categories: informal and formal. Observations, discussions and interviews are used in the informal studies (83–86). In the formal studies, quality of life scales are used (81,82,87). The majority of these informal and formal studies indicate that ventilator-dependent patients have happy, meaningful lives and a positive affect, and that professionals tend to underestimate patients' satisfaction with their lives and overestimate their dissatisfaction.

Some studies focus on specific quality of life issues. Bach (88,89) and Bach and colleagues (90) examined method of ventilation with respect to quality of life and found that noninvasive ventilatory regimens can be effective and preferable alternatives to tracheostomy.

Despite these numerous studies of quality of life in ventilator-dependent individuals, only three studies comment specifically upon the communication status of the ventilator-dependent individuals. These reports suggest that oral communication positively influences patients' perceptions about the quality of their lives. Maynard and Muth (91) described a 17-year-old male with ventilator-dependent quadriplegia after a diving accident who obtained a court order to disconnect his ventilator. The patient's parents believed that their son's decision may have been different if he had been able to speak, swallow, and breathe. Silverstein and colleagues (92) conducted a prospective survey of 38 patients with amyotrophic lateral sclerosis to identify their wishes for information, participation in decision making, and life-sustaining therapy. In their conclusion, they stated that positive reports about quality of life of patients who received mechanical ventilation usually describe individuals who are ambulatory, can speak despite having a tracheostomy, or can communicate via head or eye movements while intubated. Wang and colleagues (93) described six patients with spinal muscular atrophy, a degenerative anterior horn cell process with a variable progression. They found that the four individuals with spinal muscular atrophy who could communicate orally remained socially active, and one gainfully employed.

These studies suggest that the ability to speak is one factor that positively influences patients' perceptions about the quality of their lives. These studies address quality of life in individuals who are medically stable and have used mechanical ventilation for several months to years. There are no published studies to our knowledge that address oral communication and quality of life in the acute care setting.

Cases 4 and 5 in Appendix A are presented to illustrate quality of life issues in acute care and the speech–language pathologist's role. These cases suggest that the influence of speech on patients' perceptions of quality of life in acute care is less straightforward. Issues to consider are diagnosis, prognosis, time postonset, medical stability, and age. Further definition is needed regarding the speech–language pathologist's role in facilitating patients' abilities to convey important medical decisions (94).

Quite likely, it is necessary to develop a new quality of life assessment, which includes those aspects of quality of life which can be improved by patients being able to talk. Some of these aspects may include sense of control, ability to engage in pleasurable activities, emotional status, and degree of social support. Assessment of quality of life may be conducted pre- and postrestoration of oral communication. A trained interviewer may be needed. Some methodological concerns are the diverse etiologies and ages of this population, disposition, patients' perceptions of their deficits, habituation resulting in a decline in the subjective unpleasantness of a situation, and positive bias or the tendency of interviewees to give socially acceptable responses, thus exaggerating satisfaction with quality of life. Documentation of a positive association between oral communication and improved quality of life as perceived by patients is important to support the costly and labor-intensive treatment to teach ventilator-dependent patients how to speak.

Appendix A

CASE 1

Background

Olivopontocerebellar degeneration
  A group of similar disorders
  Sporadic and inherited forms
  Autosomal dominant and recessive
  Age 15–65 years (sporadic later)
  May be associated with some forms of cancer

  Symptoms
    Progressive ataxia: Unsteady walking, unstable use of hands
    Variety of associated symptoms
    Bulbar symptoms: Dysarthria, dysphagia
    Dementia
    Parkinsonism

A 78-year-old female with olivopontocerebellar degeneration was admitted to an intensive care unit after falling, breaking her hip, and becoming unresponsive. She underwent a total left hip replacement. Postoperatively, the patient required tracheostomy because of airway obstruction. Otolaryngology examination revealed incomplete bilateral vocal fold abduction. MRI showed atrophy of brain stem and cerebellum. The patient was transferred to a rehabilitation hospital three weeks post ICU admission. At that point, she had a no. 6 metal tracheostomy cannula, required oxygen via nasal cannula, and was alimented/hydrated via a mechanical soft diet. Treatment progress is outlined below.

Speech–Language Pathology Evaluation

Cognition/language: Mild-moderate deficits in personal/current information, short-term memory, verbal learning, word retrieval, verbal reasoning

Neurologic impairments of respiratory and laryngeal mechanisms

Speech: Mild dysarthria with harsh, occasionally wet-hoarse phonation, inspiratory stridor

Swallow: Deterioration in PO intake secondary to difficulty propelling boluses from mouth to pharynx after admission to rehabilitation hospital; NGFT placed

Speech–Language Pathology Treatment

Cognition/language: Develop compensations for learning new information and reasoning
  Strategies:
  Provide individual treatment
  Provide group treatment
  Counsel patient and husband regarding need for supervision

Speech: Facilitate oral communication
  Strategies:
  Provide unidirectional speaking valve
  Educate patient and husband regarding implications of tracheostomy and use
    of valve
  Monitor valve wearing

Swallow: Facilitate oral alimentation and hydration
  Strategies:
  Conduct a videofluoroscopic swallowing study (VFSS)
  Review VFSS with patient and husband
  Discuss compensations
  Raise issue of alternatives to PO intake

Treatment Progress

Hospital day 4
  Assessed cognitive/language abilities
  Plugging of cannula attempted; inspiratory stridor noted
  Initiated trials with Hopkins speaking valve

Hospital day 7
  Valve tolerated during all waking hours

Hospital day 18
  Cannula valved during VFSS
  Mild-moderate retention of solid boluses
  Retention cleared with multiple swallows
  Esophageal dysmotility with liquids and solids
  Conclusion: Pharyngeal and esophageal stage dysphagia
  Recommendation: PO intake with purees, decrease rate of intake, multiple
    swallows/bolus

Hospital day 28
  Valve worn regularly during all waking hours
  Mild dysphonia persisted but oral communication functional
  PO intake with compensations
  Mild cognitive/language deficits persisted
  Discharge to home with husband to supervise

CASE 2

Background

C-P angle epidermoid tumor
Epidermoids
  Most common embryonal intracranial tumors
  Commonly arise in cerebellopontine angle, skull base, brain stem,
    intraventricular cavity
  Slow growing

Symptoms
  Manifested at any age, often young adulthood
  Vary depending on site and size of tumor

A 33-year-old male underwent resection of a right C-P angle epidermoid tumor. The acute medical course was complicated by two respiratory arrests and hydrocephalus. A modified barium swallow study showed reduced motion of the soft palate, pharyngeal constrictors, epiglottis, and larynx. Six weeks after surgery, the patient was transferred to a rehabilitation hospital. At that point, he had a Shiley no. 8 tracheostomy cannula with an inflated cuff and a gastrostomy. Treatment progress is outlined below.

Speech–Language Pathology Evaluation

Cognition/language: Adequate for functional communication; additional testing required to rule out subtle deficits

Neurologic impairments of respiratory mechanism, larynx, velum/pharynx, tongue, lips/face, jaw

Speech: Severe dysphonia with low volume, harsh, breathy, wet-hoarse phonation; speech intelligibility 75% in conversation; dysphonia masked perceptual judgments of resonance and articulation

Swallow: NPO

Speech–Language Pathology Treatment

Cognition/language: Assess to rule out subtle deficits
  Strategies:
  Administer portions of the *Boston Diagnostic Aphasia Examination, Wechsler Memory Scale, Ravens Coloured Progressive Matrices, Ross Information Processing Assessment, Revised Boston Naming Test*
  Engage in treatment sessions to address auditory comprehension/short-term memory at a paragraph level, word retrieval on divergent tasks, verbal reasoning on abstract tasks

Speech: Facilitate oral communication
  Strategies:
  Obtain otolaryngology examination of laryngeal structure and function
  Provide a unidirectional speaking valve
  Educate patient/family/caregivers regarding implications of tracheostomy and use of valve
  Monitor valve use

Swallow: Facilitate oral alimentation and hydration
  Strategies:
  Conduct VFSS
  Educate patient/family/caregivers

Treatment Progress

Hospital day 1
  Cannula downsized to Shiley no. 6
  Obtained Hopkins speaking valve
  Initiated trial use

Hospital day 4
  Conducted VFSS
  Bolus was thick liquid by spoon
  Cuff deflated; valve in place
  Diminished pharyngeal constriction, epiglottic tilt, laryngeal rise, opening of
    PE segment
  Flagrant and immediate airway penetration without cough
  No benefit from head/chin tuck
  Recommendations: Continue NPO/G-tube; continue use of valve; obtain
    otolaryngology examination of laryngeal structure and function

Hospital day 8
  Obtained otolaryngology examination of laryngeal structure and function
  Impaired right vocal fold movement with fold in abducted position, edema,
    reduced sensation, pooling of secretions in valleculae and pyriform sinuses
    and covering glottis
  Continue NPO status, use of speaking valve; follow-up for improvement
    regarding laryngeal function and possible consideration of future surgical
    options
Hospital days 9 to 32
  Conducted daily SLP treatment sessions to address subtle cognitive/language
    deficits
  Readministered baseline cognitive/language testing
  Cannula changed to Shiley no. 6 cuffless tube
  Expanded valve wearing time to all waking hours
  Voice quality less wet-hoarse; improved ability to cough and clear secretions
  Provided intensive patient/family education regarding value of the speaking
    valve, rationale for NPO/G-tube status

Hospital day 33
  Conducted VFSS
  Bolus was thick liquid via spoon
  Substantial pharyngeal retention, poor pharyngeal contraction, diminished
    opening of PE segment
  Immediate subglottic laryngeal penetration/aspiration with cough
  Recommendations: Continue NPO/G-tube

Hospital day 34
  Discharge to home with outpatient therapies
  Plan for outpatient follow-up

Three months post discharge
  Conducted VFSS

Shiley no. 6 cuffless cannula

Speaking valve worn during all waking hours

Severe dysphonia with low volume, harsh, breathy, wet-hoarse phonation

Bolus was thick liquid via spoon

Subglottic laryngeal penetration/aspiration without cough, weak pharyngeal
constriction, pharyngeal retention of boluses, poor opening of PE segment

Recommendations: Continue NPO/G-tube, speaking valve

Seven months post discharge

Conducted VFSS

Low volume, breathy voice

Boluses were thick liquid, thin liquid via spoon

Weak pharyngeal constriction, marginal laryngeal elevation, diminished
cricopharyngeal opening

No subglottic laryngeal penetration with valve in place, head/chin flexed, small
bolus sizes of thick liquid

Recommendations: Initiate therapeutic feeding with thick liquid only with
valve in place, head/chin flexed; educate patient/family regarding assisted
cough and suctioning

CASE 3

Background

Ventilator-dependent quadriplegia

A 29-year-old male sustained a gunshot wound to the neck, resulting in C-1
ventilator-dependent quadriplegia, right vertebral artery occlusion, and brain
stem contusion. Glasgow Coma Scale score was 3T/15 at hospital admission. The
patient was referred for speech–language pathology intervention for
cognitive/language, speech, and swallow evaluation and treatment. As the patient progressed, a Portex no. 8 speaking tracheostomy cannula was placed to facilitate communication. Low technology alternative/augmentative communication
devices were tried. A modified barium swallow study showed reduced lingual
movement, weak pharyngeal constriction, diminished laryngeal elevation, pooling in valleculae, and laryngeal penetration/aspiration of puree consistency without cough. Gastrostomy was performed, and the patient was made NPO. The
patient was transferred to a rehabilitation hospital three months postinjury. Treatment progress is outlined below.

Speech–Language Pathology Evaluation

Cognition/language: Grossly within normal limits

Neurologic impairments of respiratory mechanism, larynx, velum/pharynx

Speech: Harsh, wet-hoarse phonation, hypernasality

Swallow: NPO; secretions pooled in patient's mouth, drooling, frequent suctioning

Speech–Language Pathology Treatment

Cognition/language: Direct treatment not indicated

Speech: Facilitate oral communication via cuff deflation; develop augmentative communication system (ACS)
    Strategies:
    Educate patient/caregivers regarding normal anatomy/physiology, cuff deflation
    Collaborate with team to investigate downsizing cannula
    Develop ACS with occupational therapist (OT)

Swallow: Facilitate oral alimentation and hydration
    Strategies:
    Conduct VFSS
    Educate patient/caregivers

Treatment Progress

Hospital day 1
    Conducted SLP evaluation
    Provided education to patient regarding cuff deflation

Hospital day 5
    Cuff deflation attempted
    Patient extremely anxious . . . session discontinued

Hospital days 6 to 7
    Intensive education provided

Hospital day 8
    Cannula changed to Shiley no. 6 cuffed cannula
    Cuff deflation trial initiated
    Phonation achieved
    Recommendations: Continue cuff deflation trials; defer swallow assessment

Hospital day 23
    Focused on improving coordination of speaking with onset of inspiratory cycle
    Tolerated cuff deflation 2 to 3 h/day
    Swallow assessment deferred secondary to need for frequent oral suctioning

Hospital day 29
    Continued to tolerate cuff deflation 2 h/day

Hospital day 37
    Tolerated cuff deflation 4 h/day

Hospital day 38
    Conducted VFSS
    Boluses were ultrathick and thick liquids via spoon
    Cuff deflated
    Pharyngeal retention, laryngeal penetration/aspiration without cough
    Conclusion: Pharyngeal stage dysphagia; continue NPO/G-tube

VFSS reviewed with patient

Hospital day 48
   Medical complications: Pneumonia, MRSA, C-difficile
   Persisting anxiety
   Tolerated cuff deflation 2 h/day consistently; 4 h/day occasionally
   Second review of VFSS
   Collaborate with OT, vendors regarding ACS

Hospital day 57
   Tolerated cuff deflation 4 h/day
   Evaluated for oral prosthesis for oral suctioning
   Patient/family/team conference conducted

Hospital day 73
   Tolerated cuff deflation 8 h/day
   Fine-tuning of oral prosthesis
   Trials with Morse code, scanning, sip and puff switches with ACS for written
      communication

Hospital day 85
   Discharge to nursing home
   Completed oral prosthesis for suctioning
   Tolerated cuff deflation for at least 8 h/day
   Able to access ACS via a variety of means

CASE 4

The patient is a 73-year-old man who fell from a golf cart, sustaining an odontoid fracture. On hospital admission, the patient's Glasgow Coma Scale score was 5/15. He was intubated, underwent a C1–C2 fusion, and had an oral gastric feeding tube placed. The patient was healthy, married, and had seven children. On day 6, the patient was referred for a speech–language pathology evaluation to facilitate speaking and swallowing. The patient and his family were instructed in the use of an electrolarynx. On day 7, a modified Evans blue dye test was conducted, and the patient was cleared for a diet of mechanical soft solids and liquids. Trials of cuff deflation were also initiated. These trials were specifically requested by the patient's physician in order to determine what the family felt to be the patient's requests to be disconnected from the ventilator. Successful oral communication was achieved via partial cuff deflation, and the patient orally expressed his desire to be disconnected from the ventilator to his family, physicians, and nurses. Consultations were obtained from psychiatry and the hospital ethics committee. Discussions were conducted with the patient and his family, including future rehabilitation options. The patient decided to delay his decision at that point until he had additional opportunities to engage in physical, occupational, and speech–language therapies. By day 25, the patient was tolerating partial cuff deflation for several hours per day, and all alimentation/hydration was oral. During visits with his family, the patient discussed his wishes regarding mechanical ventilation and communicated his desire to be disconnected from the ventilator to his attending physician. The patient's family supported his decision. On day 28 a family conference was held. On day 32, the patient met privately with his wife and each child and then was disconnected from mechanical ventilation.

CASE 5

The patient is a 74-year-old man who was involved in a motor vehicle accident. The patient sustained a C-4 fracture. On hospital admission the patient's Glasgow Coma Scale score was 6/15. He was intubated. His fracture was stabilized and an oral gastric feeding tube was placed. The patient was healthy prior to his injury, widowed, and had two daughters. On day 2 a speech–language pathology consult was initiated to facilitate communication and evaluate swallowing. Cuff deflation was initiated. The patient achieved successful oral communication. A modified Evans blue dye test was conducted which revealed aspiration with puree. On day 5 the modified Evans blue dye test was repeated and persisting aspiration was found. An otolaryngology consult was obtained, and the patient was diagnosed with tracheitis and hypopharyngeal edema. The oral gastric feeding tube was replaced with a nasogastric feeding tube. Cuff deflation was continued for oral communication trials. The patient and his family were instructed in alternatives to oral communication, including an electrolarynx and an eyegaze board. On day 26 a family conference was held to discuss rehabilitation options. On day 38 the modified Evans blue dye test was repeated. Oral intake with thickened liquids and mechanical soft solids was initiated. On day 42 the patient was reevaluated with thin liquids but aspiration persisted with this bolus. On day 46 the patient was discharged to an acute inpatient rehabilitation hospital, having progressed from an oral gastric feeding tube to a bolus modified diet and from nonoral to oral communication.

Appendix B.   Competency Regarding Cuff Deflation

Outcome

Cuff deflation is used to effect the following:

1. Facilitate oral communication
2. Facilitate upper airway clearance of secretions via cough, throat-clear
3. Complete swallow assessment at the bedside to determine if aspiration/laryngeal penetration is evident

Staff

Speech-language pathologists (may involve physicians, nurses, respiratory therapists)

Equipment

Syringe

Manometer

Core Components of Performance Criteria

The speech–language pathologist:

1. States candidacy criteria for cuff deflation
   a. Patient is alert
   b. Patient is medically stable to tolerate cuff deflation (e.g., respiratory function, cardiac function, pulmonary function)
   c. Patient demonstrates readiness to communicate, including emerging communication attempts
   d. Patient may be a candidate for assessing swallow ability

2. Assesses candidacy for cuff deflation
   a. Checks size and type of cannula
   b. Monitors oxygen saturation, heart rate, blood pressure, ventilator alarms as appropriate
   c. Consults with other professional staff, i.e., nurse, physician, respiratory therapist

3. Deflates/inflates cuff correctly
   a. Withdraws air/water from pilot balloon via syringe
   b. Is prepared to suction or has nurse present
   c. Monitors vital signs and patient's comfort
   d. Reinflates cuff if change occurs in vital signs or patient's comfort
   e. Reinflates cuff without overinflating; measured via manometry or onset of absence of phonation

4. Instructs patient regarding phonation/respiration during cuff deflation
   a. Allows patient to become comfortable with cuff deflation
   b. Performs intermittent digital occlusion of cannula if patient is not ventilator-dependent
   c. Teaches patient to phonate when cannula is occluded intermittently
   d. Teaches patient vocal fold adduction technique to compensate for leak created by deflating cuff (if patient is ventilator-dependent)
   e. Facilitates phonation during inspiratory phase if patient is ventilator-dependent

5. Assesses patient's tolerance, speech, and/or swallow (as appropriate) with cuff deflated
   a. Monitors vital signs
   b. Monitors ventilator alarms
   c. Monitors patient comfort
   d. Assesses perceptual characteristics of speech (phonation, resonance, articulation)
   e. Assesses speech intelligibility
   f. Assesses swallowing based on voice quality, presence of cough, evidence of food particles or evidence of dyed boluses in tracheal secretions

  g. Proposes possible etiologies for aphonia/dysphonia
  h. Makes recommendations for additional referrals as appropriate, e.g., assessment of laryngeal structure/function by otolaryngology

6. States contraindication to cuff deflation
    a. Patient cannot tolerate cuff deflation secondary to change in vital signs, comfort
    b. Low pressure alarm sounds when cuff is deflated
    c. Tracheostomy is performed within 24 h

7. Identifies need for suctioning

8. Performs suctioning as appropriate or alerts nurse

9. Uses appropriate infection control techniques

10. Implements a treatment plan based on performance during initial cuff deflation trial
    a. States duration and frequency of cuff deflation
    b. Establishes a schedule for cuff deflation with patient, family, team members
    c. Educates patient and family regarding cuff deflation

Appendix C.   Competency Regarding Unidirectional Tracheostomy Speaking Valves

Outcome

A unidirectional tracheostomy speaking valve is applied to a tracheostomy cannula to:

1. Restore oral communication
2. Facilitate upper airway clearance of secretions via cough, throat-clear

Staff

Speech–language pathologists (may involve physicians, nurses, respiratory therapists)

Equipment

Unidirectional tracheostomy speaking valve

Core Components of Performance Criteria

The speech–language pathologist:
1. Recognizes candidacy for a unidirectional tracheostomy speaking valve
    a. Patient is alert
    b. Patient has a tracheostomy cannula with or without mechanical ventilator dependency
    c. Patient can tolerate cuff deflation

    d. Patient has adequate inspiratory effort to open valve

    e. Patient demonstrates readiness to communicate, e.g., patient may be "mouthing" words, writing, gesturing

    f. Patient may be a candidate for assessing swallow ability

2. Assesses candidacy for a unidirectional tracheostomy speaking valve
   a. Checks size and type of tracheostomy cannula
   b. Deflates cuff of tracheostomy cannula
   c. Monitors oxygen saturation
   d. Monitors ventilation, especially low-pressure alarm
   e. Performs intermittent digital occlusion of tracheostomy cannula if patient is not ventilator-dependent
   f. Facilitates phonation during inspiratory phase if patient is ventilator-dependent
   g. Assesses voice quality via cuff deflation
   h. Teaches patient vocal fold adduction technique to compensate for leak created by deflating cuff (if patient is ventilator-dependent)
   i. Discusses candidacy with nurse, physician, and/or respiratory therapist as appropriate

3. States available unidirectional tracheostomy speaking valves e.g., Passy–Muir, Olympic, Montgomery

4. Describes the purpose, characteristics, and care of unidirectional speaking valves
   a. Purpose = facilitate speech and upper airway clearance
   b. Function = valve is unidirectional; air flows in at the level of the cannula during inspiration and then flows out through the larynx during expiration
   c. Airway resistance can be increased with a valve in place
   d. Valves usually can be cleaned with mild soap and water; see product instructions for specifics

5. Assesses patient's tolerance, speech, and/or swallow (as appropriate) with valve in place
   a. Monitors oxygen saturation
   b. Monitors ventilator alarms
   c. Monitors patient's level of comfort
   d. Assesses perceptual characteristics of speech (phonatory quality, resonance, articulation)
   e. Assesses speech intelligibility
   f. Assesses swallowing based on voice quality, presence of cough, evidence of food particles or evidence of dyed boluses in tracheal secretions

6. Assesses function of unidirectional tracheostomy speaking valve
   a. Examines valve for cleanliness
   b. Determines if valve closes upon expiration

   c.   Determines if valve opens upon inspiration

   d.   Discards valve if not operating properly

7.   States contraindications to application of unidirectional speaking valve
   a.   Tracheostomy cannula occludes airway
   b.   Patient cannot tolerate cuff deflation
   c.   Patient desaturates with cuff deflation or application of valve
   d.   Low-pressure alarm sounds when valve is applied or cuff is deflated
   e.   Secretions are copious
   f.   Airway is obstructed by vocal fold paralysis in midline, granulation tissue, tracheal stenosis, edema
   g.   Patient is uncomfortable, anxious

8.   Identifies need for suctioning

9.   Performs suctioning as appropriate or alerts nurse

10.   Educates patient/family regarding unidirectional tracheostomy speaking valve
   a.   Discusses purpose, function, characteristics of valve
   b.   Informs regarding contraindications for valve use
   c.   Explains cleaning of valve
   d.   Explains application/removal of valve
   e.   Assesses learning needs, readiness
   f.   Evaluates patient/family learning
   g.   Uses materials appropriate to cognitive/developmental level, culture

References

1. World Health Organization. *Constitution of the World Health Organization.* Geneva: World Health Organization, 1964.
2. Rogers ES. *Human ecology and health: introduction for administrators.* New York: Macmillan Company, 1960.
3. Zejdlik CP. Promoting optimal respiratory function. In: *Management of spinal cord injury.* Monterey, CA: Wadsworth Health Sciences Division, 1983:167–211.
4. Gracey DR, McMichan JC, Divertie MB, et al. Respiratory failure in Guillain–Barré syndrome: a 6-year experience. *Mayo Clinic Proceedings* 1982;57:742–746.
5. Moore P, James O. Guillain–Barré syndrome: incidence, management and outcome of major complications. *Critical Care Med* 1981;9:549–555.
6. Ropper AH, Kehne SM. Guillain–Barré syndrome: management of respiratory failure. *Neurology* 1985;35:1662–1665.
7. Ropper AH, Wijdicks EFM, Truax BT. Respiratory failure. In: *Guillain–Barré syndrome.* Philadelphia: FA Davis, 1991:253–262.
8. Sivak ED, Cordasco EM, Gipson WT. Pulmonary mechanical ventilation at home: a reasonable and less expensive alternative. *Respir Care* 1983;28:42–49.
9. Sivak ED, Gipson WT, Hanson MR. Long-term management of respiratory failure in amyotrophic lateral sclerosis. *Annals of Neurology* 1982;12, 18-23.
10. Gracey DR, Divertie MB, Howard FM. Mechanical ventilation for respiratory failure in myasthenia gravis: two-year experience with 22 patients. *Mayo Clinic Proceedings* 1983;58:597–602.
11. Bach J, Alba A, Pilkington LA, Lee M. Long-term rehabilitation in advanced stage of childhood onset, rapidly progressive muscular dystrophy. *Arch Phys Med Rehabil* 1981;62:328-331.

12. Snider GL. Historical perspective on mechanical ventilation: from simple life support system to ethical dilemma. *Am Rev Respir Dis* 1989;140:S2–S7.

13. Fischer DA, Prentice WS. Feasibility of home care for certain respiratory-dependent restrictive or obstructive lung disease patients. *Chest* 1982;82:739–743.

14. Goldberg AI, Faure EAM. Home care for life-supported persons in England: the responaut program. *Chest* 1984;86:910–914.

15. Snider GL. Thirty years of mechanical ventilation: changing expectations. *Archives of Internal Med* 1983;143:745–749.

16. Pokras R. Detailed diagnosis and procedures for patients discharged from short-stay hospitalizations, United States, 1985. Vital Health and Statistics, Series 30, No. 90. DHHS Pub. No. (PHS) 87-1751 Public Health Service. Washington, DC: US Government Printing Office (April 1987).

17. Make B, Dayno S, Gertman P. Prevalence of chronic ventilator dependency. *Am Rev Respir Dis* 1986;133:A167.

18. American Association for Respiratory Care. *A study of chronic ventilator patients in the hospital.* Dallas: AARC, 1991.

19. Swinburne AJ, Fedullo AJ, Shayne DS. Mechanical ventilation: analysis of increasing use and patient survival. *J Intensive Care Med* 1988;3:315.

20. Rosen RL, Bone RC. Financial implications of ventilator care. *Critical Care Clinics* 1990;6:797–805.

21. American Speech-Language-Hearing Association. Ad Hoc Committee on Use of Specialized Medical Speech Devices. Position statement and guidelines for the use of voice prostheses in tracheotomized persons with or without ventilatory dependence. *ASHA* 1993;35(Suppl 10):17–20.

22. Mitsuda PM, Baarsalag-Benson R, Hazel K, et al. Augmentative communication in intensive and acute care settings. In: Yorkston KM, ed. *Augmentative communication in the medical setting.* Tucson: Communication Skill Builders, 1992:25.

23. Simmons KF. Airway care. In: Scanlan CL, Spearman CB, Seldon RL, eds. *Egan's fundamentals of respiratory care. 5th edition.* St. Louis: C.V. Mosby, 1990:483–512.

24. Skelly M. *Amerind gestural code based on universal American Indian hand talk.* New York: Elsevier North Holland, 1979.

25. Sunners J. The use of the electrolarynx in patients with temporary tracheostomies. *J Speech Hear Dis* 1973;38:335–338.

26. Godwin JE, Heffner JE. Special critical care considerations in tracheostomy management. *Clinics Chest Med* 1991;12:573–583.

27. Beukelman DR, Yorkston KM, Dowden PA. *Communication augmentation: a casebook of clinical management.* San Diego: Hill Press, 1985.

28. Blackstone S, Tippett DC, Watkins C. Communication options for persons dependent on a tracheostomy or ventilator. *Augmentative Commun News* 1992;5:6.

29. Dedo HH. Tracheotomy. In: *Surgery of the larynx and trachea.* Philadelphia: BC Decker, Inc., 1990:81–110.

30. Furiel AE, Putnam JS. Patients with tracheostomies: goals of management. *Symposium Advance Pulmonary Med* 1978;5:557–567.

31. Cane RD, Woodward C, Shapiro BA. Customizing fenestrated tracheostomy tubes: a bedside technique. *Critical Care Med* 1982;10:880–881.

32. Toremalm NG. A tracheotomy speech valve. *Laryngoscope* 1968;78:2177–2182.

33. Emery FM. Speaking valve for attachment to a tracheostomy tube. *Br Med J* 1972;2:466.

34. Cowan DL. Laryngeal and tracheal stenosis: an adapted speaking aid tracheostomy tube. *J Laryngol Otol* 1975;89:531–534.

35. Saul A, Bergstrom B. A new permanent tracheostomy tube—speech valve system. *Laryngoscope* 1979;89:980–983.

36. French J, Siebens A, Kummell J, et al. Preserving communication and airway clearance in tracheostomized children and adults. *Arch Phys Med Rehabil* 1984;65:651.

37. Passy V. Passy-Muir tracheostomy speaking valve. *Otolaryngol Head Neck Surg* 1986;95:247–248.

38. French JJ, Kummell J, Siebens AA. Adapting the "Hopkins speaking valve" for use with a Shiley cannula. *Proceedings of the 14th RESNA Conference* 1991;376–378.

39. Fornataro-Clerici L, Zajac DJ. Aerodynamic characteristics of tracheostomy speaking valves. *J Speech Hear Res* 1993;36:529–532.

40. Manzano JL, Lubillo S, Henriquez D, et al. Verbal communication of ventilator-dependent patients. *Critical Care Med* 1993;21:512–517.

41. Lichtman SW, Birnbaum IL, Sanfilippo MR, et al. Effect of a tracheostomy speaking valve on secretions, arterial oxygenation, and olfaction: a quantitative evaluation. *J Speech Hear Res* 1995;38:549–555.

42. Wee M. A speaking adaptor for a tracheostomy tube. *Br J Anaesthesia* 1988;61:516.

43. Lynch CQ, Tippett DC, French JJ, et al. Tracheostomy and upper extremity paresis: restoration of oral communication. *ASHA* 1990;32:181.

44. Siebens AA, Tippett DC, Kirby N, et al. Dysphagia and expiratory air flow. *Dysphagia* 1993;8:266–269.

45. Walsh JJ, Rho DS. A speaking endotracheal tube. *Anesthesiology* 1985;63:703–705.

46. Sparker AW, Robbins KT, Nevlud GN, et al. A prospective evaluation of speaking tracheostomy tubes for ventilator dependent patients. *Laryngoscope* 1987;97:89–92.

47. Safar P, Grenvik A. Speaking cuffed tracheostomy tube. *Critical Care Med* 1975;3:23–26.

48. Whitlock RML. A means of speaking for patients with cuffed tracheostomy tubes. *Br Med J* 1967;3:547.

49. Gordan V. Effectiveness of speaking-cuffed tracheostomy tube in patients with neuromuscular diseases. *Critical Care Med* 1984;12:615–616.

50. Kluin KJ, Maynard F, Bogdasarian RS. The patient requiring mechanical ventilatory support: use of the cuffed tracheostomy "talk" tube to establish phonation. *Otolaryngol-Head Neck Surg* 1984;92:625–627.

51. Leder SB, Astrachan DI. Stomal complications and airflow line problems in the Communi-Trach I cuffed talking tracheotomy tube. *Laryngoscope* 1989;99:194–196.

52. Heffner JE, Miller KS, Sahn SA. Tracheostomy in the intensive care unit Part I: indications, technique, management. *Chest* 1986;90:269–274.

53. Leder SB, Traquina DN. Voice intensity of patients using a Communi-Trach I cuffed speaking tracheostomy tube. *Laryngoscope* 1989;99:744–747.

54. Shinnick JP, Freedman AP. Acetylcysteine and speaking tracheostomy tubes. *JAMA* 1981;246:1771.

55. Levine SP, Koester DJ, Kett RL. Independently activated talking tracheostomy systems for quadriplegic patients. *Arch Phys Med Rehabil* 1987;68:571–573.

56. Leder SB. Verbal communication for the ventilator-dependent patient: voice intensity with the Portex "talk" tracheostomy tube. *Laryngoscope* 1990;100:1116–1121.

57. Editorial. Speech with a cuffed tracheostomy tube. *Lancet* 1987;2:432.

58. Blom ED. Alternative methods of communication for intubated patients in critical care. *Indiana Med* 1988;81:398–400.

59. Auchingloss JH, Gilbert R. Mechanical aid to ventilation in the home: use of volume-limited ventilator and leaking connections. *Am Rev Respir Dis* 1973;108:373–375.

60. Lehner WE, Ballard IM, Figueroa WG, et al. Home care utilizing a ventilator in a patient with amyotrophic lateral sclerosis. *J Family Pract* 1980;10:39–42.

61. Make B, Gilmartin M, Brody JS, et al. Rehabilitation of ventilator-dependent subjects with lung diseases: the concept and initial experience. *Chest* 1984;86:358–365.

62. Bach JR, Alba AS. Tracheostomy ventilation: a study of efficacy with deflated cuffs and cuffless tubes. *Chest* 1990;97:679–683.

63. Tippett DC, Siebens AA. Using ventilators for speaking and swallowing. *Dysphagia* 1991;6:94–99.

64. Duggan M, Dory AE. Speech for the ventilator dependent patient. Poster session presented at the Annual Convention of the American Association of Spinal Cord Injury Nurses, Las Vegas, NV, 1990, September.

65. Kinnear WJM, Shneerson JM. Assisted ventilation at home: is it worth considering? *Br J Dis Chest* 1985;79:313–351.

66. O'Donohue WJ, Giovannoni RM, Goldberg AI, et al. Long-term mechanical ventilation: guidelines for management in the home and at alternate community sites. *Chest* 1970;90:1S–37S.

67. Tippett DC, Siebens AA. Preserving oral communication in individuals with tracheostomy and ventilator dependency. *Am J Speech-Language Pathol* 1995;4:55–61.

68. Hoit JD, Shea SA, Banzett RB. Speech production during mechanical ventilation in tracheostomized individuals. *J Speech Hear Res* 1994;37:53–63.

69. Hoit JD, Banzett RB. Simple adjustments can improve ventilator-supported speech. *Am J Speech-Language Pathol* 1997;6:87–96.

70. Splaingard ML, Frates RC, Harrison GM, et al. Home positive-pressure ventilation: twenty years' experience. *Chest* 1983;84:376–382.

71. Glover DW. Three years at home on an MA-1. *Resp Ther* 1981;11:69–70.

72. Prentice W, Baydur A, Passy V. Passy-Muir tracheostomy speaking valve on ventilator dependent patients. *Am Rev Respir Dis* 1989;139:A541.

73. Dikeman KJ, Kazandjian MS. *Communication and swallowing management of tracheostomized and ventilator-dependent adults.* San Diego: Singular Publishing Group, Inc., 1995.

74. Weller J, Siebens A, Marshall T, et al. The effect of position on cross sectional area of pharynx. *Proceedings of the Fifth International Conference on Pulmonary Rehabilitation and Home Ventilation* 1995;106.

75. Birdsell M. Personal communication. Baltimore, Maryland: Good Samaritan Hospital, 1992.

76. Wenger NK, Mattson ME, Furberg CD, et al. Assessment of quality of life in clinical trials of cardiovascular therapies. *Am J Cardiol* 1984;54:908–913.

77. Campbell A, Converse PE, Rodgers WL. *The quality of American life: perceptions, evaluations and satisfaction.* New York: Russell Sage Foundation, 1976:37–113.

78. Hunt SM, McKenna SP, McEwen J, et al. A quantitative approach to perceived health status: a validation study. *J Epidemiol Commun Health* 1980;34:281–286.

79. Bergner M, Bobbitt RA, Carter WB, et al. The Sickness Impact Profile: development and final revision of a health status measure. *Med Care* 1981;19:787–805.

80. Spitzer WO, Dobson AJ, Hall J, et al. A concise Q-L Index for use by physicians. *Journal of Chronic Disease* 1981;34:585–597.

81. Bach JR, Campagnolo DI. Psychosocial adjustment of post-poliomyelitis ventilator assisted individuals. *Arch Phys Med Rehabil* 1992;73:934–939.

82. Bach JR, Campagnolo DI, Hoeman S. Life satisfaction of individuals with Duchenne muscular dystrophy using long-term mechanical ventilatory support. *Am J Phys Med Rehabil* 1991; 70:129–135.

83. Alexander MA, Johnson EW, Petty J, et al. Mechanical ventilation of patients with late stage Duchenne muscular dystrophy: management in the home. *Arch Phys Med Rehabil* 1979;60:289–292.

84. Gilgoff IS. End-stage Duchenne patients: choosing between respirator and natural death. In: Charash LI, Wolf SG, Kutscher AH, Lovelace RE, Hale MS, eds. *Psychosocial aspects of muscular dystrophy and allied diseases: commitment to life, health and function.* Springfield, Illinois: CC Thomas, 1983:301–307.

85. Miller JR, Colbert AP, Osberg JS. Ventilator dependency: decision-making, daily functioning and quality of life for patients with Duchenne muscular dystrophy. *Dev Med Child Neurol* 1990;32:1078–1086.

86. Snyder RD, Goldberg NM. Use of ventilation support in the terminal care of Duchenne muscular dystrophy. In: Charash LI, Wolf SG, Kutscher AH, Lovelace RE, Hale MS, eds. *Psychosocial aspects of muscular dystrophy and allied diseases: commitment to life, health and function.* Springfield, Illinois, CC Thomas, 1983:41–44.

87. Bach JR. Ventilator use by muscular dystrophy association patients. *Arch Phys Med Rehabil* 1992;73:179–183.

88. Bach JR. Amyotrophic lateral sclerosis: communication status and survival with ventilatory support. *Am J Phys Med Rehabil* 1993;72:343–349.

89. Bach JR. A comparison of long-term ventilatory support alternatives from the perspective of the patient and care giver. *Chest* 1993;104:1702–1706.

90. Bach JR, Alba AS, Saporito LR. Intermittent positive pressure ventilation via the mouth as an alternative to tracheostomy for 257 ventilator users. *Chest* 1993;103:174–182.

91. Maynard FM, Muth AS. The choice to end life as a ventilator-dependent quadriplegic. *Arch Phys Med Rehabil* 1987;68:862–864.

92. Silverstein MD, Stocking CB, Antel JP, et al. Amyotrophic lateral sclerosis and life-sustaining therapy: patients' desires for information, participation in decision making and life-sustaining therapy. *Mayo Clinic Proceedings* 1991;66:906–913.

93. Wang TG, Bach JR, Avilla C, et al. Survival of individuals with spinal muscular atrophy on ventilatory support. *Am J Phys Med Rehabil* 1994;73:207–211.

94. Tippett DC, Sugarman J. Discussing advance directives under the Patient Self-Determination Act: a unique opportunity for speech-language pathologists to help persons with aphasia. *Am J Speech-Language Pathol* 1996;5:31–34.

6

Swallowing, Tracheostomy, and Ventilator Dependency

DONNA C. TIPPETT

Evaluation and treatment of swallowing disorders are relatively recent additions to the speech–language pathologist's scope of practice (1,2). Despite the recent advent of this role, the management of swallowing disorders now comprises a large component of speech–language pathologists' daily clinical activity in many settings, particularly in acute care hospitals. In addition to being "high volume," management of swallowing disorders can represent "high risk" clinical activity. The consequences of dysphagia, particularly aspiration or laryngeal penetration of foodway contents, can be benign or lethal. A primary concern is that aspiration or laryngeal penetration will result in aspiration pneumonia; however, a clear cause and effect relationship has not been established.

The consequences of airway penetration by foodway contents depend on many factors (e.g., chronicity of aspiration, volume of solid or liquid aspirated, pH of aspirate) (3,4). Furthermore, there are anecdotal cases of patients who eat and drink without manifesting ill health effects, despite exhibiting gross aspiration on videofluoroscopy. Recently, Langmore and colleagues (5) found that while dysphagia and aspiration are important risks for aspiration pneumonia, they are insufficient to cause pneumonia unless other factors are present. Predictive risk factors for pneumonia included dependency for feeding, dependency for oral care, number of decayed teeth, tube feeding, more than one medical diagnosis, number of medications, and smoking. This murky and multifactorial relationship between dysphagia, aspiration, and aspiration pneumonia is challenging when evaluating swallowing disorders in individuals with tracheostomy and/or ventilator dependency. These individuals are among the most ill and medically com-

Tracheostomy and Ventilator Dependency: Management of Breathing, Speaking, and Swallowing. Edited by Donna C. Tippett, MPH, MA, CCC-SLP. Thieme Medical Publishers, Inc. New York © 2000.

plex patients encountered by speech–language pathologists, and are known to aspirate.

Aspiration is common in individuals with tracheostomy. Cameron and colleagues (6) demonstrated evidence of aspiration in 42 of 61 (69%) individuals with tracheostomy. Bone and colleagues (7) studied three groups of individuals with tracheostomy. Aspiration occurred in 13 of 15 (87%) individuals with either uncuffed metal tracheostomy tubes or low-volume, high-pressure cuffed tubes with cuffs deflated, two of 12 (17%) individuals with high-volume, low-pressure cuffed tubes, and two of 13 (15%) individuals with sponge-filled cuffed tubes. Although incidence of aspiration was decreased when cuffs were inflated, this practice is neither inviolate nor inocuous. Secretions and liquefied food boluses can leak past the inflated cuff into the trachea. Cuff inflation precludes phonation, may compromise the integrity of the trachea, and can contribute to swallowing problems.

Restoration of "safe" oral alimentation/hydration (i.e., without significant laryngeal penetration or aspiration) (8,9) is a realistic and important goal for many individuals with tracheostomy and/or ventilator dependency. The ability to eat and drink is known to affect perceptions of quality of life among cancer patients (10,11), and is likely to influence perceptions of quality of life similarly in individuals with tracheostomy and/or ventilator dependency, especially if function in other areas is restricted as in ventilator-dependent quadriplegia. Safe oral alimentation/hydration in the tracheostomy population can be facilitated by cuff deflation, valving of the cannula, and the use of ventilator support during meals.

This chapter covers normal anatomy and physiology relevant to swallowing, the effects of tracheostomy on swallowing, bedside and radiographic swallowing evaluation, and techniques specific to individuals with tracheostomy and/or ventilator dependency. An algorithm for the evaluation of swallowing in the tracheostomy population is reviewed. Case studies are presented to illustrate chapter principles.

Normal Anatomy and Physiology

In order to understand dysphagia, it is necessary to review the process of normal swallowing (12–14). The process of swallowing is very intricate, requiring the integrated function of more than 50 muscles, at least six nerves, multiple brain stem nuclei, the hypothalamus, thalamus, and cerebral cortex. In addition, swallowing must be coordinated carefully with other functions (i.e., respiration and phonation). Swallowing serves two functions—intermittent alimentation and continuous airway protection. The latter is accomplished by repeated clearing of the pharyngeal airway to allow safe breathing.

The process of moving food from the lips to the stomach basically involves a transport mechanism (i.e., muscles), a monitoring system (i.e., afferent nerves), and an integrative command center (i.e., brain stem and cerebrum). The passageway is continuous as is the process of swallowing. However, the action usually is separated into three stages that vary in several important ways.

The oral stage involves preparing food for transport. Food is contained in the mouth by jaw closure and lip seal as well as apposition of the soft palate to the posterior portion of the tongue. The preparation is accomplished by decreasing particle size (mastication) and adding saliva to the food to form a bolus on the dorsum of the tongue. The tongue tip is placed against the area just posterior to the maxillary incisors (alveolar ridge) to seal the mouth just before the food bolus is propelled posteriorly to the pharynx by an anterior to posterior elevation of the tongue. All components of this stage are under voluntary control.

The pharyngeal stage involves maneuvering the food bolus downward, successfully past two other openings (nasopharynx and larynx) and into the esophagus. Retrograde flow is prevented by sealing of the two openings noted above. The nasopharynx is protected by elevation of the soft palate and contraction of the posterior and lateral nasopharyngeal walls. The larynx is sealed by a complex set of redundant actions to assure airway protection. As the food bolus fills the vallecular space, the epiglottis begins to tilt downward covering the laryngeal opening. The hyoid and larynx move forward and upward closing the laryngeal vestibule and pushing the epiglottis against the base of the tongue to close the laryngeal opening. The intrinsic muscles of the larynx contract causing it to close tightly, and respiration momentarily ceases. If food is misdirected into the larynx, a reflexive cough is elicited to clear the airway. In addition, the process of closing the larynx described above occurs in such a way as to sweep laryngeal residue toward the hypopharynx. Propulsion of the food bolus is accomplished by tongue motion and pharyngeal constriction. The tongue pushes posteriorly and downward and the pharyngeal muscles constrict sequentially producing a stripping action that propels the bolus toward the esophagus. The pharyngoesophageal sphincter is closed between swallows by the twin action of cricopharyngeus muscle contraction and soft tissue compression by the resting position of the hypopharynx. During swallowing the cricopharyngeus muscle relaxes, and the anterior laryngeal movement pulls the soft tissue (anterior pharyngeal wall) forward, opening the pharyngoesophageal sphincter and allowing passage of the bolus into the esophagus. The sphincter then returns to its usual closed position and the other structures involved return to their resting positions to be used for respiration, phonation, or another swallow. This complex stage is largely involuntary and is initiated when a bolus is sensed in the oropharynx.

The esophageal stage involves the movement of the bolus through the esophagus and into the stomach. Peristaltic action, that is, sequential contraction of the superior to inferior musculature, moves the bolus through the esophagus. Gravity assists this process when performed in the upright position. Finally, the esophagogastric junction opens and allows the bolus to enter the stomach, thus completing this totally involuntary stage (Fig. 6–1) (15).

The central nervous system control of swallowing involves sensory information from the trigeminal, facial, glossopharyngeal, and vagus nerves. This information is processed initially in brain stem sensory nuclei and, later, in ill-defined pattern generators (swallowing center) closely associated with the solitary nucleus and tract in the medulla. The sensory information is also processed in the thalamus and transmitted to the cortex. Higher cortical influence of swallowing may then be exerted in varying amounts (greatest for oral stage). The pattern generators project to discrete motor neurons in the brain stem nuclei of the trigeminal, facial, glossopharyngeal, vagus, spinal accessory, and hypoglossal nerves. The in-

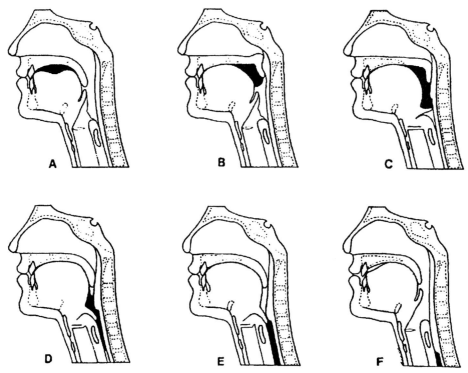

Fig. 6–1. Schematic of normal swallowing. **(A)** Bolus is confined in the oral cavity with tongue and soft palate in close approximation. **(B)** Bolus has passed into the oropharynx. The soft palate has apposed Passavant's cushion in the constrictor wall and thus closes the palatopharyngeal isthmus, preventing regurgitation into the nasopharynx. **(C)** Bolus is contained in oropharynx. The larynx has elevated and closed and the epiglottis is in a horizontal position. **(D)** Bolus has entered the oro- and hypopharynx and adjacent esophagus. The epiglottis is tilted downward and the peristaltic wave is in the midpharynx. **(E)** Bolus has passed through the pharyngoesophageal segment into the esophagus. The larynx is still closed. **(F)** Bolus is disappearing into the upper esophagus. The laryngeal airway has reopened and the epiglottic is upright. All structures have returned to the resting position. Reprinted, with permission, from Donner, Bosma, and Robertson (15).

dividual nerves transmit these intricate directions to the many muscles involved in swallowing.

Effect of Tracheostomy on Swallowing

Tracheostomy alters normal swallow function. It is well recognized that a tracheostomy cannula with an inflated cuff has adverse implications for upper airway clearance, laryngeal protection against aspiration of foodway contents, and laryngeal displacement.

Although the tracheostomy tube provides access for suctioning to clear the upper airway, this advantage is offset by the impairment of cough when the cuff is inflated. The airway protection function of the inflated cuff is imperfect as well. The presence of an inflated cuff is commonly cited as a mechanical barrier against aspiration (7,16,17). However, despite the relatively more effective barrier formed by high-volume, low-pressure cuffs as compared to small-volume, high-pressure cuffs, seepage of foodway products remains likely (6,18).

In addition to inadequate prevention against aspiration, an inflated cuff may even contribute to aspiration. "Silent penetration" (i.e., penetration of saliva or food below the level of the true vocal folds without cough or any other symptom indicating that foodway products are entering the airway) (8,9) may be enhanced by desensitization of the larynx secondary to diversion of airflow through the tracheostomy (19). Buckwalter and Sasaki (20) demonstrated that chronic upper airway bypass can lead to an uncoordinated laryngeal closure response in dogs which may allow aspiration to occur. Furthermore, according to Betts (18) and Weber (21), an inflated cuff can bulge posteriorly and compress the esophagus. Under this circumstance, foodway products may fill the proximal esophagus, overflow into the trachea to rest above the cuff, and eventually be aspirated when the cuff is deflated. Data from manometric studies in dogs indicate that the cuff compresses the esophagus. Leverment, Pearson, and Rae (22) measured intraluminal esophageal pressures in 24 dogs after tracheostomy and intubation with either uncuffed or cuffed tubes. Increased intraluminal pressures were found in the esophagus at the level of the cuff and 5 to 10 cm below the pharyngo-esophageal junction. The upper esophageal sphincter was observed to relax incompletely.

Finally, the tracheostomy tube can partially immobilize laryngeal elevation and anterior movement during swallowing (19,23,24). One may hypothesize that this tethering effect is exacerbated when the cuff is inflated.

Morbidities associated with cuff inflation are several. Secretions pool above the cuff in the proximal trachea and larynx (25). The integrity of the trachea may be lost if cuff pressure and duration of inflation interfere with blood flow to the tracheal cartilages sufficient to cause necrosis and softening (tracheomalacia). The tracheal lumen may be narrowed by granulation tissue and scarring that follows damage to the wall. A communication between tracheal and esophageal lumens (tracheoesophageal fistula) may occur, a circumstance under which either food may enter the airway and/or air may enter the foodway (26).

Evaluation of swallowing is often warranted given the multiplicity and complexity of these effects of tracheostomy. Several factors must be considered when planning and conducting a swallowing evaluation with individuals who have tracheostomy and/or ventilator dependency.

Candidacy for Evaluation and Preevaluation Considerations

The readiness of an individual with tracheostomy and/or ventilator dependency for a swallowing evaluation is determined by the patient's medical diagnosis, pulmonary and gastrointestinal issues, cognitive/language status, physical limitations, and psychosocial factors. The medical diagnosis of the individual can be obtained through review of medical records, discussion with physicians, nurses and other professional staff, and an interview with the patient, family members, and caregivers. Evaluation and treatment of swallowing may be influenced by the nature of the underlying etiology associated with tracheostomy and/or ventilator dependency. For example, use of compensations, consideration of alternatives to oral alimentation/hydration, plans for follow-up videofluoroscopic swallowing studies, and prognosis may hinge upon whether the underlying etiology is a progressive, deteriorating disease (e.g., amyotrophic lateral sclerosis) or a stable injury (e.g., spinal cord injury). Medical stability affects the timing of the swallow study. It may be appropriate to delay evaluation of swallowing until an individual is medically stable.

Information should be obtained about the individual's respiratory status, including cuff deflation trials, cannula plugging and valving trials, weaning trials, ventilator free time, ability to breathe independently, suctioning frequency, and episodes of aspiration pneumonia. It is desirable for patients to be tolerating cuff deflation and communicating orally prior to evaluation of swallowing, rather than introduce cuff deflation at the time of the swallowing evaluation. Cuff deflation allows patients the opportunity to cough, use throat clearing, and experience airflow through the larynx. Ability to speak and clear the upper airway are favorable prognostic factors for restoration of safe swallowing. Exceptions to the initiation of cuff deflation prior to evaluation of swallowing are appropriate in certain circumstances. For example, it may be acceptable to evaluate swallowing in individuals who are not expected to tolerate cuff deflation and who desire oral alimentation/hydration for pleasure (nonnutritive) purposes.

Consideration should be given to any gastrointestinal issues that may present contraindications to oral alimentation/hydration (e.g., gastritis, gastroesophageal reflux, gastrointestinal bleed, need for NPO status for pending surgery). Current means of alimentation and hydration (e.g., nasogastric feeding tube, gastrostomy feeding tube, oral alimentation/hydration) should be noted. If the individual is orally alimented/hydrated, the type of diet (i.e., bolus consistency modifications or restrictions) should be documented, and observations regarding swallow function should be solicited from the individual, family members, and/or caregivers.

Cognitive/language status must be considered as this affects the individual's ability to participate in the examination, understand the implications of the swallowing evaluation, and follow through with recommendations in subsequent treatment sessions and in all eating situations. Individuals who cannot understand commands, such as "tuck your chin and then swallow" and remember bolus restrictions and compensations must be approached differently from those who do not have cognitive/language impairments (27). Involvement of family members and caregivers is important in the management of swallowing disorders for all patients and is vital for those who will need supervision to achieve carryover of recommendations for safe swallowing.

The individual's physical limitations need to be considered in the context of feeding procedures. Collaboration with physical and occupational therapists is essential for achieving optimal positioning and using specialized devices to compensate for physical deficits.

Psychosocial factors, such as discharge disposition, family support, and depression, can influence the timing of the evaluation and recommendations regarding supervision, diet modifications, and use of nutrition supplements. For example, an individual with ventilator-dependent quadriplegia and depression may not be ready to meet nutritional needs solely via oral alimentation/hydration. Continued use of a nasogastric feeding tube or gastrostomy feeding tube may be indicated while the patient adjusts to his or her disability and until he or she demonstrates adequate oral nutrition intake as measured by calorie counts.

In general, candidacy for swallowing evaluation is optimal when the individual is medically stable and alert, has adequate cognitive/language abilities to participate in the evaluation, tolerates cuff deflation, and has had experiences producing speech via cuff deflation.

Evaluation of swallowing by speech–language pathologists is initiated by physician referral. Specifics of the evaluation should be discussed and approved by the patient's physician, particularly cuff deflation, changes to ventilator settings, and bolus trials at the bedside. Consensus is essential regarding all of the specific components of the swallowing evaluation as these may affect the individual's respiratory status. The patient's physician, nurse, and respiratory therapist should be present for the evaluation as appropriate to perform duties, such as suctioning and making ventilator setting changes.

At times, speech–language pathologists may find that a swallowing evaluation, cuff deflation and/or trials of boluses at the bedside are not appropriate for an individual, even when a referral has been received to proceed with an evaluation. Speech–language pathologists must exercise professional judgment regarding the appropriateness of their clinical interventions. Individuals with tracheostomy and/or ventilator dependency are susceptible to changes in medical status, especially during the acute stages of hospitalization that may dictate changes in planned interventions. In these circumstances, evaluation may be deferred and/or consultations or involvement of other professional staff may be recommended. Recommendations should be documented in the patient's medical record (1,2,28).

Bedside Evaluation

As with other populations, evaluation of swallow begins with clinical or bedside assessment in individuals with tracheostomy and/or ventilator dependency. The conventional bedside examination includes an interview of the patient and/or caregivers, examination of speech/swallow components, and observation of what happens when the patient is fed. Usually, the interview begins with questions regarding present complaint—duration of the problems, frequency of swallowing difficulty, factors that exacerbate or alleviate the problem, changes in oral motor function or speech quality, and weight loss. Figure 6–2 includes questions asked by speech–language pathologists when evaluating individuals admitted to the Johns Hopkins rehabilitation unit, Good Samaritan Hospital, Baltimore, Maryland. Some specific questions for individuals with tracheostomy and/or ventilator dependency are the ability to tolerate cuff deflation, comfort level with valving or plugging the cannula, progress with weaning trials, and comparison of current speech quality with premorbid function.

The speech–language pathologist should include an assessment of cognitive and language abilities (e.g., attention, memory, orientation, comprehension, ex-

Fig. 6–2. Sample speech/swallow interview questions.

1. Patient's or informant's description of the speech/swallow problem.
2. Describe duration/course of problem.
3. Describe present status compared to onset.
4. Does speech/voice sound different since illness?
5. Describe changes in what tongue, lips, jaw can/cannot do now.
6. How well is speech understood by others?
7. Does voice sound different after eating?
8. Have you experienced choking when eating? How often? On what foods?
9. Have you experienced coughing when swallowing? How often? On what foods? On own secretions?
10. Do you feel foods "catch in throat"?
11. Do you have difficulty moving food around in your mouth?
12. Do you have difficulty keeping foods in your mouth?
13. Is drooling present? Describe situations.
14. Rate the easiest to hardest foods to swallow.
15. How long does it take to eat?
16. What is your current feeding mode?
17. Has anyone ever told you that you have aspiration pneumonia? If yes, when?

pression) either through formal testing or informal observations during the bedside swallowing evaluation. A judgment is made regarding an individual's ability to participate in swallowing trials at the bedside or a videofluoroscopic swallowing study, and need for supervision with treatment, including the use of a bolus-modified or restricted diet, postural strategies, and respiratory and laryngeal maneuvers.

There are a variety of approaches to examine speech/swallow components, such as the Assessment of Intelligibility of Dysarthric Speech (29), the Frenchay Dysarthria Assessment (30), the Dysarthria Examination Battery (31), and the Dysarthria/Dysphagia Battery (DDB). The DDB is based on the functional component model described by Netsell and Daniel in the late 1970s (32,33) and originated from the clinical examination described by Linden and Shaughnessy in 1985 (34).

In Linden and Shaughnessy's clinical examination (34), the functional components of the respiratory mechanism (i.e., abdominal muscles, the diaphragm, rib cage), larynx, tongue/pharynx, posterior tongue, anterior tongue, velum/pharynx, jaw and lips are assessed. Linden and Shaughnessy (34) outlined the roles of each of these components in the processes of speaking and swallowing (Table 6–1).

Each component is assessed with a variety of nonspeech and speech tests. Assessment items are required and optional. Nonspeech tests of the respiratory mechanism include posture, breath sounds, and breathing effort at rest. Speech tests of the respiratory mechanism are maximum phonation time and habitual loudness. For individuals with tracheostomy and/or mechanical ventilation, notations are made regarding the use of mechanical ventilation, ventilator settings, cannula type and size, cannula accessories, and cuff status. Nonspeech laryngeal items are laryngeal elevation with swallowing, ability to cough, or ability to clear the throat. Perceptual characteristics of phonation are described. Gag and sensa-

Table 6–1. Roles of functional components in speaking and swallowing.

Component	Roles in speaking	Roles in swallowing
Respiratory mechanism	Supplies adequate subglottic air pressure to the vocal folds	Cessation of respiration is timed with initiation of swallow
Laryngeal mechanism	Vibrates to produce and control phonation	Vocal folds close and larynx rises to protect airway
Velum/pharynx	Responsible for resonance	Separates oral and nasal cavities and prevents nasal regurgitation
Tongue	Shapes airstream	Transports boluses from the oral cavity into the pharynx and clears the mouth
Lips	Shapes airstream	Seals boluses in mouth
Jaw	Assists in tongue carriage and shaping of oral cavity	Mastication of boluses

tion to light touch are assessed for the velopharynx. Resonance quality and velopharyngeal movement during phonation are the speech items for this component. Lingual, labial, and mandibular range of motion, strength against resistance, and sensation to light touch form the nonspeech assessment of these structures. Lingual and labial articulation are also assessed (Fig. 6–3) (33). The characteristics of speech production are described, and overall speech intelligibility is rated. The speech–language pathologist also notes any signs that indicate dysphagia. For example, abnormalities pertaining to laryngeal function (e.g., wet-hoarse phonation, reduced laryngeal elevation, abnormal voluntary cough) are associated with subglottic laryngeal penetration (Fig. 6–4) (33).

Remarkable speech and nonspeech findings, and the anticipated effects on swallowing, are recorded for each speech/swallow component. This organization assists in predicting the nature of a swallowing problem, developing a plan for a videofluoroscopic swallowing study, and preparing a preliminary treatment plan. An example regarding clinical findings for the laryngeal component, anticipated swallowing deficits, and a plan for the videofluoroscopic swallowing study is described in Figure 6–4 (35).

In addition to the examination of speech/swallow components, oral intake at the bedside may be observed. Observations of eating can give information regarding oral stage functioning, general feeding behavior, and time required to complete a meal. Bedside trials are usually performed by presenting specific bolus consistencies (e.g., puree, thick liquid, thin liquid, mechanical soft, particulate, multitextured) or by observing a meal if the patient is receiving oral alimentation/hydration. Characteristics associated with dysphagia include drooling, pocketing of food in buccal spaces, slow rate of intake, multiple swallows per mouthful, coughing during or after swallowing, wet-hoarse voice quality associated with swallowing, and/or sensation of boluses being retained in the throat (34). In individuals with tracheostomy, oral intake at the bedside may be assessed by performing a modified Evans blue dye test.

Fig. 6–3.   Dysarthria/dysphagia battery.

Patient Name (Last, First): _____

Date:_____ Tester: _____ Birth Date: _____

Sex: M F   Race: Asian Black Caucasian Other/Unknown

Type: Inpatient Outpatient   Date of Onset _____

Required Test Items

I. Assessment of respiration
  A. Required nonspeech items
    1. Posture during test
1 ☐   1 = sitting upright (≥ 80°)
      2 = reclining (30–79°)
      3 = lying (0–29°)
    2. Head externally supported during test
2 ☐   1 = no
      2 = yes
    3. Breathing effort at rest
3 ☐   1 = unlabored
      2 = labored
    4. Breathing sounds at rest
4 ☐   1 = quiet
      2 = noisy inhalation only
      3 = noisy exhalation only
      4 = noisy inhalation and noisy exhalation
    5. Mechanical ventilation during test
5 ☐   1 = no
      2 = yes
    6. Tracheostomy at time of test
6 ☐   1 = none
      2 = yes, cannula without cuff
      3 = yes, cuff inflated
      4 = yes, cuff deflated
      5 = open stoma
      6 = other
  B. Required speech items
7 ___ 1. Maximum duration of /a/ in sec
      (Enter 0 for cannot test)
    2. Respiratory support for speech
8 ☐   1 = normal
      2 = impaired
      3 = cannot test
    3. Habitual loudness
9 ☐   1 = normal
      2 = loud
      3 = soft
      4 = cannot test
    4. Inhale/exhale at appropriate linguistic
      junctures
10 ☐   1 = yes
      2 = no
      3 = cannot test

Optional Test Items

I. Assessment of respiration
  A. Optional nonspeech items
    1. Ability to take deep breath on command
      _____ yes
      _____ no
      _____ cannot test
    2. Ability to hold a deep breath
      _____ yes
      _____ no
      _____ cannot test
    3. Ability to displace 5 cm water for 5 sec or better
      _____ yes
      _____ no
      _____ cannot test
    4. Mechanical ventilator
      Comments: _____
      _____
      _____
    5. Cannula accessories at time of test
☐   1 = no cannula
      2 = plug
      3 = unidirectional speaking valve (French)
      4 = other
    6. Other cannula characteristics
☐   1 = none or no cannula
      2 = fenestrated with inner cannula
      3 = fenestrated without inner cannula
      4 = speaking "trach" tube
      5 = other
    7. Trach cannula material
☐   1 = no cannula
      2 = plastic cannula
      3 = metal cannula
    8. Tracheostomy cannula size
      _____ Enter size of cannula in mm
    9. Tracheostomy
      Comments: _____
      _____
      _____
  10. Other
      Comments: _____
      _____
      _____
  B. Optional speech items
    _____ 1. Maximum duration of /s/ in sec
      (Enter 0 for cannot test)
    _____ 2. Mean number of syllables/minute
      (Enter 0 for cannot test)
    _____ 3. Mean number of breaths/minute
      (Enter 0 for cannot test)
    4. Loudness range
      _____ Adequate _____ Unable to speak softly
      _____ Unable to speak loudly _____ Cannot test
    5. Comments: _____
      _____
      _____

Fig. 6–3. (*continued*)

Required Test Items	Optional Test Items

Required Test Items

II. Assessment of larynx
  A. Required nonspeech items
    1. Elevation during swallowing
      1 = normal
11 ☐   2 = abnormal
      3 = absent
      4 = cannot test
    2. Spontaneous cough
      a. Frequency
        1 = normal or none
12 ☐   2 = increased
        3 = unable to assess
      b. Quality
        1 = no spontaneous cough or cannot test
13 ☐   2 = dry
        3 = wet
      c. Strength
        1 = no spontaneous cough or cannot test
14 ☐   2 = strong or normal
        3 = weak
    3. Volitional cough
      a. Ability to perform
        1 = able
15 ☐   2 = unable
      b. Quality
        1 = dry
16 ☐   2 = wet
        3 = cannot test
      c. Strength
        1 = strong or normal
17 ☐   2 = weak
        3 = cannot test
  B. Required speech items
    1. Voiced/voiceless contrasts
      1 = normal
18 ☐   2 = some breakdown
      3 = never achieved
      4 = cannot test
    2. Phonatory quality
      a. Phonation
        1 = normal phonation
19 ☐   2 = dysphonic
        3 = aphonic
        4 = cannot test
      b. Has harsh phonation
        1 = no
20 ☐   2 = yes
        3 = cannot test
      c. Has breathy phonation
        1 = no
21 ☐   2 = yes
        3 = cannot test
      d. Has wet phonation
        1 = no
22 ☐   2 = yes
        3 = cannot test
    3. Habitual pitch
      1 = normal
23 ☐   2 = high
      3 = low
      4 = cannot test
    4. Overall severity of dysphonia
      1 = no dysphonia
24 ☐   2 = mild
      3 = moderate
      4 = severe
      5 = aphonic
      6 = cannot test

Optional Test Items

II. Assessment of larynx
  A. Optional nonspeech items
    1. Ability to clear throat on command
      _____ yes
      _____ no
    2. Strength of throat clearing
      _____ normal or strong
      _____ weak
      _____ cannot test
    3. Ability to perform consecutive maneuvers
      (circle one)
      Swallow/exhale   Yes; No; Cannot test
      Clear throat/swallow Yes; No; Cannot test
      Consecutive swallows Yes; No; Cannot test
      Flex neck/swallow   Yes; No; Cannot test
      Other_____   Yes; No; Cannot test
    4. Comments: _____
    _____
    _____
    5. Secretion management (drooling, spitting, etc.)
    _____
    _____
    _____

  B. Optional speech items
    1. Rapid alternating movement: /ha-ha-ha/
      (Check all that apply)
      _____ normal
      _____ voiced/voiceless contrast breakdown
      _____ reduced rate
      _____ cannot test
    2. _____/s/ to /z/ ratio
    3. Pitch range (Check all that apply)
      _____ adequate
      _____ reduced at high end of range
      _____ reduced at low end of range
      _____ cannot test
    4. Clears throat spontaneously when voice is wet
      1 = voice not wet or cannot test
☐   2 = yes
      3 = no
    5. Comments: _____
    _____
    _____

Fig. 6–3. *(continued)*

Required Test Items	Optional Test Items

Required Test Items

III. Assessment of velum and pharynx
  A. Required nonspeech items
    1. Rest position of velum/uvula

25 ☐
  1 = normal
  2 = deviated to right
  3 = deviated to left
  4 = bilateral abnormality
  5 = cannot test

    2. Palatal gag
      a. When stimulated on right

26 ☐
  1 = normal
  2 = diminished
  3 = absent
  4 = cannot test

      b. When stimulated on left

27 ☐
  1 = normal
  2 = diminished
  3 = absent
  4 = cannot test

    3. Pharyngeal gag
      a. When stimulated on right

28 ☐
  1 = normal
  2 = diminished
  3 = absent
  4 = cannot test

      b. When stimulated on left

29 ☐
  1 = normal
  2 = diminished
  3 = absent
  4 = cannot test

    4. Sensation to touch of velum

30 ☐
  1 = present on right and left
  2 = present on right only
  3 = present on left only
  4 = absent on right and left
  5 = cannot test

    5. Sensation to touch of pharynx

31 ☐
  1 = present on right and left
  2 = present on right only
  3 = present on left only
  4 = absent on right and left
  5 = cannot test

    6. Swallowing of secretions

32 ☐
  1 = all
  2 = some
  3 = none

  B. Required speech items
    1. Movement on phonation of /a-a-a-a/
      a. Range

33 ☐
  1 = normal
  2 = reduced
  3 = cannot test

      b. Symmetry on phonation

34 ☐
  1 = normal
  2 = asymmetric
  3 = cannot test

    2. Resonance

35 ☐
  1 = normal
  2 = hyponasal
  3 = hypernasal
  4 = cannot test

    3. Oral-nasal articulation

36 ☐
  1 = normal
  2 = impaired
  3 = cannot test

Optional Test Items

III. Assessment of velum and pharynx
  A. Optional nonspeech items
    1. Velar and pharyngeal motion during gag:

_____
_____
_____

    2. Comments: _____
_____

  B. Optional speech items:
    Comments: _____
_____
_____

Fig. 6–3. *(continued)*

| **Required Test Items** | **Optional Test Items** |

Required Test Items

IV. Assessment of tongue
   A. Required nonspeech items
     1. Protrusion of tongue in midline
       a. Range

37 ☐
         1 = full
         2 = diminished
         3 = none
         4 = cannot test
       b. Direction

38 ☐
         1 = midline
         2 = deviates to right
         3 = deviates to left
         4 = cannot test
     2. Intraoral elevation
       (tongue tip to alveolar ridge)

39 ☐
       1 = full
       2 = diminished
       3 = none
       4 = cannot test
     3. Atrophy (by visual inspection)

40 ☐
       1 = no atrophy
       2 = atrophy on right only
       3 = atrophy on left only
       4 = bilateral atrophy
   B. Required speech items
     1. Lingual consonant articulation
       a. Anterior

41 ☐
         1 = normal
         2 = impaired
         3 = cannot test
       b. Posterior

42 ☐
         1 = normal
         2 = impaired
         3 = cannot test

V. Assessment of lips, face and teeth
   A. Required nonspeech items
     1. Facial weakness
       a. Right side

43 ☐
         1 = no weakness
         2 = mild
         3 = moderate or severe
         4 = no voluntary movement
         5 = cannot test
       b. Left side

44 ☐
         1 = no weakness
         2 = mild
         3 = moderate or severe
         4 = no voluntary movement
         5 = cannot test
     2. Dentition during test adequate for chewing

45 ☐
       1 = yes
       2 = no
       3 = cannot test
     3. Dentures in place during test

46 ☐
       1 = none
       2 = upper only
       3 = lower only
       4 = upper and lower
       5 = cannot test
   B. Required speech items
     1. Labial articulation

47 ☐
       1 = normal
       2 = impaired
       3 = cannot test

Optional Test Items

IV. Assessment of tongue
   A. Optional nonspeech items
     1. Strength against resistance
       ___ normal or strong   ___ weak
       ___ cannot test
     2. Lateralization, range
       ___ full range, right   ___ reduced range, right
       ___ full range, left   ___ reduced range, left
       ___ cannot test
     3. Sensation to touch
       ___ present   ___ inconsistent
       ___ absent   ___ cannot test
     4. Comments: _____
       _____
       _____

   B. Optional speech items
     1. Rapid alternating movement
       a. /tâ-tâ-tâ/
         normal: ___ yes; ___ no
         rate: ___ normal; ___ reduced; ___ no./sec
         dysrhythmic: ___ yes; ___ no
         imprecise: ___ yes; ___ no
         cannot test: ___
      2. /k$_\wedge$-k$_\wedge$-k$_\wedge$/
         normal: ___ yes; ___ no
         rate: ___ normal; ___ reduced; ___ no./sec
         dysrhythmic: ___ yes; ___ no
         imprecise: ___ yes; ___ no
         cannot test: ___
      3. /p$_\wedge$-t$_\wedge$-k$_\wedge$/ or "pattycake"
         normal: ___ yes; ___ no
         rate: ___ normal; ___ reduced; ___ no./sec
         dysrhythmic: ___ yes; ___ no
         imprecise: ___ yes; ___ no
         cannot test: ___
     4. Comments: _____
       _____
       _____

V. Assessment of lips, face and teeth
   A. Optional nonspeech items
     1. Lip protrusion: _____
       _____
     2. Lip retraction: _____
       _____
     3. Labial apposition: _____
       _____
     4. Comments: _____
       _____
       _____

   B. Optional speech items
     1. Rapid alternating movement: /p$_\wedge$-p$_\wedge$-p$_\wedge$/
       normal: ___ yes; ___ no
       rate: ___ normal; ___ reduced; ___ no./sec
       dysrhythmic: ___ yes; ___ no
       imprecise: ___ yes; ___ no
       cannot test: ___
     2. Comments: _____
       _____

Fig. 6–3. *(continued)*

Required Test Items	Optional Test Items
VI. Assessment of jaw	VI. Assessment of jaw

VI. Assessment of jaw
  A. Required nonspeech items
    1. Opening, range
48 ☐
      1 = full
      2 = diminished
      3 = cannot test
    2. Opening, direction
49 ☐
      1 = midline
      2 = deviation to right
      3 = deviation to left
      4 = cannot test

VII. Assessment of parenteral feeding
  A. Required nonspeech items
50 ☐
    1 = none
    2 = nasal tube
    3 = gastrostomy tube
    4 = other

VI. Assessment of jaw
  A. Optional nonspeech items
    1. Strength
      ___ strong or normal   ___ weak
      ___ cannot test
  2. Comments: _____
_____
_____

  B. Optional speech items
    1. Are lingual/labial articulations compromised
      when jaw is immobilized, e.g., in "bite-block"
      position?
☐
      1 = no
      2 = yes
      3 = cannot test
    2. Comments: _____
_____
_____

VII. Assessment of parenteral tube
  A. Comments: _____
_____
_____

VIII. Assessment of drooling
  A. Comments: _____
_____
_____

Source: Reprinted, with permission, from Linden, Kuhlemeier, and Patterson, 1993 (33).

Modified Evans Blue Dye Test

The patient with tracheostomy presents a unique opportunity for identifying the presence of airway contamination. This examination is conducted by dyeing what is swallowed and examining the color of what is suctioned from the trachea. The modified Evans blue dye test may be an appropriate method to assess swallowing when patients are unable to be transported to the radiology suite for a videofluoroscopic swallow study (e.g., patients who fatigue easily and/or have multiple intravenous lines and catheters).

The modified Evans blue dye test is based on the Evans blue dye test. The Evans blue dye test was described by Cameron and colleagues (6) and named after the respected anatomist and physiologist Herbert McClean Evans (1882–1971) who used the dye in the determination of blood volume. Swallowing is assessed by placing four drops of aqueous solution of Evans blue dye on a patient's tongue every 4 h. Routine tracheostomy care is performed, and tracheal secretions are monitored for bluish discoloration for 48 h. Any evidence of blue dye in tracheal secretions is judged to indicate aspiration.

The modified Evans blue dye test is performed by first deflating the cuff of the cannula, performing suctioning as needed, facilitating speech production during cuff deflation, and then presenting dyed boluses in order of anticipated difficulty (easiest to hardest). The patient is observed while swallowing for signs and symp-

Fig. 6–4.   Sample summary of clinical findings for the larynx.

Laryngeal Component

Nonspeech: decreased laryngeal elevation with swallow (upon palpation and visual
   inspection)
Speech: wet-hoarse phonation
Implications: compromised laryngeal closure; pooling in the pyriform sinuses;
   aspiration or laryngeal penetration of boluses

Prediction of Nature of Swallowing Problem (Check those that apply):

___Slow oral stage
___Delayed swallow response
___Nasal regurgitation
___Supraglottic laryngeal penetration
✓Laryngeal penetration with cough
✓Laryngeal penetration without cough
✓Reduced laryngeal elevation
___Reduced epiglottic tilt
✓Reduced pharyngeal constriction
___Bolus specific dysphagia

Plan for Videofluoroscopic Swallowing Study

First bolus consistency, amount: thick liquid, 5 cc
Method of delivery: spoon
Compensations to be tried (Check those that apply):

___Multiple swallows per bolus
___Alternation of liquids and solids
✓Neck flexion/rotation/extension
✓Supraglottic swallow
✓Volitional cough or throat clear after swallow
___Mendelsohn maneuver

---

toms of dysphagia. Suctioning is performed after each bolus consistency. Suctioned material is examined for evidence of blue tint. If there is no evidence of bluish discoloration, the bedside examination may proceed with additional boluses. If blue discoloration is present, then testing should be discontinued. A competency for the modified Evans blue dye test is in Appendix A.

Value of the Conventional Bedside Assessment

The value of the bedside examination has been studied extensively in the nontracheostomy population. Investigators have looked at the information gained from the bedside assessment to see how well clinicians can predict aspiration and if there are findings that are associated with aspiration. Others have examined the kinds of management decisions made on the basis of the bedside examination.

Studies indicate that clinicians are poor predictors of aspiration based on bedside observations. Logemann and colleagues (36) studied 75 patients with dysphagia secondary to neoplastic diseases or neurologic disorders and found that even the most experienced clinicians failed to identify approximately 50% of patients who aspirated on videofluoroscopy. Similarly, Splaingard and colleagues (37) studied 107 patients with neurogenic etiologies and found that only 42% of patients who aspirated on videofluoroscopy were identified as aspirators during bedside evaluation of swallowing. Scales, Patterson, and Linden (38) reported that 42% of their subjects with aspiration on videofluoroscopy were identified from clinical examination ($n = 26$). Linden and colleagues (33) found that subglottic penetration could be predicted 66% of the time ($n = 249$). Given these data, the bedside examination is felt to be inadequate in assessing pharyngeal function. Videofluoroscopy is commonly said to be justified because clinicians are not able to predict swallowing abnormalities reliably, thereby exposing patients to the risk of aspiration and its consequences.

For over a decade, studies have been aimed at identifying specific characteristics that would improve clinicians' predictive abilities at the bedside (8,33,39–41). Although populations and methods varied in these studies of clinical correlates, two findings emerge consistently: abnormal cough and abnormal phonation quality. Both reflect impaired laryngeal functioning. One implication is that those patients who evidence impaired laryngeal function are those who should be referred for videofluoroscopic swallowing studies as this cluster of signs is associated with aspiration.

Investigators have also examined the influence of the bedside examination on direct treatment decisions—those decisions pertaining to actual oral intake. Splaingard and colleagues (37) and Sorin and colleagues (42) found that diet recommendations generally cannot be made on the basis of the bedside examination, supporting the videofluoroscopic swallowing study as the "gold standard" for the evaluation of swallowing in most patient populations.

Value of the Modified Evans Blue Dye Test

Less is known about the value of the bedside assessment with tracheostomy and ventilator dependency. Thompson-Henry and Braddock (43) examined the use of the modified Evans blue dye test in five patients with tracheostomy. They found that none of their five patients had evidence of aspiration on the modified Evans blue dye tests, but that all of these individuals had evidence of aspiration on follow-up modified barium swallow studies or fiberoptic endoscopic evaluations of swallow. They concluded that the modified Evans blue dye test fails to detect aspiration in patients with tracheostomy. The implication is that the modified Evans blue dye test is of questionable value in determining whether someone should be fed by mouth. However, the methodology and interpretation of the Thompson-Henry and Braddock study have been challenged (44,45).

Tippett and Siebens (46) investigated speech–language pathologists' ability to detect aspiration by the modified Evans blue dye test and use test results in making appropriate recommendations regarding alimentation/hydration. Specifically, they wanted to determine whether the recommendations stemming from the modified Evans blue dye tests were validated by subsequent observations of pa-

Table 6–2. Etiologies of patients' diagnoses.

Etiologies	No. of patients
Motor vehicle accidents	21
Falls	6
Gunshot wounds	5
Motor cycle accidents	4
Pedestrian/motor vehicle accidents	4
Stab wounds	2
Smoke inhalation/CO poisoning	1
Assault with a blunt instrument	1
Systemic ailments	9
Total	53

tients who were fed. Their study included 53 patients with a variety of etiologies (Table 6–2).

Of the 53 patients who received modified Evans blue dye tests, 24 (45%) had test results that were positive for aspiration, and 29 (55%) had test results that were negative for aspiration. Of these 29 patients with negative tests, six were not fed after the speech–language pathologist's evaluation because of a change in medical status or a scheduled medical procedure requiring that the patient remain NPO. The remaining 23 patients were fed meals that contained the recommended bolus consistencies dyed blue. Of these 23 patients, two patients (9%) had evidence of blue-tinged tracheal secretions after meals with dyed foods, and 21 patients (91%) did not have evidence of blue-tinged tracheal secretions after meals with dyed foods. The patients with aspiration were retested by the speech–language pathologist; both were found to aspirate on the repeat modified Evans blue dye tests. At discharge, 20 of the 21 (95%) patients without aspiration were being alimented/hydrated orally at discharge, and one patient was lost to follow-up. Results are summarized in Figure 6–5.

A clinical implication of these results is that modified Evans blue dye tests generally lead to appropriate recommendations regarding oral alimentation/hydration when test results are negative. When results of modified Evans blue dye tests are positive, these tests should be supplemented by radiographic or endoscopic evaluation of swallowing in order to identify the presence or absence of effective compensatory strategies to minimize aspiration/laryngeal penetration, thereby facilitating return to oral alimentation/hydration.

Approaches other than postprandial inspections of tracheal secretions may be superior in validating the modified Evans blue dye test. For example, modified Evans blue dye tests and videofluoroscopy or endoscopy could be conducted simultaneously, in a manner similar to studies comparing results of fiberoptic endoscopic and videofluoroscopic examinations of swallowing (47).

The modified Evans blue dye test appears to be a reliable, low-cost bedside technique for detecting aspiration/laryngeal penetration. It requires no expensive equipment and is relatively noninvasive (i.e., no exposure to radiation, no insertion of an endoscope). There are obvious limitations of the modified Evans blue dye test. For example, pharyngeal swallowing events are not observable as they

Fig. 6–5.   Modified Evans blue dye test results.

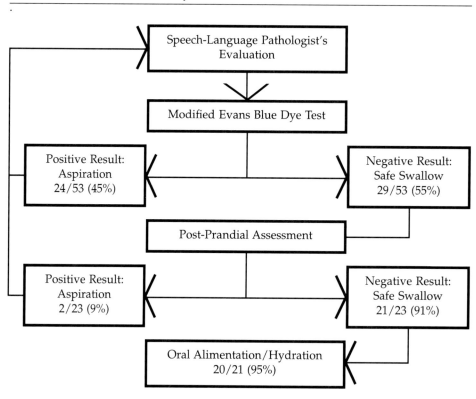

are during videofluoroscopic and endoscopic evaluations, therefore the underlying mechanism of the dysphagia remains unknown. Nevertheless, the modified Evans blue dye test may allow clinicians to evaluate swallowing in individuals with tracheostomy at the bedside, determine appropriate means of alimentation/hydration, and identify the need for videofluoroscopic or endoscopic evaluations of swallowing. This practice may decrease unnecessary delays in initiating oral alimentation/hydration and facilitate appropriate referrals for more sophisticated procedures in individuals with tracheostomy. Cases 1 through 5 in Appendix C illustrate treatment progress in speaking and swallowing following modified Evans blue dye tests in individuals with a variety of diagnoses. Positive and negative results of modified Evans blue dye tests are described.

Fiberoptic Endoscopic Evaluation of Swallowing

A well-established technique for evaluating swallowing at the bedside is the fiberoptic endoscopic evaluation of swallowing. Langmore and colleagues (48) developed the fiberoptic endoscopic examination of swallowing safety (FEESS). A flexible fiberoptic laryngoscope is used to view the hypopharynx, laryngeal vestibule, and glottis while the patient is eating. Boluses are dyed blue or green to distinguish them from secretions. Langmore (49) reported that the FEESS is an alternative to videofluoroscopic swallowing studies for those patients who cannot be transported to radiology easily because of their medical status, including ventilator-dependent individuals, and for individuals in nursing facilities where videofluoroscopy is not available. Advantages of this technique include objective documentation of pharyngeal stage swallowing events, visualization of actual structures, appreciation of anatomic configuration of structures within the hypopharynx, localization of secretions and bolus materials, assessment of laryngeal airway closure and protective movements, ability to assess swallowing without requiring the patient to eat or drink, and ability to perform this procedure in a clinic or at the bedside. Limitations of FEESS include obliteration of the view from the endoscope during actual swallow and need to place an endoscope transnasally (49).

Videofluoroscopic Swallowing Studies

Videofluoroscopy is a radiographic study of swallowing recorded on videotape. This technology was introduced in the early 1980s and has been written about extensively over that past 10 years (4,50–52). In general, the two primary objectives of videofluoroscopic swallowing studies (VFSS) are to assess pharyngeal and esophageal structural and functional components and plan swallow treatment. The first objective may include studying airway and foodway relationships. The second objective includes assessing optimal head/neck position, utilizing clearance and respiratory/laryngeal maneuvers during swallowing, and monitoring the patient's ability to handle different bolus consistencies, bolus amounts, and rate of intake.

As previously discussed, videofluoroscopy has been considered essential in the identification of aspiration primarily because clinicians have been reported to be poor predictors of aspiration at the bedside in the nontracheostomy population; prediction of aspiration being complicated in this situation by the occurrence of "silent" aspiration—that is, penetration of saliva or food below the level of the true vocal folds without cough or any other symptom indicating that foodway products are entering the airway (8,9).

Palmer and colleagues (53) described a protocol for conducting a videofluoroscopic swallowing study. Their protocol includes clinical evaluation of patients by physicians and speech–language pathologists, preparation of standardized foods, use of a prescribed sequence for fluoroscopy of speaking and swallowing in lateral and posteroanterior views, and documentation of specific swallowing events. This protocol is applicable to individuals with tracheostomy and/or ventilator dependency.

Videofluoroscopic swallowing studies are feasible in medically stable individuals with tracheostomy and/or mechanical ventilation. The evaluation should be interdisciplinary and should include the physician, nurse, respiratory therapist, radiology technician, and speech–language pathologist. It is useful to outline the responsibilities of each team member during the VFSS in order to insure an optimal study. The physician and speech–language pathologist are responsible for the VFSS plan, including bolus consistencies to be tested, order of presentation, bolus size, and modifications to be tried. They also discuss the VFSS results and recommendations, and document these in the medical record. The radiology technician prepares the suite for fluoroscopy, including setting up the video equipment, preparing the barium boluses, gathering feeding supplies, and obtaining lead aprons. Responsibilities of the nurse include preparing the patient for transport to radiology, including positioning on a specialized swallow study chair if one is to be used, escorting the patient to radiology, insuring that suction equipment accompanies the patient, and "bagging" and suctioning the patient as needed. The respiratory therapist provides the portable ventilator to be used during the VFSS, places the patient on the portable ventilator in the radiology suite, insures that the portable ventilator is operational and that settings are correct, adjusts the ventilator settings as appropriate during the VFSS, inflates and deflates the tracheostomy cuff, and suctions and "bags" the patient as needed.

As stated above, the protocol described by Palmer and colleagues (53) is appropriate for studying individuals with tracheostomy and/or ventilator dependency. The VFSS is more likely to yield favorable results if individuals have had opportunities to have airflow restored through the larynx and pharynx, enabling them to speak and cough. Individuals who breathe independently and have a tracheostomy should have opportunities to experience cannula valving or plugging prior to VFSS. Individuals who are ventilator-dependent should have opportunities to have their tracheostomy cuffs deflated and utilize ventilator-supported oral communication. The steps to facilitate speech via valving a tracheostomy cannula and/or deflating the tracheostomy cuff are described in Chapter 5. A competency for the VFSS is in Appendix B.

Treatment of Swallowing Problems

The treatment of swallowing impairments involves the participation of the patient, family, nurse, dietitian, speech–language pathologist, and physician. Many variables can be manipulated to facilitate oral alimentation and hydration (9,12,50). Treatment can include bolus restrictions, bolus modifications, postural changes, and compensatory techniques. In some cases, it may be necessary to eliminate a bolus type from an individual's diet. For example, particulate or multitextured solids (e.g., hamburger, beef stew) may need to be restricted when boluses of these characteristics are precariously retained in the pharyngeal recesses, placing an individual at risk for airway obstruction. In other instances, slow rate of intake, reduced bolus size, multiple swallows per bolus, or alternation of liquid and solid swallows may be used to clear pharyngeal collection of boluses. Postural changes may also facilitate clearance of boluses from the pharyngeal recesses (e.g., neck rotation) and improve airway protection (e.g., neck flexion). Commercial thickeners can modify liquids, if laryngeal penetration occurs with swallows of thin liquids.

Direct speech–language pathology treatment as well as compensatory swallowing strategies have been shown to yield improvements in swallowing safety. Logemann and colleagues (54) found that head rotation toward the paretic side increased the amount of bolus swallowed and upper esophageal sphincter opening diameter in patients with lateral medullary syndrome. Horner and colleagues

(40) showed that exercises for oral and pharyngeal muscles helped to restore oral intake in individuals with neurogenic dysphagia.

For individuals with tracheostomy, valving or plugging of the cannula may facilitate a safe swallow. Valving and plugging both restore cough and throat clearing. Unlike plugging, valving has the advantage of allowing *unidirectional* airflow through the larynx, thereby sweeping the airway clear of secretions and foodway contents. Because inspiration does not occur through the larynx, secretions and food boluses are not penetrated further into the airway during inspiration (25).

The effect of tracheostomy tube occlusion during swallowing has been studied in nonsurgical and surgical patients with tracheostomy (55–57). In the first study, Leder and colleagues (55) studied the effect of tracheostomy tube occlusion on aspiration during fluoroscopy in 20 consecutive, nonsurgical patients. They found no aspiration in 10 of 20 patients with and without occluded tracheostomy tubes, aspiration of liquid and puree in nine with and without occluded tubes, and aspiration of liquid in one with and without an occluded tube. In the second study, Leder and colleagues (56) found aspiration of both liquid and puree boluses in 10 of 16 consecutive, early, postsurgical head and neck cancer patients regardless of whether their tracheostomy tubes were occluded or unoccluded, no aspiration of liquid or puree in four patients when their tubes were first occluded then unoccluded, and aspiration of liquid in two patients with and without occluded tracheostomy tubes but no aspiration of puree in these individuals under either occlusion condition. In the third study, Leder (57) studied the incidence of aspiration after valve use in 20 consecutive patients with documentation of previous aspiration via fiberoptic endoscopic examinations. Incidence of aspiration was not affected by the use of a tracheostomy valve; patients either continued to aspirate with valve use or did not exhibit aspiration for both valve-on and -off conditions.

Leder and colleagues (55–57) concluded that occlusion status of the tracheostomy tube did not influence the incidence of aspiration in nonsurgical and surgical patients with tracheostomy tubes. They argued that factors other than restoration of subglottic pressure via valving are important in facilitating a safe swallow (e.g., tongue propulsive forces, contraction of the pharyngeal walls, negative suction pressure generated by laryngeal rise and opening of the pharyngoesophageal segment). Leder (57) pointed out, however, that subglottic pressure can aid in the clearance of residual bolus from the upper airway after swallow.

Duration was limited of tracheostomy tube occlusion. In one study, tracheostomy tubes were occluded three to five min prior to videofluoroscopic swallowing studies (55). In another study, tracheostomy tubes were occluded for several hours prior to the videofluoroscopic examinations if tolerated, or for three to five min prior to the video studies. In Leder's most recent study (57), time off mechanical ventilation is narrow, and patients appear to have had limited opportunities to experience airflow through the upper airway, speak, and cough. These factors may have limited the value of valving in this study. In contrast to Leder's and colleagues results (55–57), our experiences show that results of swallowing evaluations and return to oral alimentation/hydration are facilitated by allowing individuals the opportunity to have cuffs deflated, wear valves, speak and clear the upper airway for several days before initiating swallowing evaluations.

For those patients who are ventilator-dependent, cuff deflation may be appropriate to facilitate upper airway clearance and laryngeal protection against entry of foodway products. Clinical trials with five ventilator-dependent, cognitively intact individuals (including one patient with a motor neuron disease) with glottic control have documented that a deflated cuff is compatible with ventilation, preserves oral communication, and restores safe alimentation by mouth (58). Cases 6 through 8 in Appendix C illustrate the valve of valving and cuff deflation to facilitate safe swallowing.

Swallowing Algorithm

A challenge for speech–language pathologists in today's health care environment is the emphasis placed on cost savings by reducing the variance in patient care. Critical pathways indicate the preferred pattern of service delivery and are intended to help organize, sequence, and time the major events in patient care. Critical pathways are usually organized along diagnostic groups (DRG) such as stroke and hip replacement, but can be developed for conditions such as failure to wean (59,60). It is incumbent upon speech–language pathologists to contribute to the development of critical pathways for their areas of clinical practice, especially "high-risk" and "high-volume" populations, such as those with tracheostomy and ventilator dependency.

Vogelman and colleagues (61) proposed a pathway for the assessment of swallowing in individuals with tracheostomy and/or ventilator dependency. Their pathway sequences available tests for the following circumstances: independent ventilation with cuffed cannula, independent ventilation with cuffless cannula, and positive pressure ventilation/cuffed cannula. The diagnostic tools included in the pathway are the Evans blue dye test, modified Evans blue dye test, fiberoptic endoscopic evaluation of swallowing, and the videofluoroscopic swallowing study. (Figs. 6–6 through 6–8). Rationales are provided for each test under each circumstance. It is the authors' experience that swallowing function of critically ill patients is often delayed until discharge is imminent. Without an organized approach, patients may be discharged without evaluation of swallowing, unnecessarily prolonging NPO status or requiring transportation to a facility for swallowing evaluation. The adoption of a critical pathway allows reasonable consistency among different members of a speech–language pathology department and informs the medical team of what to expect when a swallowing evaluation is ordered. By marshaling the expertise of team members, including the nurse, physician, radiologist, and speech–language pathologist, intervention can be initiated in a timely manner and evaluation can proceed in a structured and well-planned progression.

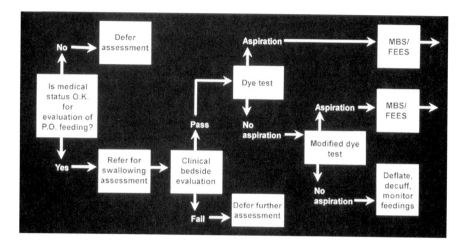

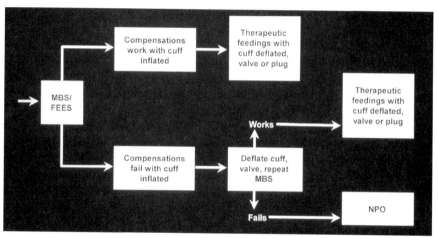

Fig. 6–6. Algorithm for assessment of dysphagia in tracheotomized patients: Independent ventilation, cuffed tube.

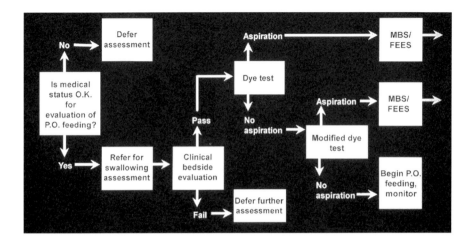

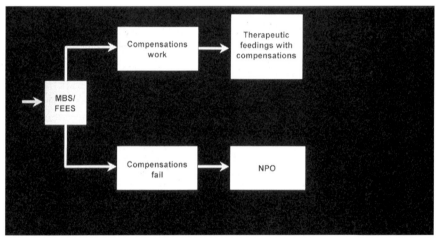

Fig. 6–7. Algorithm for assessment of dysphagia in tracheotomized patients: Independent respiration, cuffless tube.

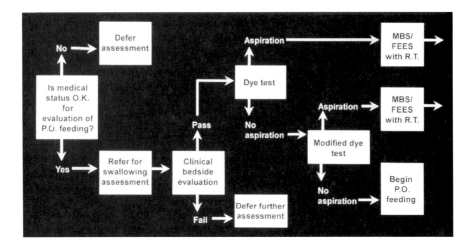

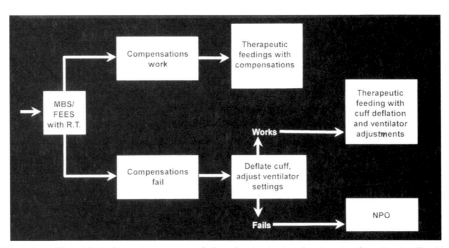

Fig. 6–8.   Algorithm for assessment of dysphagia in tracheotomized patients: Positive pressure ventilation, cuffed tube.

Appendix A. Competency Regarding Modified Evans Blue Dye Test (MEBDT)

Outcome

The modified Evans blue dye test (MEBDT) is conducted to effect the following:

1. Determine the presence or absence of laryngeal penetration/aspiration of foodway contents in individuals with tracheostomy and/or ventilator dependency;

2. Determine recommendations for alimentation/hydration, including safe (i.e., without laryngeal penetration/aspiration) bolus consistencies for oral alimentation/hydration;

3. Identify the need for instrumental procedures or other consultations to assess swallowing.

Staff

Speech–language pathologists (may involve nurses, respiratory therapists, physicians)

Equipment

Blue food coloring/dye

Food items (purees such as pudding, applesauce; honey- and nectar-thickened liquid; thin liquid; solids such as bread, cookies)

Cups

Straws

Spoons

Tongue blades

Penlight

Napkins

Oral swabs

Suction

Syringes

Gloves

Pulse oximetry as indicated

Stethoscope (optional)

Core Components of Performance Criteria

The speech–language pathologist:

1. States candidacy criteria for a MEBDT
   a. Patient is alert

    b. Patient has a tracheostomy cannula with or without ventilator dependency

    c. Patient is a candidate for cuff deflation

    d. Patient has no medical contraindications for oral alimentation/hydration

2. States risk of aspiration/laryngeal penetration in individuals with tracheostomy

    a. Cameron and colleagues (1973) (6): 42/61 (69%) individuals with tracheostomy

    b. Bone and colleagues (1974) (7): 13/15 (87%) individuals with either uncuffed metal tracheostomy tubes or low-volume, high-pressure cuffed tubes with cuffs deflated; 2/12 (17%) individuals with high-volume, low-pressure cuffed tubes; and 2/13 (15%) individuals with sponge-filled cuffed tubes

    c. Tippett and Siebens (1995) (46): 24/53 (45%) individuals with tracheostomy

3. States possible effects of tracheostomy on swallowing

    a. Access for suctioning

    b. Impairment of cough

    c. Mechanical barrier

    d. Desensitization of larynx

    e. Compression of esophagus

    f. Tethering of laryngeal elevation and anterior movement

    g. Pooling of secretions in proximal trachea and larynx

    h. Tracheomalacia

    i. Granulation, scarring

    j. Tracheoesophageal fistula

4. Obtains background information from the medical record and documents information on the data collection sheet and in the consultation report, for example

    a. Size and type of tracheostomy cannula

    b. Method of mechanical ventilation

    c. Duration of intubation and/or tracheostomy

    d. Cuff status

    e. Current method of alimentation/hydration

    f. Signs/symptoms of dysphagia

    g. Secretion management

    h. "Free time" from mechanical ventilation

    i. Communication status

5. Interviews patient, family, caregivers regarding speaking/swallowing as appropriate

6. Assesses patient's readiness for a MEBDT
   a. Determines the patient's ability to participate given alertness, cognitive/language status, endurance, comfort
   b. Monitors oxygen saturation, heart rate, blood pressure, ventilator alarms as appropriate
   c. Explains procedure to the patient
   d. Consults with other professional staff as needed

7. Assesses structure and function of speech/swallow components
   a. Respiratory mechanism
   b. Laryngeal mechanism
   c. Velum/pharynx
   d. Tongue
   e. Lips/face/teeth
   f. Jaw

8. Deflates/inflates cuff correctly
   a. Withdraws air/water from the pilot balloon via syringe
   b. Is prepared to suction or has nurse present to do so
   c. Monitors vital signs and the patient's subjective comfort
   d. Reinflates cuff if a change occurs in vital signs or the patient's comfort
   e. Reinflates cuff without overinflating; measured via manometry or onset of absence of phonation

9. Instructs the patient regarding phonation/respiration
   a. Allows patient to become comfortable with cuff deflation
   b. Performs intermittent digital occlusion of cannula if the patient is not ventilator dependent
   c. Teaches the patient to phonate when the cannula is occluded intermittently
   d. Teaches the patient to phonate during the inspiratory cycle of the ventilator if the patient is ventilator-dependent
   e. Teaches the patient vocal fold adduction to compensate for the leak created by deflating the cuff

10. Assesses speech production
    a. Describes perceptual characteristics
    b. Rates speech intelligibility
    c. Proposes possible etiologies for dysphonia/aphonia
    d. Makes recommendation for additional referrals as appropriate, e.g., assessment of laryngeal structure/function by otolaryngology

11. States rationale for bolus hierarchy, for example
    a. Purees and thick liquids are safest when patients present with neurogenic dysphagia

  b. Thin liquids are easier to swallow than thick for patients with mechanical dysphagia

12. Observes the patient for signs/symptoms of dysphagia, for example
    a. Loss of bolus through lips
    b. Retention in buccal space
    c. Wet-hoarse voice quality
    d. Throat-clearing or coughing after swallow
    e. Reduced laryngeal rise
    f. Expectoration or suctioning of food particles or blue-tinged tracheal secretions

13. Identifies the need for suctioning

14. Performs suctioning as appropriate

15. Uses appropriate infection control techniques

16. Proceeds with or terminates MEBDT based on
    a. Evidence of aspiration/laryngeal penetration
    b. Vital signs
    c. Subjective comfort

17. Develops recommendations for alimentation/hydration
    a. positive MEBDT: NPO, alternative to oral alimentation/hydration
    b. negative MEBDT: oral intake with appropriate boluses; dye meals blue for 24 to 48 h
    c. Monitors for signs/symptoms of laryngeal penetration/aspiration
    d. Discontinues oral intake if signs/symptoms of laryngeal penetration/ aspiration are evidenced
    e. Contacts nurse or other caregivers as appropriate regarding post-prandial suctioning
    f. Advances diet as appropriate

18. Educates the patient, family, caregivers regarding MEBDT
    a. Explains results
    b. Discusses plan for alimentation/hydration
    c. Assesses learning needs
    d. Evaluates the patient's/family's learning
    e. Uses materials appropriate to cognitive/developmental level, culture

19. States advantages and limitations of MEBDT
    (See Thompson-Henry and Braddock (1995) (43) and Tippett and Siebens (1996) (45))

Appendix B.   Competency Regarding Videofluoroscopic Swallowing Studies (VFSS)

Outcome

The videofluoroscopic swallowing study is conducted to:

1. Assess pharyngeal and esophageal structural and functional components;

2. Assess the value of compensatory techniques;

3. Determine recommendations for alimentation/hydration;

4. Plan swallow treatment.

Staff

Speech–language pathologists (may involve physicians, nurses, respiratory therapists)

Equipment

Swallow study chair

Food items (puree such as pudding, applesauce; honey-thick liquid; nectar-thick liquid; thin liquid; solid such as bread, cookie)

Cups

Straws

Spoons

Tongue blades

Penlight

Napkins

Oral swabs

Gloves

Suction as indicated

Syringes as indicated

Pulse oximetry as indicated

Barium liquid, paste, powder

Fluoroscopy equipment

Video equipment

Core Components of Performance Criteria

The speech–language pathologist:

1. States candidacy criteria for a VFSS
    a. Patient is alert
    b. Patient has no medical contraindications for oral alimentation/hydration, e.g., gastrointestinal, pulmonary

2. States ability to predict laryngeal penetration/aspiration at the bedside from literature, for example

Linden and colleagues,	1993 (33)	66%
Logemann and colleagues,	1982 (36)	50%
Splaingard and colleagues,	1988 (37)	42%
Scales and colleagues,	1988 (38)	42%

3. States clinical correlates of aspiration from literature, for example

Linden and Siebens (1983) (8)
N = 15 with neurogenic dysphagia

Laryngeal penetration on videofluoroscopy	11/15
"Silent" laryngeal penetration	9/11
Wet-hoarse voice quality	10/11
Impaired pharyngeal gag reflex	10/11

Horner and Massey (1988) (39)
N = 21 stroke patients

Aspiration on videofluoroscopy	11/21
"Silent" aspiration	8/11

Aspirators: lower prevalence of subjective complaints, higher prevalence of weak cough, and dysphonia

Horner and colleagues (1988) (40)
N = 47 stroke patients

Aspiration on videofluoroscopy	24/47

Aspirators: abnormal sputum, noncardiac chest pain, fever, dysphonia

Horner and colleagues (1990) (41)
N = 70 patients with bilateral CVAs

Aspiration on videofluoroscopy	34/70

Aspirators: abnormal gag reflex, abnormal cough, abnormal phonation

Linden and colleagues (1993) (33)
N = 249

Significant relationships with subglottic penetration: reclining or lying posture, dysphonia, aphonia, inability to test phonation, abnormal or absent laryngeal elevation, wet spontaneous cough, abnormal palatal gag, some or no swallowing of secretions

4. Identifies medical diagnoses that place patients at risk for swallowing disorders

Central nervous system (e.g., CVA, traumatic brain injury); peripheral nervous system (e.g., amyotrophic lateral sclerosis); neuromuscular junction (e.g., myasthenia gravis); muscle (e.g., muscular dystrophy); head/neck cancer; inflammation, e.g., pharyngitis; trauma to oral-pharyngeal area (e.g., gunshot wound, intubation trauma)

5. States limitations of videofluoroscopy

   a. Radiographic assessment may not be feasible because patients may be weak, lethargic, easily agitated require multiple catheters, intravenous lines need monitoring equipment

   b. Radiographic assessment is a "snapshot" of feeding/swallowing behavior and therefore may not represent what the patient does in his/her natural environment.

6. Obtains background information from the medical record and documents information on the data collection sheet and in the consultation report, for example

   a. Current method of alimentation/hydration

   b. Signs/symptoms of dysphagia

   c. Secretion management

   d. Speech/communication status

7. Interviews patient, family, caregivers re: speaking/swallowing as appropriate. See sample questions (Fig. 6–2)

8. Assesses patient's readiness for a VFSS

   a. Determines the patient's ability to participate given alertness, cognitive/language status, behavior, endurance, comfort

   b. Monitors oxygen saturation, heart rate, blood pressure, and ventilator alarms as appropriate

   c. Explains procedure to the patient

   d. Consults with other professional staff as needed

9. Assesses structure and function of speech/swallow components

   a. Respiratory mechanism

   b. Laryngeal mechanism

   c. Velum/pharynx

   d. Tongue

   e. Lips/face/teeth

   f. Jaw

10. Assesses speech production

    a. Describes perceptual characteristics

    b. Rates speech intelligibility

    c. Makes recommendation for additional referrals as appropriate, e.g., assessment of laryngeal structure/function by otolaryngology

11. Develops prediction regarding nature of swallowing problem anticipated during VFSS

12. States rationale for bolus hierarchy, consistency, size/amount, for example

    a. Purees and thick liquids are safest when patients present with neurogenic dysphagia

    b. Thin liquids are easier to swallow than thick for patients with mechanical dysphagia

13. Develops a plan for therapeutic and compensatory maneuvers to try during VFSS for example,
    a. Multiple swallows per bolus
    b. Alternation of liquids and solids
    c. Neck flexion/rotation/extension
    d. Supraglottic swallow
    e. Volitional cough or throat clear and swallow
    f. Mendelsohn maneuver

14. Makes observations re: structure/function during VFSS (Palmer and colleagues, 1991) (53)
    a. Anatomy
    b. Mastication and oral food transport
    c. Velopharyngeal apposition
    d. Position of bolus at onset of pharyngeal swallow
    e. Laryngeal displacement
    f. Epiglottic tilt
    g. Closure of laryngeal vestibule
    h. Occurrence of laryngeal penetration
    i. Pharyngeal constriction
    j. Opening of PE segment
    k. Occurrence of retention in pharynx after swallow
    l. Occurrence of retention in esophagus after swallow
    m. Peristaltic activity in esophagus
    n. Opening of gastroesophageal sphincter

15. Identifies the need for suctioning

16. Performs suctioning as appropriate

17. Uses appropriate infection control techniques

18. Proceeds with or terminates VFSS based on
    a. Evidence of aspiration/laryngeal penetration
    b. Vital signs
    c. Subjective comfort
    d. Response to therapeutic and compensatory maneuvers

19. Develops recommendations for alimentation/hydration as appropriate
    a. NPO
    b. Alternative feeding method
    c. Specific boluses, techniques, compensations

20. Refers for additional testing, therapy or other consultations as appropriate
    a. Nutrition consultation, calorie count
    b. Observation at meal
    c. Otolaryngology consultation

21. Educates the patient, family, caregivers regarding VFSS
    a. Explains results
    b. Discusses plan for alimentation/hydration
    c. Assesses learning needs
    d. Evaluates the patient's/family's learning
    e. Uses materials appropriate to cognitive/developmental level and culture

Appendix C

CASE 1

Background

A 20-year-old female was admitted to a trauma center status post motor vehicle accident, resulting in a closed head injury, aortic tear, liver and spleen lacerations, left femur fracture, and right knee contusions and lacerations. There was a questionable loss of consciousness. At admission, her Glasgow Coma Scale score was 13/15. Head CT was negative. She was extubated on day 7, reintubated on day 10, and a tracheostomy was performed on day 16.

Past medical history: Allergic to bee stings; gastric ulcer

Social history: Single; college sophomore; works as a waitress; enjoys basketball and softball

Cognition/language: Initial evaluation: Ranchos Los Amigos Scale IV. Received SLP intervention daily

Swallow Assessment

Modified Evans blue dye test (MEBDT) conducted on hospital day 18
NGFT
Portex no. 8 cuffed tracheostomy cannula
Trach collar
Cuff deflated for MEBDT; no phonation with intermittent digital occlusion of cannula

Remarkable findings for speech/swallow components were limited laryngeal rise with dry swallows, reduced lingual and labial range of movement, slow lingual movements, and open mouth posture at rest

Boluses such as pudding, orange juice
Slow bolus manipulation, reduced laryngeal rise with swallow, inconsistent cough after liquids

MEBDT results: Negative

Recommendations:
Initiate PO intake with liquids, mechanical soft solids
Dye boluses blue for 24 h
Monitor tracheal secretions for evidence of blue tint
Discontinue PO intake if + blue tint
Deflate cuff during meals
Downsize tracheostomy cannula

24 to 48 h post:
Negative

Hospital Course

<u>Day 20</u>
  Cannula downsized to Shiley no. 6 fenestrated cuffed tube
  Moderate to severe dysphonia with low volume and breathy quality

<u>Day 30</u>
  Metal no. 4 cannula

<u>Discharge</u>
  Day 36 to home with outpatient speech–language pathology intervention
  RLAS VII
  Decannulated; persisting dysphonia
  Regular diet

CASE 2

Background

A 32-year-old male was admitted to a trauma center status post motor vehicle accident resulting in facial and pelvic fractures. There was loss of consciousness. Glasgow Coma Scale score was 15/15 at admission. Head CT was negative. Tracheostomy was performed on day 1.

Past medical history: Right knee surgery; HTN; hepatitis; headaches; indigestion; unspecified "emotional problems"

Social history: Married; two children; 9th grade education; self-employed; enjoys bowling and pool; ETOH use/abuse; tobacco use; PCP

Cognition/language: Initial evaluation: Ranchos Los Amigos Scale VI to VII. Received SLP intervention daily

Swallow Assessment

Modified Evans blue dye test (MEBDT) conducted on hospital day 11
NPO
Portex no. 9 cuffed tracheostomy cannula
Cannula plugged
Face mask
Speech was 100% intelligible in conversation
Boluses such as thick liquid Shake-up, fruit punch via straw
No cough or wet-hoarse voice after thick liquid; cough and wet-hoarse voice after thin liquid

MEBDT results: Negative

Recommendations:
Initiate PO intake with thick liquids, purees through straw or syringe/tubing
Dye boluses blue for 24 h
Monitor tracheal secretions for evidence of blue tint

Discontinue PO intake if + blue tint

24 to 48 h post:
Negative

Hospital Course

Day 19
  PO intake with blenderized solids, all liquids

Discharge
  Day 25 to acute rehabilitation hospital
  RLAS VIII

CASE 3

Background

A 31-year-old male was transferred to a trauma center 38 days post stab wound to the chest resulting in laceration of the right lung, pericardium, and right atrium. There was no loss of consciousness. Glasgow Coma Scale score and head CT were not reported. Tracheostomy and PEG were performed at the outside facility.

Past medical history: Healthy

Social history: Married; two children

Cognition/language: GWNL

Swallow Assessment

Modified Evans blue dye test (MEBDT) conducted on hospital day 16
Portex no. 8 cuffed tracheostomy cannula
Trach collar
Cuff deflated for MEBDT; no phonation with intermittent digital occlusion of cannula
Boluses such as pudding, thick liquid Shake-up, apple juice, graham cracker
Intermittent coughing throughout evaluation; copious white, frothy secretions expectorated through cannula

MEBDT results: Negative

Recommendations:
Initiate PO intake with regular diet
Dye boluses blue for 24 h
Monitor tracheal secretions for evidence of blue tint
Discontinue PO intake if + blue tint
Downsize tracheostomy cannula

24 to 48 h post:
Possible aspiration; patient with nausea and vomiting

Hospital Course

<u>Day 18</u>
  Reevaluated swallow
  Phonation achieved
  Negative MEBDT with applesauce

<u>Day 19</u>
  No evidence of aspiration with purees

<u>Day 22</u>
  Diet advanced to mechanical soft
  Cannula plugged

<u>Day 23</u>
  Regular diet

<u>Discharge</u>
  Day 32 to acute rehabilitation hospital

CASE 4

Background

A 46-year-old male was transferred to a trauma center three days post respiratory failure and pulmonary hemorrhage associated with systemic lupus erythematosus. His Glasgow Coma Scale score was 3T/15. MRI showed hemorrhagic contusions in right frontal region with ischemic changes throughout both hemispheres, right > left. At admission he required mechanical ventilation and was weaned by hospital day 54. A Portex no. 8 cuffed tracheostomy cannula and NGFT were in place on arrival.

Past medical history: Left CVA; HTN; SLE.

Social history: Married; one son; ETOH use/abuse

Cognition/language: Lethargic, crying, and minimally responsive to auditory/ tactile stimuli on initial evaluation. Received speech–language pathology intervention daily

Swallow Assessment

Modified Evans blue dye test (MEBDT) conducted on hospital day 61
Shiley no. 6 cuffed tracheostomy cannula
Trach collar
Cuff deflated for MEBDT
Phonation was low volume, harsh, breathy, occasionally wet-hoarse
Remarkable findings for speech/swallow components were maximum sustained phonation = 4 s (GWNL is greater than or equal to 10 s), reduced velopharyngeal movement on left, reduced lingual range of movement, bilateral facial droop (left > right), edentulous

Boluses such as applesauce, fruit punch
Wet-hoarse voice and coughing after liquid

MEBDT results: Positive

Recommendations:
Continue NGFT/NPO; SLP to reevaluate

Hospital Course

Day 63
   Repeat MEBDT with applesauce, juice
   Negative result
   Initiated PO intake with purees, thin liquids
   Dye boluses blue for 24 h
   Discontinue PO intake if + blue tint

Day 64
   Particulate boluses received at breakfast
   Coughing with meal
   Diet clarified
   Correct boluses received at lunch; negative result
   Decannulated

Discharge
   Day 68 to acute rehabilitation hospital
   Moderate cognitive/language deficits
   PO intake with purees, liquids

CASE 5

Background

A 74-year-old male was admitted to a trauma center status post motor vehicle accident resulting in cervical spinal cord injury. There was loss of consciousness. Admission Glasgow Coma Scale score was 6/15. Head CT was negative. There were airway problems at the accident scene; cricothyroidotomy was performed in the field.

Past medical history: CAD; hernia repair

Social history: Retired; widowed; two daughters

Cognition/language: Followed directions and expressed a variety of intentions during initial evaluation. Received speech–language pathology intervention daily

Swallow Assessment

Modified Evans blue dye test (MEBDT) conducted on hospital day 3
OGFT
Portex no. 8 cuffed tracheostomy cannula

Trach collar

Speech 100% intelligible in conversation with intermittent digital occlusion of cannula

Bolus = pudding

MEBDT results: Positive

Recommendations:
Continue OGFT/NPO
Refer to otolaryngology for evaluation of laryngeal structure/function

Hospital Course

Day 6
  Repeat MEBDT; positive with pudding despite benefit of upright positioning, more neutral position of head/neck, removal of OGFT

Day 7
  Diagnosed with displaced retropharynx posterior pharyngeal wall, tracheitis

Day 37
  Mechanical ventilation
  Shiley no. 8 cuffed tracheostomy
  Negative blue-tinged tracheal secretions when tongue coated with blue dye

Day 40
  Repeat MEBDT
  Negative with pudding, juice, water
  Initiate PO intake with mechanical soft solids, all liquids
  Dye boluses blue for 24 h
  Monitor tracheal secretions for evidence of blue tint
  Discontinue PO intake if + blue tint

Day 41
  Positive result with thin liquid
  Diet modified to mechanical soft solids, thickened liquids
  Negative result with these boluses

Day 44
  Repeat MEBDT
  Positive result with thin liquids

Discharge
  Day 48 to acute rehabilitation hospital Bolus restricted diet
  Oral communication with cuff deflation/intermittent digital occlusion of cannula

CASE 6

Background

Myotonic dystrophy
  Muscle disorder with wasting, weakness, and myotonia
  Autosomal dominant
  15/100,000 births
  Cause not known—a defect in muscle membrane
  Symptoms
    Myotonia—sustained involuntary contraction of muscle
    Intellectual impairment
    Falls
    Weakness—predilection for neck muscles
    Dysarthria
    Dysphagia—usually mild
    Somnolence
    Other organ involvement

A 56-year-old male was admitted to an acute care hospital with complaint of weakness and falling. He was diagnosed with adenocarcinoma of distal esophagus and myotonic dystrophy. A transhiatal total esophagectomy with cervical esophagogastrostomy and pyloromyotomy was performed. The patient received a jejunostomy tube and a tracheostomy. There were multiple postoperative complications, including bilateral vocal fold paralysis with a 3 mm gap. A modified barium swallow study showed no peristalsis, pooling in valleculae and pyriform sinuses, absence of swallow response, reverse peristalsis when the patient was bent over at the waist. He was transferred to a rehabilitation hospital two months postop. Treatment progress is outlined below.

Speech–Language Pathology Evaluation

Cognition/language: GWNL

Neurologic impairments of respiratory mechanism, larynx, velum/pharynx, tongue, lips/face

Speech: Moderate dysarthria with reduced vocal intensity, wet-hoarse phonation, hypernasality, articulatory imprecision

Swallow: NPO

Speech–Language Pathology Treatment

Cognition/language: Direct treatment not indicated

Speech: Facilitate oral communication
  Strategies:
  Investigate possibility of changing from Bivona to Shiley cannula
  Provide unidirectional speaking valve if appropriate
  Educate patient re: implications of tracheostomy and valve use

Swallow: Facilitate PO intake for pleasure with compensations
  Strategies:
  Conduct a videofluoroscopic swallowing study (VFSS)
  Discuss results with patient

Treatment Progress

Hospital day 2
  Assessed cognitive/language abilities
  Cuff deflated on Bivona for phonation trial

Hospital day 14
  Introduced electrolarynges; rejected by patient
  Cannula downsized to Bivona no. 6
  Initiated trial of cuff deflation/intermittent digital occlusion
  Cuff deflation tolerated 1 h/day
  Excellent speech intelligibility achieved
  Patient education regarding need maintain upright positioning with cuff
      deflation

Hospital day 23
  Cannula changed to Shiley no. 6
  Hopkins speaking valve worn 7 to 8 h/day
  Conducted VFSS
  Absence of laryngeal rise, absence of epiglottic tilt, retention of boluses,
      supraglottic penetration with liquids; foodway contents were swept out of
      the airway with throat clear after swallow
  Conclusion: pharyngeal stage dysphagia
  Recommendation: trial of PO with liquids and purees with compensations of
      cuff deflated, valve on, upright positioning, slow rate of intake, small
      portions

Hospital day 29
  Discharge to home
  PO intake with bolus-restricted diet
  Plan for outpatient follow-up

Two months postdischarge
  Continued to wear Hopkins valve
  Conducted VFSS
  Reduced laryngeal rise, reduced epiglottic tilt, bilateral retention in pyriform
      sinuses, no laryngeal penetration/aspiration with valve in place
  Conclusion: persisting pharyngeal stage dysphagia
  Recommendation: expand diet to soft mechanical boluses in small quantities
      with compensations noted above

CASE 7

Background

Arnold-Chiari malformation

Congenital anomaly of the hindbrain characterized by elongation of the brain stem and cerebellum into the cervical portion of the spinal cord

Described by Arnold in 1894 and Chiari in 1895

Often associated with spina bifida occulta or presence of a meningocele (displacement of brain stem and cerebellum secondary to fixation of the spinal cord at the site of spinal defect early in life, or developmental arrest and overgrowth of the neural tube in embryonic life)

Small number of cases in literature

Symptoms

Ataxia; leg weakness

Visual complaints

Onset of symptoms rarely delayed until adulthood

The patient was a 34-year-old male status post decompressive surgery of the brain stem secondary to Arnold-Chiari malformation. He had a complicated acute medical course. A modified barium swallow study at the acute care hospital showed leakage of boluses over the base of the tongue, no coordinated pharyngeal constriction, pharyngeal retention of boluses, aspiration of thick liquids without cough, and reduced gastric emptying 48 h after study. He was transferred to a rehabilitation hospital three months postop. He had a halo for immobilization of cervical spine, a nasogastric feeding tube, and a Shiley no. 6 cuffed tracheostomy cannula. He required positive pressure mechanical ventilation at night and oxygen throughout the day.

Speech–Language Pathology Evaluation

Cognition/language: Intact

Neurologic impairments of respiratory mechanism, larynx, velum/pharynx

Speech: Mild to moderate dysarthria with reduced vocal intensity, breathiness, occasional wet-hoarseness, hypernasality and nasal emissions

Swallow: NPO; unable to swallow all secretions; frequent oral suctioning

Speech-Language Pathology Treatment

Cognition/language: Direct intervention not indicated

Speech: Facilitate oral communication

Strategies:

Initiate cuff deflation for speech with positive pressure mechanical ventilation

Provide unidirectional speaking valve

Educate patient/family re: implications of tracheostomy and valve use

Monitor valve wearing

Swallow: Facilitate oral alimentation and hydration
  Strategies:
  Conduct a videofluoroscopic swallowing study (VFSS)
  Educate patient/family

Treatment Progress

Hospital day 11
  Conducted VFSS
  Boluses were ultra-thick liquid, particulate solid
  Cuff deflated
  Studied with and without positive pressure mechanical ventilation
  Airway contamination prevented by positive pressure mechanical ventilation
    with tidal volume and inspiratory/expiratory ratio increased
  Recommendations: therapeutic feeding with ultrathick liquids, purees,
    particulate solids with compensations of double swallows, small bolus sizes,
    self-assessment of voice quality

Hospital day 18
  Diet expanded to include thick liquids
  Calorie count adequate; NGFT discontinued

Hospital day 32
  Discharge to home
  PO intake with ventilator support
  Plan for outpatient follow-up

One month post discharge
  Conducted VFSS
  Continue positive pressure mechanical ventilation during meals
  Expand diet to include thin liquids and all solids

CASE 8

Background

Guillain-Barré syndrome
  Acute inflammatory demyelinating polyradiculoneuropathy
  Children and adults
  Both sexes
  Cause unknown
  Usually preceded by a minor viral illness
  May be associated with AIDS, Lyme disease, vaccines (Swine Flu 1976)
  Symptoms
    Minor tingling in feet and hands
    Symmetrical weakness evolves over several days

Usually legs involved first

Can progress to total paralysis

Death from respiratory failure

A 70-year-old male was admitted with tingling of hands and feet and weakness which progressed to ventilator-dependency and quadriplegia. The patient had a complicated acute medical course over nine months. When he was transferred to a rehabilitation hospital, he remained ventilator-dependent and quadriplegic. He had a nasogastric feeding tube.

Speech–Language Pathology Evaluation

Cognition/language: Intact

Neurologic impairments of respiratory mechanism, larynx, velum/pharynx, tongue, lips/face

Speech: Profound dysarthria with reduced vocal intensity, wet-hoarse phonation, hypernasality, reduced phrase length, and imprecise lingual articulation

Swallow: NPO, NGFT

Speech–Language Pathology Treatment

Cognition/language: Direct intervention not indicated

Speech: Facilitate oral communication
  Strategies:
  Downsize tracheostomy cannula
  Deflate cuff
  Modify ventilator settings
  Increase cuff deflation time/day gradually

Swallow: Facilitate oral alimentation and hydration
  Strategies:
  Conduct periodic videofluoroscopic swallowing studies (VFSS)
  Defer gastrostomy tube placement
  Expand range of bolus consistencies gradually

Treatment Progress

Hospital day 20
  Shiley no. 8 plastic cuffed tracheostomy cannula
  Cuff deflation for speech initiated
  Cuff inflated for VFSS
  Silent subglottic laryngeal penetration with ultrathick and thick liquids
  Conclusion: pharyngeal stage dysphagia
  Recommendation: continue NGFT

Hospital day 48
  Cuff deflation × 4 h/day

Mild to moderate dysarthria with hypernasality, imprecise lingual articulation
Cuff inflated during VFSS; subglottic laryngeal penetration of thick liquid
Cuff then deflated during VFSS
Airway contaminants swept orally by ventilator outflow
Conclusion: pharyngeal stage dysphagia persisted, but "safe" swallowing possible
Recommendations: ventilator-supported oral alimentation/hydration; bolus-restricted diet

Hospital days 76 to 92
Tolerated 9 h/day free time from ventilator
Communicated with no. 6 metal cannula plugged
Progressed to 3 meals/day
NGFT removed

Hospital day 134
Cannula plugged/valved during VFSS
Subglottic laryngeal penetration of ultrathick and thick liquids
Conclusion: persisting pharyngeal stage dysphagia
Recommendation: continue ventilator-supported PO intake

Hospital day 153
Discharged to an extended care facility
Achieved goals of oral communication and oral alimentation/hydration

References

1. American Speech-Language-Hearing Association. Knowledge and skills needed by speech-language pathologists providing services to dysphagic patients/clients. *ASHA* 1990;32(Supplement 2):7–12.
2. American Speech-Language-Hearing Association. Scope of practice in speech-language pathology. *ASHA* 1996;38(Supplement 16):16–20.
3. Teabeaut JR. Aspiration of gastric contents: an experimental study. *Am J Pathol* 1952;28:51–67.
4. Logemann J. *Evaluation and treatment of swallowing disorders.* San Diego: College Hill Press, Inc., 1983.
5. Langmore SE, Terpenning MS, Schork A, et al. Predictors of aspiration pneumonia: how important is dysphagia? *Dysphagia* 1998;13:69–81.
6. Cameron JL, Reynolds J, Zuidema GD. Aspiration in patients with tracheostomies. *Surgery, Gynecol Obstet* 1973;136:68–70.
7. Bone DK, Davis JL, Zuidema GD, et al. Aspiration pneumonia: Prevention of aspiration in patients with tracheostomies. *Annal Thoracic Surg* 1974;18:30–37.
8. Linden P, Siebens AA. Dysphagia: predicting laryngeal penetration. *Arch Phys Med Rehabil* 1983;64:281–284.
9. Siebens AA, Linden P. Neurogenic pharyngeal swallowing disorders. In: Bayless TM ed. *Current therapy in gastroenterology and liver disease.* Philadelphia: BC Decker, Inc., 1984:32–36.
10. Beeken L, Claman F. A return to normal eating after curative treatment for oral cancer: what are the long-term prospects? *Eur J Cancer* 1994;30B:387–392.
11. Schliephake H, Neukam FW, Schmelzeisen R, et al. Long-term quality of life after ablative intraoral tumour surgery. *J Cranio-Maxillo-Facial Surg* 1995;23:243–249.
12. Siebens AA. Rehabilitation for swallowing impairment. In: Kottke FJ, Lehmann JF, eds. *Krusen's handbook of physical medicine and rehabilitation.* Philadelphia: W.B. Saunders, Inc., 1990:765–777.
13. Cunningham ET, Donner MW, Jones B, et al. Anatomical and physiological overview. In: Jones B, Donner MW, eds. *Normal and abnormal swallowing: imaging in diagnosis and therapy.* New York: Springer-Verlag 1991:7–32.
14. Palmer JB, DuChane AS. Rehabilitation of swallowing disorders due to stroke. In: Goldberg G, ed. *Physical medicine and rehabilitation clinics of North America.* Philadelphia: WB Saunders, Inc., 1991:529–546.
15. Donner MW, Bosma JF, Robertson DL. Anatomy and physiology of the pharynx. *Gastrointest Radiol* 1985;10:196–212.
16. Kinnear WJM, Shneerson JM. Assisted ventilation at home: is it worth considering? *Br J Dis Chest* 1985;79:313–351.
17. O'Donohue WJ, Giovannoni RM, Goldberg AI, et al. Long-term mechanical ventilation: guidelines for management in the home and at alternate community sites. *Chest* 1986;90:1S–37S.
18. Betts RH. Post-tracheostomy aspiration. *New Engl J Med* 1965;273:155.
19. Feldman SA, Deal CW, Urquhart W. Disturbance of swallowing after tracheostomy. *Lancet* 1966;1:954–955.
20. Buckwalter JA, Sasaki CT. Effect of tracheotomy on laryngeal function. *Otolaryngol Clin of North Am* 1984;17:41–48.
21. Weber B. Eating with a trach. *Am J Nursing* 1974;74:1439.
22. Leverment JN, Pearson FG, Rae S. A manometric study of the upper oesophagus in the dog following cuffed-tube tracheostomy. *Br J Anaesthesia* 1976;48:83–89.
23. Bonanno PC. Swallowing dysfunction after tracheostomy. *Annals Surg* 1971;174:29–33.
24. Muz J, Mathog RH, Nelson R, et al. Aspiration in patients with head and neck cancer and tracheostomy. *Am J Otolaryngol* 1989;10:282–286.
25. Siebens AA, Tippett DC, Kirby N, et al. Dysphagia and expiratory air flow. *Dysphagia* 1993;8:266–269.
26. Cooper JD, Grillo HC. Analysis of problems related to cuffs on intratracheal tubes. *Chest* 1972;62:21S–27S.
27. Tippett DC, Palmer J, Linden P. Management of dysphagia in a patient with closed head injury. *Dysphagia* 1987;1:221–226.

28. American Speech-Language-hearing Association. Code of ethics. *ASHA* 1994;40(Suppl 18):43–45.

29. Yorkston KM, Beukelman DR. *Assessment of intelligibility of dysarthric speech.* Tigard, Oregon: CC Publication, Inc., 1981.

30. Enderby PM. *Frenchay dysarthria assessment.* Austin, TX: Pro-Ed, Inc., 1983.

31. Drummond SS. *Dysarthria examination battery.* Tucson, AZ: Communication Skill Builders, 1993.

32. Netsell R, Daniel B. Dysarthria in adults: physiologic approach to rehabilitation. *Arch Phys Med Rehabil* 1979;60:502–508.

33. Linden P, Kuhlemeier KV, Patterson C. The probability of correctly predicting subglottic penetration from clinical observations. *Dysphagia* 1993;8:170–179.

34. Linden P, Shaughnessy A. Evaluating and treating the neurogenic dysphagic patient: an individual approach. *ASHA* 1985;27:179.

35. Linden P. Practical approaches in the rehabilitation of swallowing. Paper presented at the Johns Hopkins Symposium on Dysphagia, Baltimore, Maryland, February 1986.

36. Logemann J, Lazarus C, Jenkins P. The relationship between clinical judgment and radiographic assessment of aspiration. Paper presented at the Annual Convention of the American Speech-Language-Hearing Association, Toronto, November 1982.

37. Splaingard ML, Hutchins B, Sulton LD, et al. Aspiration in rehabilitation patients: videofluoroscopy vs bedside clinical assessment. *Arch Phy Med Rehabil* 1988;69:637–640.

38. Scales KD, Patterson CS, Linden PL. Correlation between clinical and motion fluoroscopy observations of swallowing. *ASHA* 1988;30:197.

39. Horner J, Massey EW. Silent aspiration following stroke. *Neurology* 1988;38:317–319.

40. Horner J, Massey EW, Riski JE, et al. Aspiration following stroke: clinical correlates and outcome. *Neurology* 1988;38:1359–1362.

41. Horner J, Massey EW, Brazer SR. Aspiration in bilateral stroke patients. *Neurology* 1990;40:1686–1688.

42. Sorin R, Somers S, Austin W, et al. The influence of videofluoroscopy on the management of the dysphagic patient. *Dysphagia* 1988;2:127–135.

43. Thompson-Henry S, Braddock B. The modified Evan's (sic) blue dye procedure fails to detect aspiration in the tracheostomized patient: five case reports. *Dysphagia* 1995;10:172–174.

44. Leder S. Comment on Thompson-Henry and Braddock: the modified Evan's (sic) blue dye procedure fails to detect aspiration in the tracheostomized patient: five case reports. *Dysphagia* 1996;11:80–81.

45. Tippett DC, Siebens AA. Reconsidering the value of the modified Evans blue dye test: a comment on Thompson-Henry and Braddock (1995). *Dysphagia* 1996;11:78–79.

46. Tippett DC, Siebens AA. Validating the modified Evans blue dye swallowing test. *ASHA* 1995;37:84.

47. Langmore SE, Schatz K, Olson N. Endoscopic and videofluoroscopic evaluation of swallowing and aspiration. *Annal Otol Rhinol Laryngol* 1991;100:678–681.

48. Langmore SE, Schatz K, Olsen N. Fiberoptic endoscopic examination of swallowing safety: a new procedure. *Dysphagia* 1988;2:216–219.

49. Langmore SE, Logemann JA. After the bedside clinical swallowing examination: what next? *Am J Speech-Language Pathol* 1991;1:13–20.

50. Siebens AA, Linden P. Dynamic imaging for swallowing reeducation. *Gastrointest Radiol* 1985;10:251–253.

51. Linden P. Videofluoroscopy in the rehabilitation of swallowing dysfunction. *Dysphagia* 1989;3:189–191.

52. Palmer JB, DuChane AS, Donner MW. Role of radiology in rehabilitation of swallowing. In: B Jones, Donner MW, eds. *Normal and abnormal swallowing: imaging in diagnosis and therapy.* New York: Springer-Verlag 1991:215–225.

53. Palmer JB, Kuhlemeier KV, Tippett DC, Lynch C. A protocol for the videofluorographic swallowing study. *Dysphagia* 1993;8:209–214.

54. Logemann JA, Kahrilas PJ, Kobara M, et al. The benefit of head rotation on pharyngoesophageal dysphagia. *Arch Phys Med Rehabil* 1989;70:767–771.

55. Leder SB, Tarro JM, Burrell MI. Effect of occlusion of a tracheotomy tube on aspiration. *Dysphagia* 1996;11:254–258.
56. Leder SB, Ross DA, Burrell MI, et al. Tracheotomy tube occlusion status and aspiration in early postsurgical head and neck cancer patients. *Dysphagia* 1998;13:167–171.
57. Leder SB. Aspiration following use of one-way tracheostomy speaking valve in previously aspirating patients. *ASHA Leader* 1998;3:133.
58. Tippett DC, Siebens AA. Using ventilators for speaking and swallowing. *Dysphagia* 1991;6:94–99.
59. Hofman P. Critical path method: an important tool for coordinating clinical care. *J Quality Improve* 1994:235–246.
60. Shekim L. Critical pathways. *Quality Improve Digest* 1994:1–10.
61. Vogelman L, Siebens A, Saunders J, et al. Algorithm for dysphagia assessment in tracheotomized patients. Poster presented at the Fourth Annual Dysphagia Research Society Meeting, McLean, Virginia, October 1995.

7

Pediatric Considerations

LYNN E. DRIVER

Continued, rapid advances in medical technology have resulted in a dramatic increase in the survival rate of medically fragile infants and children over the past decade. Based on information reported in three separate studies with relatively large subject groups (n = 101, 130, 155), the mortality rate for children with tracheostomy and ventilator dependence ranges from 22% to 30% (1). The majority of these deaths (70% to 84%) occur during the first year following surgery, are primarily due to illness, and are slightly higher among the ventilator-dependent group. Following the second year, the percentage of deaths attributed to airway and mechanical difficulties increases to approximately one-half. Children under 13 months of age who require either tracheostomy or ventilator assistance for more than one month are generally considered to be long-term or chronic tracheostomy and/or ventilator users (1). The combination of increased survival rate and growth of managed care has resulted in earlier hospital discharge of these children. This, in turn, has resulted in the need for increased education and training of all medical professionals as well as families in the specialized care needs of children with tracheostomy and ventilator dependence. Critical aspects of this care include facilitation of functional oral communication, feeding, and swallowing abilities.

Estimates from the U.S. Congress in their 1987 report on technology-assisted children are that the annual number of children in the United States requiring long-term (one month or longer) mechanical ventilation is between 680 and 2,000. Although similar estimates for children with long-term tracheostomy are not available, the number is likely to be at least as large considering that the majority

Tracheostomy and Ventilator Dependency: Management of Breathing, Speaking, and Swallowing. Edited by Donna C. Tippett, MPH, MA, CCC-SLP. Thieme Medical Publishers, Inc. New York © 2000.

of long-term ventilator users have tracheostomies, and an additional number of children exist with long-term tracheostomies who do not require mechanical ventilation (2).

It has been reported that 85% of children who require tracheostomies are less than one year of age at the time they receive them (3). There is evidence that the presence of a chronic tracheostomy during critical periods of speech and language acquisition can alter the normal course of development (4–9). In addition to the tracheostomy, the conditions necessitating it (e.g., bronchopulmonary dysplasia (BPD), craniofacial anomalies) often have an adverse impact on the development of oral motor skills critical for normal feeding, swallowing, and articulation (10).

This chapter addresses the impact of tracheostomy and ventilator dependence on oral communication, feeding, and swallowing abilities in children, with a focus on the developmental aspects of each. It is divided into three main sections: Respiratory Considerations; Oral Communication; Feeding and Swallowing. The first section includes a brief review of normal anatomy and physiology of respiration, highlighting those aspects unique to pediatrics. A short discussion of medical conditions commonly associated with chronic tracheostomy and ventilator dependence is also provided. This section concludes with an overview of respiratory management, including tracheostomy tube selection and types of ventilation. The next section addresses the impact of tracheostomy and ventilator dependence on oral communication and emphasizes the importance of an interdisciplinary model. It includes a thorough description of assessment, including advantages and disadvantages of specific types of tracheostomy tubes, protocols for tracheostomy tube selection and use, and manipulation of ventilator parameters to promote oral communication. In addition, the specialized needs of prelinguistic ventilator-assisted children are reviewed, including a discussion of treatment and outcome. The final section addresses the impact of tracheostomy and ventilator dependence on feeding and swallowing. It reviews aspects of anatomy and physiology of swallowing unique to pediatrics, highlights typical conditions associated with dysphagia in children with tracheostomy and ventilator dependence, and addresses the impact of respiratory compromise, including prolonged intubation, tracheostomy, and ventilation on the development of feeding and swallowing, concluding with a discussion of assessment and treatment.

Anatomy and Physiology of Respiration

The respiratory system is composed of the upper and the lower airways. The upper airway consists of the nose, mouth, pharynx, and larynx. The lower airway consists of the tracheobronchial tree and the lungs.

Upper Airway

The upper airway has many functions. Its primary role in respiration is to warm, filter, and humidify inspired air while conducting it to the lower airway. In addition, it has an integral role in the processes of speech, taste, and smell. The mucous membranes covering much of the upper airway structures are softer, looser, and more fragile in infants and young children than in older children and adults, and more susceptible to edema and injury from trauma.

Nose

All passageways within the nasal cavity allow for filtration and humidification of air entering the upper airway, as well as detection of odors. All children are obligate nasal breathers during the first six months of life, during which time the soft palate is in close anatomic approximation with the epiglottis. This factor combined with the large size of the tongue relative to the oral cavity at this age renders nasal patency essential for maintaining an airway. Those children with nasal obstructions such as choanal atresia (11) are at risk for respiratory compromise (cyanosis) during feeding.

Mouth

The lips, mandible, maxilla, cheeks, teeth, tongue, and palate are the most important components of the oral cavity with regard to manipulation of airflow for respiration and speech production. The infant tongue takes up a larger area in the mouth and rests more anteriorly in the oral cavity than that of the adult (Fig. 7–1). There are numerous congenital craniofacial anomalies, often associated with syndromes, that have an adverse impact on airflow. Some anomalies, such as cleft palate, prevent sufficient valving of the air stream, resulting in inaccurate production of speech sounds. Other anomalies, such as glossoptosis (oropharyngeal or hypopharyngeal obstruction during feeding caused by tongue retraction, and common in Pierre Robin Sequence), can result in blockage of the air stream and subsequent respiratory distress.

Pharynx

The pharynx, a muscular tube shared by the respiratory and digestive tracts, is sometimes referred to as the aerodigestive tract, and serves vital functions for both respiration and swallowing. It is divided into three portions: the nasopharynx, oropharynx, and the hypopharynx. The pharynx in an infant is gently curved, and as the child grows and develops the angle increases to approximately 90° (Fig. 7–1).

The nasopharynx is the portion of the pharynx directly behind the nasal cavity, extending from the roof of the nasal cavity to the roof of the mouth. In addition to conducting air, the nasopharynx also acts as a resonator for voice. The eustachian tubes from the middle ear open into the nasopharynx. The eustachian tubes in an infant and young child run horizontally, changing to a more vertical plane as the child matures. The adenoids are located in the roof of the nasopharynx, and can interfere with air passage when enlarged. The adenoids increase in size during the first year of life and atrophy by puberty. In some children the adenoids can act to compensate for velopharyngeal incompetence by completing closure. For this reason it is important to assess velopharyngeal structure and function prior to removing the adenoids.

The oropharynx is that portion of the pharynx directly behind the oral cavity, extending from the roof of the mouth (pharyngeal aspect of the soft palate) down

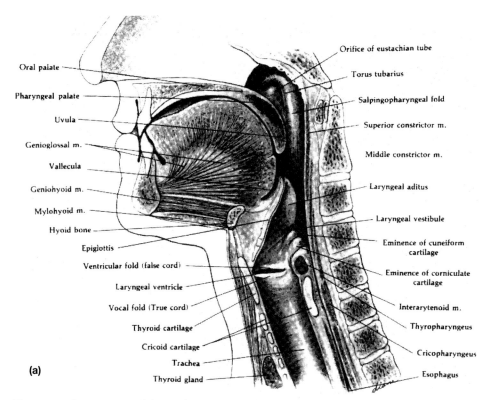

Oral palate

Pharyngeal palate

Uvula

Genioglossal m.

Vallecula

Geniohyoid m.

Mylohyoid m.

Hyoid bone

Epiglottis

Ventricular fold (false cord)

Laryngeal ventricle

Vocal fold (True cord)

Thyroid cartilage

Cricoid cartilage

Trachea

Thyroid gland

(a)

Orifice of eustachian tube

Torus tubarius

Salpingopharyngeal fold

Superior constrictor m.

Middle constrictor m.

Laryngeal aditus

Laryngeal vestibule

Eminence of cuneiform cartilage

Eminence of corniculate cartilage

Interarytenoid m.

Thyropharyngeus

Cricopharyngeus

Esophagus

Fig. 7–1. Comparison of the oral cavity and pharynx of the infant with that of the adult. **a:** Anatomy of adult oral cavity and pharynx. Reprinted, with permission, from Bosma, Donner, Tanaka, et al. (47).

to the base of the tongue, at the level of the tip of the epiglottis. Movement of the pharyngeal walls in this portion, together with elevation of the soft palate and the posterior portion of the tongue, are crucial for velopharyngeal closure. Inadequate closure, or velopharyngeal incompetence, can result in disordered speech production.

The hypopharynx extends from the base of the tongue at the level of the hyoid bone and tip of epiglottis down to the entrance to the larynx and esophagus.

Larynx

The larynx is a complex structure that serves a variety of functions for both respiration and communication. It is composed of cartilage, muscle, and ligaments, and functions as the entrance to and protection for the lower airway, as well as provides for phonation. The infant's larynx is situated higher in the neck at birth, much closer to the base of the tongue, with the thyroid cartilage directly under the hyoid bone (Fig. 7–1). The cricoid cartilage is the lowest portion of the larynx. It is at the level of the second or third cervical vertebra in infants, forms a complete ring, and represents the narrowest portion of the larynx in infants and small children. For this reason, it is particularly susceptible to damage from

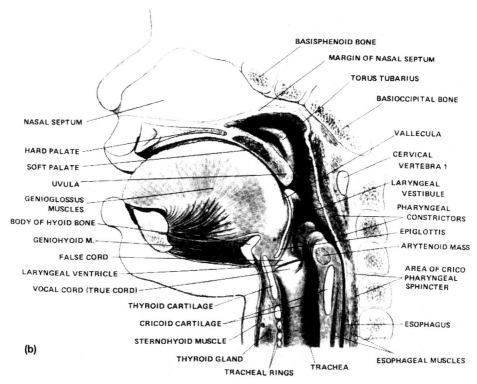

Fig. 7–1 *(continued)* **b:** Anatomy of infant oral cavity and pharynx. Reprinted, with permission, from Kramer (48).

trauma (e.g., from passage of endotracheal tubes) which can result in subglottic stenosis, scarring, or granuloma formation. At birth the larynx has a wider, more funnel-like shape, becoming straighter and more elongated with age, as it descends. The epiglottis is a thin, broad, u-shaped cartilage which serves to protect the open airway by descending to cover the glottis or opening between the vocal folds, during swallowing. The infant's epiglottis and soft palate are in direct approximation, providing added protection against aspiration and promoting coordination of the suck–swallow pattern with respiration (Fig. 7–1). The passage of air through the vocal folds creates vibration, producing sound.

Lower Airway

The lower airway consists of the tracheobronchial tree and the lungs. The tracheobronchial tree consists of a system of connecting tubes that conduct airflow in and out of the lungs and allow for gas exchange.

Trachea

The trachea is situated anteriorly to the esophagus, beginning at the cricoid cartilage and extending inferiorly to the carina, where it bifurcates into the right and

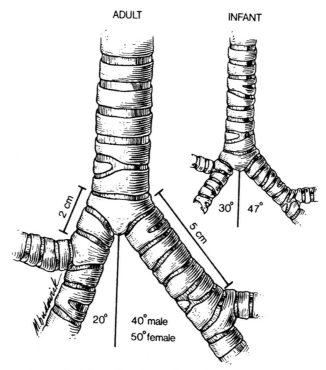

Fig. 7–2. Comparison of adult and pediatric bronchi. Reprinted, with permission, from Finucane and Santora (49).

left mainstem bronchi. The infant carina angulates at the mainstem bronchi fairly symmetrically, whereas the adult right and left mainstem bronchi angulate at 20° and 40° to 50°, respectively (Fig. 7–2). The infant tracheal diameter is approximately 0.55 cm, compared to 1.5 to 2.5 cm in the adult. It is composed of C-shaped cartilage rings joined by connective tissue. These cartilage rings assist in keeping the trachea open during breathing. As noted above, the mucous membranes of the trachea are softer, looser, and more fragile than those of the adult, and more susceptible to damage, increasing the risk of obstruction from edema or inflammation.

Lungs

The lungs are situated in the thoracic cavity, enclosed by the rib cage and diaphragm, the major muscle of ventilation, which separates the thoracic cavity from the abdominal cavity. The diaphragm in an infant is flatter than an adult's, resulting in less efficient functioning for respiration (Fig. 7–3). The lungs consist of five lobes. The right lung has three lobes: the upper, middle, and lower. The left lung has two lobes: the upper and lower. The primary function of the lungs is gas exchange in the form of absorption of oxygen and elimination of carbon dioxide. The air passages in infants and small children are much smaller, increasing their

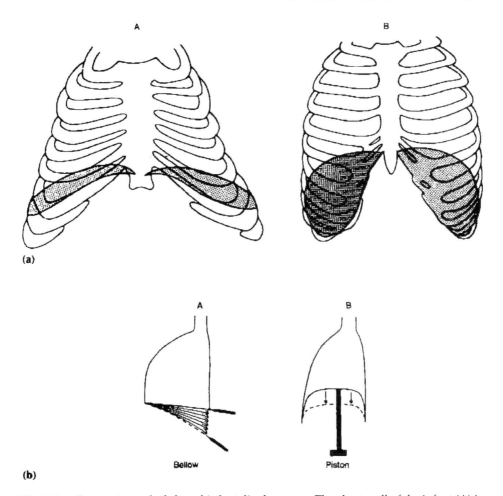

Fig. 7–3. Comparison of adult and infant diaphragm. **a:** The chest wall of the infant (A) is triangular shaped compared to that of the adult (B). **b:** Ventilation in the infant is due to a bellows-like action (A) compared to the piston effect of the diaphragm in the adult (B). Reprinted, with permission, from Greenough, Milner, and Robertson (50).

susceptibility to obstruction. The respiratory bronchioles, alveolar ducts, and alveoli grow in number until about eight years of age, after which they continue to grow in size. The chest wall of an infant is more compliant than that of an older child or adult.

As illustrated above, there are a number of important differences between the pediatric and adult respiratory systems. Many of these differences contribute to increased susceptibility of infants and children to respiratory dysfunction in the presence of illness or injury, with subsequent need for tracheostomy and/or mechanical ventilation. The following section provides a brief description of medical conditions commonly associated with tracheostomy and ventilator dependence, as well as an overview of respiratory management in these cases.

Etiologies in Children

The primary diagnoses of children requiring chronic tracheostomy and/or ventilator dependence include trauma, congenital conditions, progressive neurologic disorders, and acquired nontrauma. Common traumatic injuries resulting in the need for tracheostomy and/or ventilator dependence include high-level spinal cord injuries (SCI) and severe traumatic brain injuries. Common congenital conditions requiring mechanical ventilation include congenital central hypoventilation syndrome (CCHS), bronchopulmonary dysplasia (BPD), tracheomalacia, congenital heart defects, diaphragmatic hernia, and Chiari malformation (12). Progressive neurologic disorders such as Friedreich's ataxia, muscular dystrophy, and certain myopathies also can result in eventual ventilator dependence. Finally, tracheostomy and/or ventilator dependence can become a necessity in acquired nontraumatic conditions such as cancer and meningitis. The actual medical conditions resulting in the need for tracheostomy and/or mechanical ventilation within these diagnostic groups are diverse, but can be grouped according to type of respiratory insufficiency or systems. Primary types of respiratory insufficiency include bellows failure (e.g., SCI, myopathy), congenital central hypoventilation, chronic lung disease, and airway problems (e.g., tracheomalacia). The primary causes of respiratory insufficiency may originate in the respiratory, cardiovascular, neurologic, or musculoskeletal systems. It is important to note that the causes of respiratory failure and subsequent need for mechanical ventilation are not always respiratory disease or disorder. The lungs themselves may be healthy, but the access to them or the systems that contribute to their function may be impaired.

Respiratory Management

A primary means of airway management in the presence of chronic respiratory insufficiency is a tracheostomy. As noted above, common conditions requiring tracheostomy include airway obstruction, chronic lung disease, and neurologic impairment resulting in bellows failure or central hypoventilation. Tracheostomy provides a secure airway, long-term airway access, and a means for interface with mechanical ventilatory devices, and as such is the most frequently used method of airway management (13).

Tracheostomy

A tracheostomy is an artificial opening created between the outer surface of the neck and the trachea between the second and third tracheal rings. The opening itself is referred to as the stoma, and the tracheostomy tube inserted into the trachea through the stoma serves to maintain the opening as well as provide a means for connecting mechanical ventilatory devices (for more detailed discussion of tracheostomy procedure and medical complications, see Chapter 4). Placement of the tracheostomy tube diverts airflow away from the trachea through the tube and out the neck, bypassing the upper airway. Depending on the size and type of tracheostomy tube, a portion of the airflow may still pass around the tube and through the vocal folds; this may or may not be sufficient to produce sound.

Tracheostomy Tube Selection

Once the decision has been made to place a tracheostomy, a number of decisions must be made regarding type of tracheostomy tube, often related to the original reason for the procedure. Information necessary to make these decisions includes the child's age and weight (14), diameter of the trachea, respiratory requirements, distance from the tracheal opening to the carina, type of neck plate or flange, use of adapters, use of inner cannula, flexibility of cannula, and presence of cuff.

Determining the child's age and weight allows for an estimate of the basic size of tracheostomy tube needed. For more accurate selection, bronchoscopy can be performed to determine the diameter of the trachea. This procedure is used more routinely in children than in adults to avoid placement of a tube that is too large, potentially damaging the developing tissue in the trachea.

The respiratory requirements of a child can also affect the decision regarding diameter of the tracheostomy tube. If a child has significant ventilatory and/or tracheobronchial demands requiring high-ventilator pressures or frequent suctioning, selection of a tube with a relatively large diameter may be optimal. If these are not issues, use of a smaller diameter tube may be possible. Because this decision will determine the degree of leakage of air around the tube and through the upper airway, affecting ability to achieve voicing, it is a critical aspect of the decision-making process.

It is important to determine the distance from the tracheal opening to the carina, as this will determine the optimal length of the tube. This can be assessed through chest x-ray. The tube should not be in direct contact with the carina, as this can result in severe bronchospasm due to the high innervation and tactile sensitivity of the carina. For this reason, neonatal tracheostomy tubes are significantly shorter than pediatric tubes.

The anatomic configuration of the infant's or child's neck, as well as the anticipated need for mechanical ventilation, assists in determining the appropriate neck plate or flange. Because the neck plate rests against the child's skin at the proximal end of the tracheostomy tube, it must fit well to avoid skin breakdown or air leakage around the stoma. For infants, who have shorter necks, a flange such as the Bivona Aberdeen-style neck plate (Bivona Medical Technologies, Gary, Indiana) is chosen due to its unique V-shape allowing better fit and increased comfort (Fig. 7–4).

If the tracheostomy tube is connected to a ventilator, the proximal end, or hub, needs to have an outer diameter of 15 mm. If the tracheostomy tube itself does not have a 15 mm hub or adapter as a component, an external adapter is needed. The type of adapter selected depends on the needs of the child; in the case of infants or children who are mobile, a swivel connector or adapter with multiple articulations is often used to allow freedom of movement while minimizing danger of excessive torque or accidental decannulation.

An inner cannula, a removable insert that fits inside the outer cannula of the tracheostomy tube, is sometimes used to allow for easier cleaning of the tube. The inner cannula can be removed and cleaned as often as needed to prevent build up of secretions and reduce likelihood of mucus plugging. This also reduces the frequency of required tracheostomy tube changes. Use of an inner can-

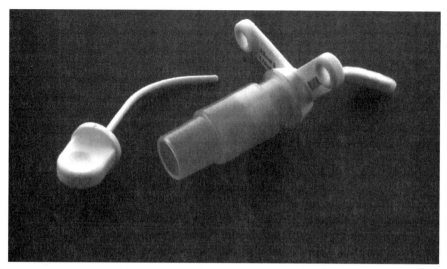

Fig. 7–4. Bivona pediatric cuffless tracheostomy tube, with Aberdeen-style neck plate. Photo courtesy of Bivona Medical Technologies, Gary, Indiana.

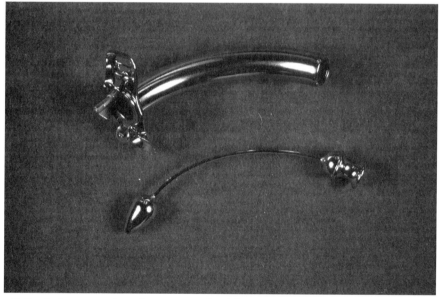

Fig. 7–5. Jackson metal tracheostomy tube. Photo courtesy of Pilling Weck, Research Triangle Park, North Carolina.

nula reduces the inner diameter of the tube, decreasing the amount of airflow through the tube. For this reason, it is typically not used in pediatric tracheostomy tubes, as the reduction in inner diameter for such a small cannula represents a significant proportion of the overall passageway and can impede airflow.

Tracheostomy tubes are available in different materials of varying pliability. They can be composed of metal, polyvinylchloride (PVC), or silicone. Metal tra-

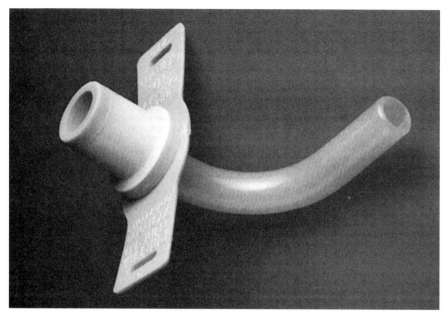

Fig. 7–6. Portex cuffless tracheostomy tube, composed of polyvinylchloride (PVC). Photo courtesy of SIMS Portex, Inc., Keene, New Hampshire.

cheostomy tubes are rarely used in children due to increased likelihood of pressure necrosis due to weight, greater risk of tissue erosion due to rigidity, reduction in airway diameter due to presence of inner cannula, increased potential for skin irritation due to oxidation and heat/cold reactivity, tendency to promote increased production of mucus, and absence of 15 mm hub (Fig. 7–5). Because metal tubes do not have a hub that protrudes beyond the stoma, the external adapter must be inserted into the tracheostomy cannula, resulting in a narrowing of the lumen at the point of insertion. PVC tubes are somewhat flexible, nontoxic, lightweight, soften at body temperature, and are less irritating to the skin than metal tubes (Fig. 7–6). The plastic material is smoother and has less surface tension than a metal tube, reducing potential accumulation of secretions. Silicone tubes are softer and more flexible than PVC tubes and are reported to be less irritating and potentially less damaging to the tracheal tissue (Fig. 7–7). They are also a good option for those children who experience an allergic reaction to PVC.

With few exceptions, the use of cuffed tracheostomy tubes is not recommended in infants and young children because of the potential damage the inflated cuff can cause to the delicate mucosa of the developing trachea. Typically, due to the relatively small diameter of the pediatric trachea, cuffs are not necessary to maintain ventilation. In certain instances, however, when a child is unable to be adequately ventilated with a cuffless tube, a cuff may be necessary. There are several different types of cuffs available depending on the needs of the child (Fig. 7–8). If a cuff is necessary for chronic ventilation, either a high-volume, low-pressure air cuff or a foam cuff are acceptable options. Unfortunately, the foam cuff does not allow for maintenance of partial deflation over time, making it a poor choice for a child with a potential for oral communication. For those children who are nonoral and have high ventilation needs, the Bivona Fome cuff tracheostomy tube

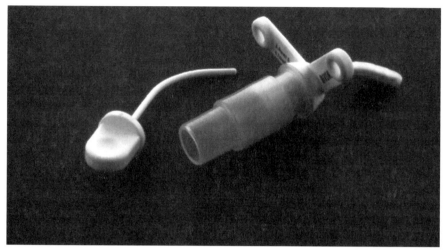

Fig. 7–7. Bivona pediatric cuffless tracheostomy tube, composed of silicone. Photo courtesy of Bivona Medical Technologies, Gary, Indiana.

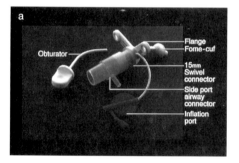

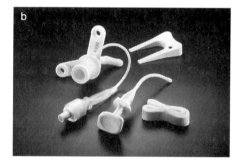

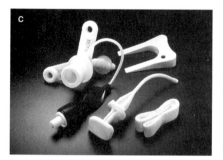

Fig. 7–8. Cuffed tracheostomy tubes. **a:** Bivona pediatric Fome cuff tracheostomy tube (cuff made of soft foam with silicone covering). **b:** Bivona Tight-to-the-Shaft (TTS) cuffed tracheostomy tube (high-pressure, low-volume air cuff made of silicone which approximates a cuffless tube when deflated). **c:** Bivona cuffed tracheostomy tube (low-pressure, high-volume air cuff). Photos courtesy of Bivona Medical Technologies, Gary, Indiana.

(Bivona Medical Technologies, Gary, Indiana) is an excellent option because the pilot balloon of the cuff can be integrated into the ventilator circuitry such that the cuff inflates and deflates with the inspiratory and expiratory cycles of the ventilator, respectively, thereby providing automatic pressure relief to minimize risk of tracheal damage. In addition to the inflated cuff, the presence of a cuffless tracheostomy tube that is large enough to prevent airflow around the tube may also

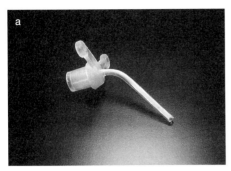
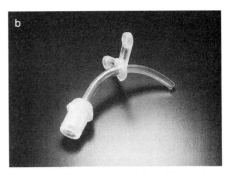

Fig. 7–9. Bivona custom tracheostomy tubes. **a:** Tracheostomy tube with cuffless, elongated precurved shaft to accommodate unique anatomy and tracheomalacia distal to a standard length shaft. **b:** Tracheostomy tube with precurved shaft, proximal extension to reduce risk of obstruction from chin flexion, and wire reinforcement to prevent kinking. Photos courtesy of Bivona Medical Technologies, Gary, Indiana.

increase the risk of tracheal injury in the form of stenosis or fistula. Thus, careful consideration and thorough knowledge of all potential contributing factors is critical to successful airway management.

It should be noted that standard, commercially available tracheostomy tubes sometimes do not meet the requirements for a particular child. For example, the optimal diameter or length of the tracheostomy tube may be in between standard sizes. When this happens, it is possible to order a custom tracheostomy tube which is made to meet whatever specifications are given (Fig. 7–9). Because such tubes are significantly more expensive and often require additional time to fabricate, standard tracheostomy tubes are preferable to custom tubes whenever possible.

Before discussing the potential impact of tracheostomy on oral communication, mechanical ventilation will be reviewed as it relates to airway management in children.

Mechanical Ventilation

Once it is determined that a child will require chronic mechanical ventilation, factors to be assessed include the most appropriate type of ventilation, degree of dependence, level of support, and ability and acceptance to wean (15). The most common types of mechanical ventilation include positive pressure ventilation (PPV) via nasal mask or tracheostomy tube, and negative pressure ventilation (NPV). PPV is the more common of these methods and refers to the act of applying positive (above atmospheric) pressure to force air into the lung, requiring either an artificial airway such as an endotracheal (ET) tube or tracheostomy tube to connect to the ventilator, or use of a nasal mask or mouthpiece, as with Bi-Pap (r) (Bi-Level Positive Airway Pressure, Respironics, Inc., Murrysville, PA). NPV refers to a noninvasive method involving the use of negative (below atmospheric) pressure within a chamber surrounding the chest and abdomen (Fig. 7–10). This negative pressure creates a vacuum which results in airflow into the chest and expansion of the lungs (see Chapters 3 and 4). This method works well with children who have relatively normal airways and mobile chests. The two major types of negative pressure ventilation devices are the body tank respirator, or iron lung, and the chest shell, or cuirass.

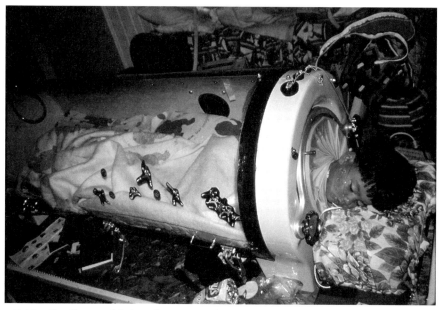

Fig. 7–10. Small, portable iron lungs are often used for negative pressure ventilation of children who require nighttime ventilation, but do not have a tracheostomy.

The degree of dependence of a child on mechanical ventilation assists in determining the type of ventilation used as well as the level of support needed. As noted above, for those children with significant respiratory disease or rigid chest walls, negative pressure is not sufficient to ventilate them. For a child with high tetraplegia and no ability to breathe above the ventilator, positive pressure ventilation via tracheostomy tube is the best option (Fig. 7–11). Positive pressure ventilation can be delivered via two types of ventilators, pressure ventilators and volume ventilators. With pressure ventilators, the pressure at which the air is forced into the lungs is preset, and the volume is variable depending on the lung compliance. With volume ventilators, the volume of air delivered with each breath is preset, allowing variable pressure to achieve this set volume.

In addition to pressure and volume, other variables to consider in assessing a child's ventilatory needs include the mode and rate. Mode may be determined by the child's ability to initiate a breath and refers to how the ventilator functions with respect to that ability. Common modes used with children include assist-control (AC) and synchronized intermittent mandatory ventilation (SIMV). Assist-control refers to a setting whereby the ventilator delivers a breath at regular, set intervals, but can be triggered to deliver additional breaths at the full tidal volume when initiated by the child. SIMV refers to a mode whereby the ventilator responds to the child's inspiratory effort and adjusts its timing of delivered breaths to coordinate with the child's rhythm in order to prevent breath stacking.

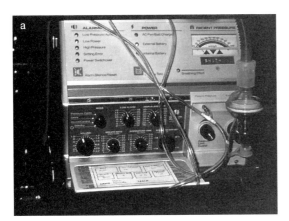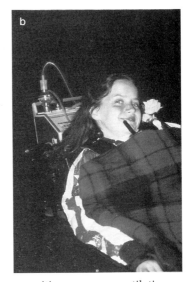

Fig. 7–11. Children with high tetraplegia are typically on positive pressure ventilation. **a:** Portable volume ventilators such as this one are often mounted on a solid tray on the back of the power wheelchair. **b:** Children who are dependent on power mobility use portable volume ventilators mounted on the rear of their wheelchairs.

Rate refers to the number of breaths delivered in 1 min, and can be a function of the volume per breath delivered, or tidal volume, and the total volume required per minute, referred to as minute ventilation. For example, if a child requires 6 L of air delivered per minute (minute ventilation of 6 L) and the tidal volume is set at 600 ml, the rate would need to be 10. This would also mean that 6 s would be available per breath (including both inspiratory and expiratory phases). In order to prevent breath stacking, the ratio of inspired to exhaled air cannot exceed a 1:1 ratio (that is, the time for inspiration cannot exceed the time for exhalation). Thus, the inspiratory time for this child would be a maximum of 3 s. For those children who are speaking while on a ventilator, it is important to maximize their inspiratory time, as this is the phase during which they are able to phonate. This is most commonly accomplished by increasing the tidal volume and/or reducing the rate, resulting in fewer breaths per minute, and longer time per breath.

By this point in our discussion it should be clear that management of children requiring tracheostomy tubes and mechanical ventilation is a complex task with many variables, and involving a number of specialists. Critical members of the management team include the pediatrician, otolaryngologist, respiratory care specialist, pulmonologist, speech–language pathologist, clinical nurse specialist, child, and family/caregiver. Throughout the management process, all decisions must be discussed with the child (if appropriate) and with the family. Their input as well as understanding and acceptance are critical to successful management. Any decisions to be made that may affect the child's medical as well as psychosocial well-being should be a product of team concensus.

Assessing Oral Communication Needs

The two critical components of oral communication (aside from certain cognitive prerequisites) are a sound source for phonation and ability to articulate sufficiently to produce intelligible speech. As noted above, the presence of a tracheostomy tube often reduces or eliminates the movement of air critical for producing sound, hindering oral communication. The extent to which phonation is affected depends in part on the type of tracheostomy tube. If the child requires mechanical ventilation, this can further compromise the ability to phonate. The primary components of oral communication assessment, then, are oral motor function, upper airway status, type of tracheostomy tube, and ventilation parameters if the child is using a ventilator.

Oral Motor Function

Oral motor ability is the first component of oral communication requiring assessment. If a child is severely dysarthric or anarthric secondary to neurologic involvement, with poor prognosis for intelligible speech production, continued assessment of oral communication options is not warranted at that time. Consideration of nonoral options, such as augmentative or alternative communication (AAC) systems is appropriate, with periodic reassessment of oral motor function to monitor any changes over time.

Upper Airway Status

Once adequate oral motor function is established, the upper airway must be assessed as it relates to oral communication. Consultation with the appropriate medical staff on the team, typically, the otolaryrngologist and/or pulmonologist, is necessary at this juncture to obtain information on laryngeal and tracheal structure and function, noting abnormalities such as vocal fold paresis/paralysis, tracheal stenosis, granulation tissue or other obstruction, tracheomalacia, or fistula which might have an impact on oral communication. Presence of any of these complications may limit available options, and medical clearance must be obtained prior to implementing any changes in tracheostomy or ventilator status that might alter respiratory function.

Tracheostomy Tubes

Once a child's potential for oral communication has been established through assessment of oral motor function, vocal fold function, and upper airway status, one can proceed to evaluate the child's tracheostomy tube with regard to communication options. It is important to become familiar with the various types of tracheostomy tubes available, know the advantages and disadvantages of each, be aware of any contraindications, be able to troubleshoot problems effectively, and understand how they interface with the ventilator in production of voice. Comparison charts and protocols for use of specific tracheostomy tubes or adaptations are useful in making decisions and recommendations. An example of these, developed for use at University of Michigan Mott Children's Hospital, is included in Appendix 1. As mentioned previously, an interdisciplinary model is optimal to best meet the complex needs of this population for achieving oral communication.

The primary goal in selecting a tracheostomy tube for purposes of communication is to choose the smallest, simplest tube that will allow for adequate ventilation (see flow chart, Appendix 2, as an example of a decision-making model). Advantages of a small, cuffless tube include a larger "functional" leak of air around the tube and through the vocal folds to produce voice, as well as a reduced risk of tracheal injury secondary to prolonged pressure against the tracheal wall.

An uncuffed tube also allows use of a unidirectional flow valve such as the Passy-Muir Tracheostomy Speaking Valve (Passy-Muir, Inc., Irvine, California) or the Montgomery(r) Tracheostomy Speaking Valve (Boston Medical Products, Inc., Westborough, Massachusetts). This type of valve utilizes a thin silicone membrane that opens on inhalation, allowing air to enter the lungs through the tracheostomy tube, and closes on exhalation, diverting air upward around the tracheostomy tube, through the larynx and out the nose and mouth, providing the airflow necessary for phonation. A byproduct of valve usage includes creation of a variable degree of back pressure in the lungs, commonly known as positive end-expiratory pressure or PEEP. Because increased pressure is necessary to push the air through the small space between the tracheostomy tube and the tracheal wall, some of that pressure exerts in a downward direction toward the lungs. This is often considered a positive feature, particularly in a child for whom distal airway opening is a concern. A unidirectional flow valve should NEVER be used with a cuffed tracheostomy tube unless the cuff is completely deflated. Risks include buildup of excess air, or air stacking, which can result in accumulation of CO_2 and/or damage to the lungs due to overinflation. If a child requires mechanical ventilation, undirectional flow valves that can be placed in the ventilator circuitry are also available [Montgomery (r)Ventrach (TM) Speaking Valve (Boston Medical Products, Inc., Westborough, Massachusetts) and Passy-Muir Ventilator Speaking Valve (Passy Muir, Inc., Irvine, California)]. Use of these valves can potentially double the amount of time that a child on a ventilator can phonate, as voice can now be achieved both on inhalation and exhalation (see Appendix 3 for further information on benefits, contraindications, and troubleshooting related to use of the unidirectional flow valve).

It is important to obtain prior medical clearance for placement of unidirectional flow valves. It is also beneficial to work closely with respiratory care specialists, as they are able to assist with determining the presence of ample airflow around the tracheostomy tube, measuring inner tracheal pressures, monitoring oxygen saturation and carbon dioxide levels, and adjusting the ventilator parameters as needed to compensate for changes in airflow direction and pressure with valve placement for those children requiring mechanical ventilation. Use of a standard protocol for placement of a unidirectional flow valve is common in many institutions, and is strongly recommended (see Appendix 4).

When a child is unable to maintain adequate ventilation with an uncuffed tube, voicing may be achieved through partial cuff deflation. Again, medical clearance should be obtained prior to beginning a trial of cuff deflation. The type of cuff used should also be determined, as cuff materials vary in rate and degree of air diffusion over time, affecting subsequent ability to maintain stable cuff pressures. For example, cuffs made from materials such as soft foam or silicone allow diffusion of air back into the cuff over time (Fig. 7–8). For the child who requires maximal cuff inflation and is at risk for tracheal injury, these cuffs are an excellent option. For the child who can tolerate at least partial cuff deflation and is a candidate for voicing through this means, a more traditional air cuff with the ability to maintain a given cuff pressure over time is recommended. This type of cuff is particularly important for children requiring mechanical ventilation, because any changes in cuff pressure potentially require changes in ventilator settings. This is another instance in which close collaboration with a respiratory care specialist is important for determining pressures and settings optimal for both communication and ventilation. When cuff pressures are manipulated frequently for purposes of voicing, it is important to obtain objective measures of air pressures or volumes both prior to and following cuff deflation; in this way, overinflation of the cuff can be avoided. For those children who require frequent suctioning to manage secretions, there may be a buildup of secretions on the upper surface of the cuff. For this reason, to avoid potential aspiration, suctioning should be done both prior to and immediately following cuff deflation.

When a child has a cuffed tube which must remain maximally inflated at all times to maintain adequate ventilation, airflow through the larynx is not sufficient for phonation. In this instance, for older children or adolescents using adult-size tracheostomy tubes, a "talking" tracheostomy tube may be considered as an option. This type of tube functions just as any other tracheostomy tube for purposes of ventilation. The cannula is equipped with either an extra tube running along its external surface and ending with an opening above the cuff or with multiple small holes or fenestrations in the upper surface. For purposes of communication, they are designed to operate independently of the ventilator cycle, employing an external air source for purposes of communication. In one type (e.g., Portex), air is delivered through the tube running along the external surface of the tracheostomy tube and exits through a port above the level of the cuff, passing through the larynx to permit phonation (Fig. 7–12). Another available type (e.g., Communitrach) delivers air from an external air source through a tube which connects to the tracheostomy tube at the hub, where air exits and travels between the inner and outer cannulae, exiting up through the multiple fenestra-

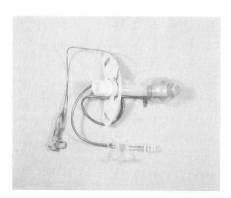

Fig. 7–12. Portex talking tracheostomy tube (Inner cannula not shown). Photo courtesy of SIMS Portex, Inc., Keene, New Hampshire.

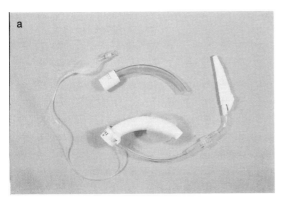
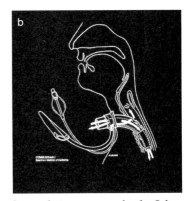

Fig. 7–13.   **a:** Communitrach Talking Tracheostomy Tube with inner cannula. **b:** Schematic of Communitrach in place, illustrating path of diverted airflow from external air source. Photo courtesy of Boston Medical Products, Westborough, Massachusetts.

tions and passing through the larynx to produce voice (Fig. 7–13). In order to activate the external air source for voicing with either type, a port at the external end of the tubing must be occluded, typically accomplished using the thumb. This requires the child to possess adequate cognitive ability and alertness to learn and remember to occlude the port, as well as the motoric capability to do so. For those children with motoric deficits such as high-level spinal cord injury, either the conversational partner must learn to occlude the port when the child wishes to speak or a switch-activated system must be developed which the child can operate independently using an intact motor movement (16).

The voice quality achieved using a "talking" tracheostomy tube is often hoarse, sometimes not much louder than an audible whisper. A relatively common complaint of individuals using "talking" tracheostomy tubes is dryness and tickling sensation in the throat due to the continuous passage of air through the vocal folds. The higher the pressure of air required to produce phonation, the more frequent the complaint of discomfort. Another common difficulty associated with use of the "talking" tracheostomy tube is the buildup of secretions in the fenestrations and/or air tubing, precluding passage of air for phonation. Diligence in keeping these areas free of secretions is essential to successful use of these tubes. Frequent irrigation of the tubing, optimally every time the child is suctioned, is essential to maintain a clear passage for air. "Talking" tracheostomy tubes are not available in pediatric sizes, and are not typically recommended for individuals with poor speech intelligibility or copious secretions. (For further information on benefits, contraindications, and troubleshooting related to use of the "talking" tracheostomy tube, see Appendix 3 and Chapter 5.)

Ventilator Parameters

Throughout assessment of oral communication options for children requiring mechanical ventilation, many of the recommended changes require alterations in the ventilator settings. When there is some potential for variation in ventilator settings, it is important to select the option that promotes the best communication while maintaining adequate ventilation. Through close collaboration with the respiratory care specialist, optimal parameters for achieving this can best be determined.

External Options

When voicing cannot be achieved through any of the options or adaptations described above, external options for voice need to be considered. Alternatives include use of an external sound source such as an electrolarynx or development of an augmentative or alternative communication system.

For those children unable to achieve voice, but with motoric and cognitive ability sufficient to activate a hand-held device, and with oral motor ability adequate for intelligible speech production, a neck or intraoral electrolarynx may be an option. These were originally developed for use with adult laryngectomy patients, and thus are not optimal for use with children. The hand-held devices such as the Servox (TM) (Siemens Hearing Instruments, Inc., Piscataway, NJ) or the Tru-Tone(TM) (Griffin Laboratories, Inc., Temecula, CA) are often too large to hold and operate with one hand, and optimal neck placement is often difficult to determine, partly due to altered resonance from the presence of the tracheostomy tube. Children are often resistant to use of an artificial sound source because of its robotic quality, which can be frightening to some.

In cases where oral communication is not possible, alternative communication options must be considered. For those with temporary loss of oral communication ability, low-technology solutions such as communication boards, simple keyboard-driven electronic voice output devices, or pen and paper may be ample to meet their immediate needs. For those with poor prognosis for oral communication, more sophisticated options may be appropriate. Detailed discussion of AAC assessment and specific devices is beyond the scope of this chapter (17–19).

In summary, the assessment of oral communication in children with tracheostomy and/or ventilator dependence is potentially complex, requiring coordination of input from many sources, including the speech–language pathologist, the pulmonologist, the respiratory care specialist, the otolaryngologist, and the family/primary caregiver. When assessment must be done on an outpatient basis, such coordination becomes difficult. Many facilities have specialty outpatient clinics staffed by multiple disciplines to meet this need. Our facility, University of Michigan Mott Children's Hospital, for example, has developed a multidisciplinary outpatient clinic for ventilator-assisted children. Regardless of the setting in which the assessment takes place, close coordination among members of disciplines appropriate to the child's needs is critical to achieve success while ensuring the safety and well-being of the child.

Tracheostomy and Ventilator Dependence in the Prelinguistic Child

It is widely accepted that the presence of a tracheostomy tube interferes with a child's ability to communicate orally. Several research studies have examined the nature and extent of this interference (4,8,20), with the general consensus that there is no significant long-term effect on the development of speech and language. Birth through five years of age is considered to be the critical period for acquisition of language. In the studies cited, at five years of age the majority of children studied who had previously undergone tracheostomy or received mechanical ventilation had language development commensurate with nonverbal intelligence, and over 80% had speech abilities on a par with their level of language development. Although these children displayed relatively normal verbal skills compared to their own nonverbal abilities, many appeared delayed in comparison to same-age peers. Comparisons of communication outcome both across children within studies and across studies should be done with caution, as the type and intensity of speech-language intervention received by the subjects during periods of tracheostomy was not documented. Further longitudinal research needs to be done which takes a systematic, prospective look at communication development in these children. The larger question, which has only begun to be addressed in the literature, concerns the long-term outcome for language and learning as academic demands increase.

During the first 12 months of life, long before the emergence of first words, infants exhibit intent to communicate using a broad range of prelinguistic exploratory behaviors. Through the use of vocalization, crying, facial expressions, and eye contact, they are developing and refining both oral motor movements that will emerge into intelligible speech, and physiologic and social cues that will develop into social, interactive communication. Interruption of this early prelinguistic development can result in delayed acquisition of critical precursors to expressive communication. Without the ability to vocalize, infants must rely on the patience and willingness of the caregiver to discern needs and wants through nonverbal signals. Caregivers, in turn, must develop the ability to recognize, interpret, and reinforce these nonverbal signals (21). With recent advances in technology providing the means for successful home ventilator management, many infants are being discharged from the hospital setting much earlier in the course of their recovery. The benefits of this earlier discharge are clear, most importantly the removal from a sterile, artificial, overstimulating environment to a more natural, comfortable, familiar setting. The challenges are also clear, placing additional burden on the caregiver to provide for the child's comprehensive physical, emotional, and social needs. Ability of these caregivers to foster the development of prelinguistic communication skills is an important aspect of these responsibilities. This most often requires education and intervention by speech–language pathologists with training in prelinguistic communication development. Ideally, this training and intervention can begin during the period of hospitalization. For example, teaching parents to recognize and respond to a variety of nonverbal communication signals (e.g., facial expressions, body posture, gesture, eye gaze) should begin as early as tolerated by the infant, as such early intervention has been demonstrated to have a significant positive impact on later cognitive and communicative abilities (22).

Hospitalization of an infant for a prolonged period (one month or more) is known to have an adverse effect on overall development (23–25). For those infants requiring tracheostomy and/or mechanical ventilation, the alterations in environment resulting from medical interventions can have a profound negative impact

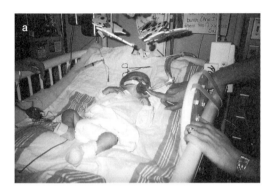
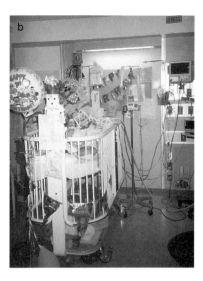
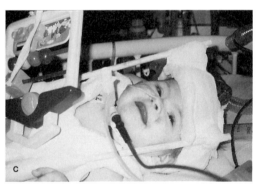
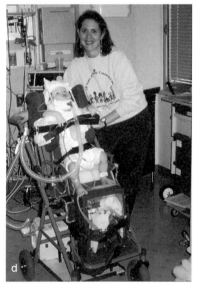

Fig. 7–14. Children in the ICU setting. **a:** Oral intubation and nasogastric tubes have a negative impact on normal development of oral motor and feeding skills, often resulting in oral aversion and hypersensitivity. **b,c:** It is important to provide colorful, positive environmental stimulation to help counteract the negative surroundings of an ICU setting. **d:** Even children with limited mobility and on mechanical ventilation in the ICU setting can be given some degree of mobility with customized seating, typically provided by physical therapy.

on acquisition of critical prelanguage experiences (3) (Fig. 7–14). For example, the frequent alarms and monitor noises can delay auditory awareness. According to Marsh and Handler (26), there is a high incidence of middle ear disease in ventilator-dependent infants. This, combined with a higher than average potential for sensorineural hearing loss in premature infants, may result in reduced auditory experiences. The presence of multiple monitors and tubes often limits the ability of the caregiver to hold the infant, reducing positive tactile input. The additional negative tactile input from repeated intubations, suctioning, oral feeding tubes, and tape to hold tubes in place can result in severe oral and tactile hypersensitivity and defensiveness. This combination of tactile deprivation and trauma, in turn, inhibits oral exploration and positive oral experiences and can impede the natural development of oral motor skills crucial to the acquisition and development of communication and feeding skills.

Prolonged intubation interferes with the natural progression of an infant's oral motor skills from early experiences of sucking on a pacifier, bottle, or breast feeding and mouthing toys, to using those developing lingual and labial movements to experiment with sounds that will later form words. Additional negative sequelae of prolonged intubation include restricted mandibular, lingual, and labial movements, unusually high vaulted palate, and vocal fold injury. Many of these sequelae are not temporary, but persist following removal of the adverse stimulus. Oral–tactile defensiveness can persist long after extubation and result in chronic feeding disorders.

Intervention Strategies

Infants who require tracheostomy and/or mechanical ventilation may not be ready to vocalize until seven or eight months of age, and will be significantly older before being able to time vocalization with the ventilator cycle. Spontaneous vocalizations may occur earlier if sufficient air leakage occurs around the tracheostomy tube. Some infants may be candidates for use of a one-way valve (3), but this should be carefully assessed by the entire team, including the respiratory care specialist, physician, and speech–language pathologist, prior to implementation.

Children who require tracheostomy and/or ventilator dependence for a prolonged period prior to the development of spoken language are at significant risk for delayed language development (6,27,28). For this reason, intervention to stimulate prelinguistic development should begin early. Intervention strategies should incorporate both indirect means such as modification of the environment and care routines to minimize negative stimuli, and direct means such as provision of positive oral experiences for the infant. Because the tracheostomy may prevent the infant from vocalizing, the typical experience of vocal play and experimentation with sounds is not possible. The parent or caregiver needs to anticipate the impact of this inability to vocalize on social interaction and be alert for nonverbal communicative signals. In the intensive care or hospital setting, interactions are typically brief, or the infant's needs are easily anticipated, limiting opportunities for the infant to develop and practice alternative means of communicating messages regarding hunger, discomfort, desire for attention, likes, and dislikes. Parents and caregivers require education regarding ways to initiate interaction with their infant, as well as how to recognize attempts on the part of the infant to respond. For example, the first step in establishing intentional communication involves identifying and promoting mutual attention, first between infant and parent, and then jointly on an object or activity. The environment can be structured to encourage such behaviors, for example, placement of a desired object just out of reach but within the visual field of the infant. Another important step in the development of communication involves recognition of certain nonverbal signals of the infant as intentional, for example, eye gaze, facial expression, or movements of head or body to signal desire or rejection. The final, most important step is the consistent, interactive response on the part of the parent or caregiver to the infant's signals, for example, waving back, verbal acknowledgment (e.g., "you want your bottle, don't you?"), or completion of a nonverbal request (e.g., giving the infant the requested object). In this way, the parent or caregiver reinforces the infant's attempts to communicate and assists in the development of intentional communication.

Establishment of these early communication skills lays the groundwork critical for further development of language skills. The primary challenge facing the parent or caregiver may be finding new opportunities and contexts in which to promote continued expansion of language skills. An important aspect of our role as speech–language pathologists is to assist parents and caregivers in meeting this challenge.

Feeding and Swallowing

This section addresses the impact of tracheostomy and ventilator dependence on feeding and swallowing. It reviews aspects of anatomy and physiology of swallowing unique to pediatrics, highlights typical conditions associated with dysphagia in children with tracheostomy and ventilator dependence, and addresses the impact of respiratory compromise, including prolonged intubation, tracheostomy, and ventilation, on the development of feeding and swallowing.

Tracheostomy and ventilator dependence can have a significant impact on feeding and swallowing abilities in children (11,29). This is true both for infants whose development of functional oral motor and swallowing abilities is just beginning, as well as for older children who have acquired functional feeding and swallowing abilities. Infants with congenital conditions requiring tracheostomy and/or prolonged mechanical ventilation frequently exhibit impaired feeding and swallowing skills. Older children can also experience swallowing difficulty as the result of acquired deficits secondary to illness or injury. In order to better understand the origin and nature of these swallowing difficulties, it is necessary to become familiar with the anatomy and physiology of pediatric swallowing, its relationship to respiration, and the impact of tracheostomy and mechanical ventilation on this relationship.

Anatomy and Physiology of Pediatric Swallowing

By the time children reach the age of three years, their ability to chew and swallow has matured, and, with the exception of laryngeal position, their anatomy and physiology closely approximate those of the adult. (For an explanation of adult anatomy and physiology of swallowing, see Chapter 6) From birth through 12 months of age, the infant anatomy and development of feeding and swallowing abilities are unique in several important respects. Infants are born with a number of anatomic features that have an impact on swallowing, and that gradually diminish with age, growth, and maturation. The larynx in infants is positioned higher in the neck, at the level of cervical vertebrae 3 and 4 (Fig. 7–1). As a result, the soft palate and epiglottis are in close approximation, protecting the entrance to the airway and allowing food to pass directly into the esophagus. This is important when one recalls that infants are obligate nasal breathers for the first few months of life, as this approximation allows them to complete the suck–swallow pattern without interfering with respiration. Because the suck–swallow–breathe sequence requires precise coordination in infants, any abnormality in upper airway structure or function is likely to have an impact on successful feeding. Another unique feature is the presence of sucking pads in the cheeks of infants, providing additional stability to assist with establishing and maintaining an adequate suck. Finally, the infant tongue is large with respect to the oral cavity, occupying most of the space and restricting tongue movement to the anterior–posterior direction characteristic of suckling.

In addition to anatomic differences, there are a number of important physiologic aspects unique to infant feeding and swallowing. Primary among these are the presence of reflexes that assist with development of feeding. The suck–swallow reflex is present at or soon after birth and is elicited through light touch to the lips or tongue. The rooting reflex is the turning of the head in the direction of stimulation in the perioral region. Phasic bite reflex is the automatic bite-release response that is elicited with tactile stimulation to the lower gums or molar surfaces. These automatic reflexes gradually evolve into more volitional actions as cortical development proceeds, generally beginning the transition during the period from four to six months of age (30). Development and refinement of the suck is thought to consist of two phases, distinguished by their distinctive patterns of movement. The first phase, suckling, is characterized by a backward and forward movement of the tongue, pronounced jaw opening and closing, and loose approximation of the lips. The second phase, sucking, is characterized by increased up-and-down movement of the tongue, smaller jaw excursion, and firmer lip approximation. The changes in direction of tongue movement and strength of lip closure provide the forces necessary to increase negative pressure in the mouth, enabling the infant to achieve a stronger, more efficient suck. The transition from suckling to sucking begins to occur at approximately six months of age and is made possible through anatomic and neurologic maturation, with gradual lowering of the jaw allowing more space for tongue movement, and gradual increase in volitional control permitting increased refinement and control of movements.

Impact of Tracheostomy and Mechanical Ventilation on Swallowing

Because of the close relationship between the structures of swallowing and those of respiration, anatomic or physiologic abnormalities affecting one process are likely to affect the other. By definition, then, the need for tracheostomy or mechanical ventilation as the result of anatomic or physiologic abnormalities of the respiratory system is likely to have an impact on swallowing function. For the newborn or developing infant, there are numerous airway abnormalities that can result in swallowing difficulties, including BPD, subglottic stenosis, tracheo-malacia, choanal atresia, tracheoesophageal fistula, vocal fold paralysis, laryngeal cleft, and a variety of other craniofacial anomalies (11). For the older child, ac-quired neurologic disease, progressive degenerative disease, spinal cord injury, laryngeal or vocal fold trauma, or a variety of other illnesses, injuries or acquired conditions which affect respiration can result in dysphagia.

For purposes of our discussion, the focus of this section is limited to the de-scription of swallowing difficulties directly related to tracheostomy and mechani-cal ventilation, regardless of the etiology. Although dysphagia associated with tracheostomy and mechanical ventilation occurs in older children secondary to acquired illness or injury as noted above, our discussion focuses on the infant and younger child, as the description of assessment and treatment of the former is comparable to that of adults and is addressed in detail elsewhere in this text book.

Coordination of respiration and swallowing are critical to successful oral feed-ing. There are many factors that influence feeding and swallowing abilities in chil-dren who require tracheostomy and mechanical ventilation. Feeding and swallowing difficulties in this population may be thought of as "primary," "sec-ondary," or "mixed." Primary difficulties consist of structural or functional abnor-malities resulting in pharyngeal dysphagia (e.g., vocal fold paralysis or reduced laryngeal elevation), while secondary difficulties refer to abnormal processes or patterns that affect feeding and swallowing and result in oral dysphagia (e.g., ab-normal oral motor patterns, oral–tactile hypersensitivity, or oral motor immatu-rity). Many children with no structural or functional abnormalities who require prolonged mechanical ventilation prior to developmental acquisition of oral mo-tor patterns prerequisite for feeding exhibit secondary dysphagic characteristics. Those children who have structural or functional abnormalities resulting in dys-phagia prior to acquisition of oral motor patterns prerequisite for feeding present with a mixed dysphagia, a combination of primary and secondary characteristics.

Primary Dysphagia

As noted above, primary dysphagia refers to swallowing problems resulting from structural or functional abnormalities of the aerodigestive tract, and typically is limited to the pharyngeal phase of the swallow. For example, repeated intubation can result in trauma and damage to the vocal folds. If this damage is sufficient to prevent complete glottic closure, risk of aspiration is significantly increased. The presence of the tracheostomy tube itself can have a negative impact on swallow-ing. The tracheostomy tube can anchor the larynx, resulting in reduced laryngeal elevation and epiglottic closure during the swallow (31). In addition, the diver-sion of air away from the larynx and pharynx can result in desensitization of both areas, leading to increased risk of aspiration. A further complication of the tra-cheostomy tube is the change in air pressures above and below the epiglottis, and the resulting interference with normal swallowing (32). (See Chapter 6.)

There are a number of respiratory conditions in infants that can result in tra-cheostomy. Pulmonary compromise necessitating prolonged ventilatory support, as in the case of BPD, airway anomalies resulting in obstruction of the upper airway, such as tracheomalacia or subglottic stenosis, or neurologic disorders affecting ability to manage secretions, can require tracheostomy. For those children without underlying pulmonary dysfunction, placement of a tracheostomy may be performed to bypass upper airway obstruction, and have limited impact on feeding. However, for those children with pulmonary compromise, tracheostomy may be performed to provide for mechanical support, but may not improve pulmonary function. In these instances, poor endurance and limited reserve may persist, interfering with the coordination of sucking, swallowing, and breathing. Infants who develop swallowing skills with tracheostomy tubes in place may experience increased swallowing difficulty due to reduced airway protection secondary to desensitization of the larynx, less effective cough, and "tethering" of the larynx during the swallow. Due to these "tracheostomy-induced" alterations in swallowing, those infants who learn to swallow successfully with tracheostomy tubes in place may initially have difficulty with coordination of respiration and swallowing following decannulation and may require some assistance.

Secondary Dysphagia

Secondary dysphagia refers to oral phase swallowing problems caused by adverse environmental factors that affect feeding and swallowing and result in development of abnormal oral motor patterns, oral–tactile hypersensitivity, or oral motor immaturity. Infants who require prolonged intubation or tracheostomy with mechanical ventilation commonly develop secondary dysphagia. Environmental factors responsible for this may include negative oral stimuli such as repeated passage of the endotracheal (ET) tube, prolonged presence of the ET tube, prolonged presence of an oral or nasal gastric tube for feeding, frequent oral or nasopharyngeal suctioning, and repeated placement and removal of tape on the face to secure tubes. All of these factors contribute to the development of oral defensiveness and oral–tactile hypersensitivity of the infant. In addition to the presence of negative environmental stimuli, the absence of positive, pleasurable oral experiences also has a negative impact on the development of oral motor patterns prerequisite to successful oral feeding. When children are orally intubated or have oral gastric feeding tubes in place, it is difficult for them to receive positive oral stimulation such as sucking on a pacifier, drinking from a bottle or breast, or mouthing toys and objects in exploration of their environment. Finally, the prolonged presence of the ET tube can result in structural and functional changes in the oral cavity, including unusually high, vaulted palate, and reduced strength and range of motion of the tongue, lips, and mandible.

Infants who experience this combination of repeated negative stimuli and oral deprivation over time develop hypersensitive reactions to any oral stimulation. These aversive responses are learned behaviors and as such do not necessarily disappear with the removal of the negative stimulation.

Mixed Dysphagia

Mixed dysphagia refers to the presence of both primary and secondary dysphagia characteristics, and is probably the most frequent type of swallowing difficulty seen in the infant population requiring tracheostomy and/or mechanical ventilation. The need for tracheostomy and ventilation typically is the result of structural or functional abnormalities of the aerodigestive tract; when this occurs prior to the development of oral motor skills prerequisite for feeding and swallowing, it often results in both oral and pharyngeal dysfunction, with components of both primary and secondary dysphagia as described above.

Assessment of Swallowing Function

Assessment of swallowing function in infants and children has been addressed thoroughly elsewhere in the literature, and the reader is referred to those excellent resources for discussions relating to general issues of assessment (30,33–37). With regard to evaluation of children requiring tracheostomy and ventilator dependence, as with any swallowing assessment, critical components include a detailed history, a thorough review of the medical record, prefeeding assessment, and oral feeding evaluation. Within each of these components, there are a number of unique aspects to assessment, and these will be the focus of discussion here.

History/Parent Interview

Children who require tracheostomy tubes and/or mechanical ventilation prior to three years of age may not have fully developed the oral motor movements necessary for normal oral feeding. Thus, knowledge regarding the nature and extent of their feeding experiences prior to onset of ventilation is especially important in determining the child's degree of readiness for feeding. In conducting the parent interview and obtaining a detailed history, then, information regarding premorbid diet consistencies, mode of presentation, and independence with feeding should be obtained.

Medical Background

Review of the child's medical record and medical status should note the presence of any contraindications to oral feeding. For example, oxygen saturation should be greater than 90%, and respiratory rate should be no higher than 65–70 breaths per minute at rest. The child should be able to manage secretions and tolerate bolus feeds if on tube feeding. Presence of gastroesophageal reflux, tachycardia, bradycardia, respiratory infection, vocal fold dysfunction, or multiple abdominal injuries are additional examples of possible contraindicators to oral feeding. Inability to produce a cough, pulmonary disease such as BPD, or history of pneumonia are factors that place the child at greater risk for aspiration and may limit ability to feed orally. Cranial nerve involvement affecting innervation of the tongue or pharynx would also interfere with ability to eat orally.

Prefeeding Assessment

In addition to indirect assessment through parent interview and chart review, direct observation of the child prior to introducing food should address alertness, ability to tolerate oral stimulation, and presence of a nonnutritive suck or ability to manipulate a bolus. Oxygen saturation and respiratory rate during these activities should be closely monitored. Positioning restrictions secondary to physical limitations or medical interventions should also be identified, as these may have an impact on the child's ability to feed.

Oral Feeding Evaluation

Because of the potentially complex nature of feeding with a tracheostomy tube and mechanical ventilation, it is recommended that a team of professionals trained to provide medical assistance be present at the bedside during this phase of the assessment. Key team members in addition to the speech–language pathologist include the respiratory care specialist and the nurse. They can provide assistance with adjusting ventilator settings; positioning the infant; monitoring oxygenation, respiration, and heart rate; suctioning; and other aspects of medical care that might arise.

Regarding oral presentation of materials, there are a number of aspects to consider. Many clinicians advocate the use of the Evans blue dye test or modified Evans blue dye test (MEBDT) to detect aspiration at the bedside (38). A recent report in the literature of a retrospective study comparing results from the use of MEBDT, fibreroptic endoscopic evaluation of swallowing (FEES), and videofluoroscopic swallowing (VFSS) documents low sensitivity of this measure to aspiration (39) and cautions the clinician regarding false-negative results. This study, although useful in illustrating the potential shortcomings of any single clinical bedside swallowing evaluation in detecting aspiration, failed to specify or describe a number of factors felt to be critical for objective comparison of these three procedures (40). Another study, reported by Tippett and Siebens (40), notes 90% sensitivity of the MEBDT in detecting aspiration of dyed foods for a group of 34 consecutive patients with tracheostomies. Thus, although the validity of the study for determining aspiration remains controversial and requires further objective study, it remains a useful component of the bedside swallowing assessment in determining safety for oral intake.

When using foods during the bedside assessment, a number of variables can be manipulated, including the presenter, the consistency, the mode of presentation, and the bolus size (41). The clinician, the parent, or the child can present the food. This decision is often based on the readiness and medical stability of the child, and the availability and willingness of the parent. If controlled amounts are critical or if the parent is reluctant or anxious, sometimes it is preferable for the clinician to present the food initially. Decisions regarding consistency, mode of presentation, and bolus size will depend on the child's age, current oral motor status, and premorbid feeding abilities.

If aspiration occurs during the bedside assessment, the decision to continue the evaluation depends on a number of factors, including the child's response and respiratory status. Any significant changes in oxygenation, heart rate, or respiratory rate may preclude continued feeding. If it is determined that the child is able to continue, the clinician may wish to proceed to assess ability to handle different consistencies, different modes of presentation, or bolus size, and manipulate variables accordingly. Whenever aspiration is documented during a bedside evaluation, a videofluoroscopic swallowing study (VFSS) is generally indicated. Such a study enables further determination of when the aspiration occurs (e.g., before, during, after the swallow), what factors influenced/caused the aspiration (e.g., premature spillage, unprotected airway, cricopharyngeal dysfunction, etc.), and what compensations, if any (e.g., food consistency, positioning, presentation) improve the swallow. Should the child demonstrate aspiration clinically on more than one consistency, the VFSS may be deferred until the child is better able to tolerate oral feeding.

If there is no evidence of aspiration during the bedside assessment, recommendations are made for oral feeding based on the results of the trial feeding, the child's level of ability to PO feed, and the child's nutritional needs. If there is clear evidence of aspiration on bedside evaluation (e.g., consistent cough with presentation of food, wet/gurgly voice quality immediately following presentation of food) and the decision is made to perform further objective assessment of swallowing, a VFSS is typically recommended. Because of concerns regarding relatively high levels of radiation exposure with this procedure for infants, physicians are often reluctant to order this study. An alternative procedure, fiberoptic endoscopic evaluation of swallowing (FEES) is another objective assessment measure available (42). It involves passage of a flexible fiberoptic endoscope transnasally to the area of the nasopharynx superior to the epiglottis, allowing observation of the swallowing mechanism from the base of the tongue downward. FEES has been performed in the adult population for several years and is well established in the literature as a safe, effective method of assessing swallowing. Use of FEES in the pediatric population is less well established, although it has been reported recently in the literature as a "practical and effective means of evaluating swallowing in children of all ages" (43, 44).

The procedures for conducting VFSS with infants and children differ from those used with adults in several respects. Seating and positioning needs for conducting the VFSS are unique. If unable to use their own seating systems due to space restrictions of the radiology equipment, infants and young children should be positioned in a molded infant seat or other specially designed pediatric VFSS seating system to allow optimal positioning during feeding (Fig. 7–15). The position in which the infants or children are initially viewed during VFSS should approximate as closely as possible that in which they will routinely be fed. If position is varied during the study to improve swallowing function, this same position should be adopted for routine feeding.

Infants and many younger children are unable to follow directions, thus certain volitional components routinely performed with adults such as oral manipulation of the bolus (e.g., hold in oral cavity until given command to swallow) and compensatory strategies (e.g., supraglottic swallow, Mendelsohn maneuver, chin tuck) are not possible. Furthermore, the parents or caregivers are the primary feeders and as such should be involved in presentation of the food during the study if at all possible. If not possible, they should be given the opportunity to review the tape with the clinician after the study, ask questions, and receive instruction regarding recommendations as approved by the referring physician. Another difference in procedures for pediatric VFSS is the lack of routine anterior-posterior (A-P) view. Due to concerns regarding radiation exposure, A-P views should be obtained only in those cases where deemed essential to further identi-

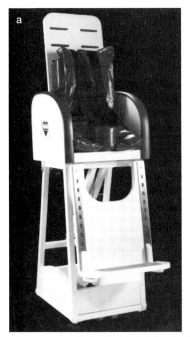
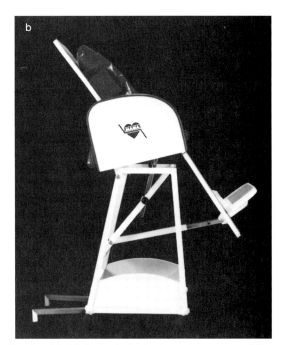

Fig. 7–15.   a,b: MAMA (Multiple Application Multiple Articulation) seating system, fully adjustable to accommodate children from birth through childhood. Photo courtesy of MAMA Systems, Inc., Oconomowoc, Wisconsin.

fication and diagnosis of suspected dysfunction. Another obvious difference regarding infants is the nature of the swallow during feeding. The process is dynamic and must be observed over time to allow adequate assessment of coordination, as opposed to observation of isolated swallows.

In addition to the above differences in VFSS procedure for infants and children, in general, there are further adaptations that must be considered when evaluating children with tracheostomy and ventilator dependence. Regarding seating and positioning, the need for portable ventilation may present a challenge and often requires assistance from a respiratory care specialist. The child requires seating or transport options that accommodate a ventilator. Once in the radiology suite, seating and positioning options need to incorporate space for the ventilator. Team members attending the VFSS should include the respiratory care specialist and the child's primary nurse or trained caregiver when possible. Suctioning equipment should be readily available during the study, and the ventilator should be positioned for easy access by the respiratory care specialist when adjustments are needed. Monitors similar to those available at the bedside swallowing evaluation should be used to note any changes in cardiac or respiratory parameters. During presentation of food, presence of tracheostomy tube and mechanical ventilation may require additional steps. Many of these measures can and should be assessed prior to the study to determine if they are feasible. For example, when evaluating a child with a tracheostomy tube in place, the tracheostomy tube should be occluded during the swallow when possible to restore the natural pressures inherent in a closed system. This can be achieved either by using a cap when tolerated or a one-way valve. For children who have cuffed tracheostomy tubes, swallowing should be assessed with the cuff deflated when possible. Although it is commonly believed that cuff inflation protects against aspiration, it has been shown that an inflated cuff can further impede the swallow through additional resistance to upward movement of the larynx or impingement on the anterior wall of the pharynx (45). Any changes in cuff pressures may necessitate changes in ventilator settings by the respiratory care specialist. If the child cannot tolerate full cuff deflation, partial deflation may still be possible, and can result in similar improvement in swallowing function. As noted with positioning, those conditions or adaptations that can be achieved and maintained during regular feeding should be the focus of assessment during the VFSS. Another potential difference in studying swallowing in infants and children with tracheostomy and ventilator dependence concerns the fatigue factor. The pulmonary dysfunction which necessitates the tracheostomy or ventilator assistance may also render the infant or child more susceptible to the influence of fatigue while feeding. For this reason, it may be necessary to assess initial swallows under fluoroscopy, and if no evidence of swallowing dysfunction is noted, continue feeding without fluoroscopy for a specified period or until fatigue becomes apparent. The VFSS would then be resumed to note any changes in swallowing resulting from fatigue.

If aspiration occurs during the study, the decision whether to continue to assess further consistencies, presentation modes, or other variables should be the result of team consensus regarding ensuring safety and well-being of the child. For children with intact respiratory function, trace aspiration may be tolerated with little or no consequence; for children with already compromised respiratory systems, trace aspiration may place them at more significant risk. Factors such as medical history, current medical status, and physical response to the aspiration as noted through direct observation of the child as well as objective changes in respiratory or cardiac status assist the team in making the decision.

Upon completion of the study, further recommendations regarding feeding are made based on the findings. In addition to diet recommendations, which may range from NPO (nothing by mouth) to a regular diet, recommendations should be made when appropriate regarding positioning; method, amount, and rate of presentation; feeders; tracheostomy tube adaptations; ventilator adjustments; and any other conditions needed to promote the safety of the child during feeding.

When swallowing function appears normal based on objective assessment, but the child continues to exhibit signs and symptoms consistent with aspiration (e.g., episodes of gagging, choking, coughing, or vomiting during feedings, frequent respiratory infections), other sources should be considered, and the child should be referred for additional assessment. A common problem associated with recurrent aspiration in infants and children is gastroesophageal reflux (GER) or the backing up of the stomach contents into the esophagus. When severe enough, materials can be refluxed into the pharynx and aspirated (for an excellent discussion of diagnosis and treatment of GER, see reference 37). When surgical intervention is warranted for control of GER, a procedure commonly performed is the Nissen fundoplication, in which the stomach opening or fundus is wrapped around the distal esophagus (46).

Treatment

Management options for feeding and swallowing problems in infants and children with tracheostomy and mechanical ventilation are selected based on the source of the problem. In those children presenting with a primary dysphagia, direct treatment techniques to improve swallowing efficiency and safety may be indicated, such as oral motor intervention to increase strength, range of motion, endurance, and coordination of oral structures for feeding. Use of a one-way valve such as the Passy-Muir speaking valve has been shown to improve swallowing function through normalization of air pressures above and below the epiglottis as well as increased sensation in the oral and pharyngeal cavities (32). Changes or adaptations in mode, rate, or amount of presentation may be indicated, such as use of different nipples to control bolus flow or frequent feedings of shorter duration to avoid fatigue.

For those children presenting with secondary dysphagia, management typically involves a program of indirect techniques designed to establish prerequisites to oral feeding, including reducing hypersensitivity to touch and taste, establishing a nonnutritive suck, and encouraging lingual cupping (36). As noted above, many ventilator-assisted children exhibit severe oral hypersensitivity due to a combination of frequent or prolonged intubation and oral deprivation. Because many of these children continue to reside in an over-stimulating environment with frequent negative orofacial input, this phase of management can be challenging. When possible, the clinician should work closely with the nursing staff and families to modify the environment and care routines to minimize aversive responses. For example, care should be taken to avoid association of negative stimuli with pleasurable experiences, such as performing painful procedures during feeding or other parent–child bonding times (21). The infant should be held during feeding when at all possible, even if being tube fed. This is a good time to encourage the nonnutritive suck, as the infant will come to associate this pleasurable oral experience with the feeling of becoming full. Because of negative early experiences, the infant may be slow to accept any stimulation in the area of the face and mouth. This should be introduced very gradually, providing opportunities for the infant to explore and mouth toys prior to introduction of food. Throughout this phase of management, the parent or caregiver should be the primary provider of pleasurable oral experiences to promote development of the infant–caregiver bond and reaffirm the role of the caregiver as nurturer and provider of their child's basic needs.

When an infant or child presents with a mixed dysphagia, the management approach typically proceeds with the indirect techniques described above, followed by the direct techniques as indicated by the infant's readiness to begin oral feeds. Education of the parent or primary caregiver should be provided for all appropriate aspects of management, and direct participation encouraged, supported, and reinforced throughout all phases of dysphagia management.

Follow-up

Assessment and management of feeding and swallowing abilities in children with tracheostomy and ventilator dependence is not a one-time event, but rather an ongoing process which must adapt to meet the changing needs of the child. As children age, their ventilation needs may change as a function of growth and medical status. These changes may result in altered swallowing function and require periodic monitoring by a dysphagia clinician experienced in recognizing and addressing the impact of such changes. This monitoring can be done during regular outpatient clinic visits or can be arranged as separate visits to the dysphagia clinician, as determined by the individualized needs of the child as well as the options available through the outpatient facility.

Case Studies

1. Infant Feeding and Swallowing

History

Adam is a 5-month-old boy born at 38 weeks gestation, with a medical history of congenital diaphragmatic hernia, bronchomalacia, and gastroesophageal reflux. Adam was mechanically ventilated from birth and was placed on extracorporeal membrane oxygenation (ECMO) from days 1 to 12. He underwent tracheostomy and gastrostomy tube placement (with fundoplication) at five months of age. Adam was weaned from the ventilator at seven months of age, put on Bi-Pap at night, and discharged from the hospital. He was subsequently weaned from Bi-Pap at 17 months of age.

Initial Presentation

Adam was initially referred to speech-language pathologyy for assessment and treatment of feeding and swallowing needs s/p tracheostomy at five months of age. He was NPO at that time, exhibiting severe oral hypersensitivity, hyperactive gag reflex, disorganized lingual movements, absent nonnutritive suck, and aversive response to all attempts at feeding.

Treatment Program

Treatment goals included decreasing oral hypersensitivity and aversion to oral experiences; promoting movement of gag reflex to a more posterior position on the tongue; increasing pleasurable, actively sought oral experiences; increasing tolerance for food tastes and textures; improving lingual function to allow efficient management of bolus; and educating family and home nursing staff in techniques to achieve goals. VFSS completed at 10 months of age revealed mild oral-phase dysphagia, with no penetration or aspiration noted.

Outcome

Reassessment at 30 months of age found Adam to no longer exhibit oral–tactile defensiveness. Gag reflex was triggered posteriorly at the base of tongue, oral-stage bolus management was efficient, and he was eating junior foods and mashed table foods. He was able to lateralize food with his tongue, and a rotary chew was beginning to emerge. Adam was using his lips to assist with removing food from the spoon, and his swallow response was immediate. He continued to demonstrate some gagging with initial presentation of increased texture.

Implications

Prolonged/chronic mechanical ventilation impedes normal oral motor/feeding development. Early intervention to minimize negative oral experiences and responses, increase pleasurable oral experiences, and educate caregivers in techniques to achieve this is critical to the development of successful oral feeding in ventilator-assisted children.

2. Child Feeding, Swallowing, and Voicing

History

Sam is an 11-year-old boy with a C_{1-2} quadriplegia status post pedestrian/motor vehicle accident at seven years of age. He underwent rehabilitation at an outside hospital for six months prior to transfer to our rehabilitation unit. At time of admission here, he was on 24-h mechanical ventilation, had a Shiley no. 5 cuffed tracheostomy tube, gastrostomy tube, no documented reflux, and intact vocal folds. VFSS performed at four months post injury had revealed aspiration, and NPO status had been maintained. He had one documented episode of pneumonia at six months post injury.

Initial Presentation

Sam was referred to speech–language pathology for speech and swallowing needs at six months post injury. He had intermittent voice with a functional leak around his trachestomy tube, and exhibited strained, hypernasal voice quality. Oral motor function was intact. Sam had a Shiley no. 5 tracheostomy tube with cuff at minimal leak. He had recently had pneumonia and was NPO. Reassessment of swallowing via VFSS revealed penetration of liquids. The cuff was inflated during the study, as medical clearance could not be obtained for cuff deflation. There was clinical evidence of aspiration of liquids (suctioning of Hawaiian Punch from the tracheostomy).

Treatment Program

Treatment goals included restricted PO diet; tolerance for partial-full cuff deflation; improved voicing through adjusted ventilator settings and cuff deflation; ability to time swallowing with ventilator cycle; ability to tolerate full cuff deflation while eating; education of family and caregivers regarding diet, tracheostomy adjustments (e.g., cuff deflation), ventilator settings, and swallowing modifications. Reassessment of swallowing via VFSS and FEES was completed when Sam was able to tolerate partial cuff deflation (two weeks following initial assessment). Results of both FEES and VFSS indicated mild residue in both valleculae and pyriform sinuses, but no penetration or aspiration of any substance.

Outcome

Upon hospital discharge two months later, Sam had a Portex tracheostomy tube of slightly smaller diameter to facilitate voicing. He was tolerating partial cuff deflation (approximately 3 cc of air in cuff), and cuff deflation to less than 2 cc during eating. He was able to time his swallow with the expiratory cycle of the ventilator. Sam's voice was improved, with greater volume and less strained quality. There was no clinical evidence of aspiration, and upon 12-month followup, no documented episodes of pneumonia.

Implications

The presence of a cuff can impede the swallow and result in aspiration. Adjustments can be made to tracheostomy and ventilator status to facilitate successful swallowing and voicing in ventilator-assisted children. VFSS results should be interpreted cautiously as representing a one time event, and should be combined with a thorough clinical assessment and history prior to making recommendations.

Appendix 1. Tracheostomy Tube Advantages (+) and Disadvantages (−)

1. Uncuffed Tracheostomy Tube
   + Easy insertion
   + Best vocalization
   + Simplest tube

   − Danger of aspiration
   − No cuff to inflate/open system

2. Low-Volume/High-Pressure Air Cuff Tracheostomy Tube
   + Minimal bulk on shaft
   + Easier insertion
   + Helps prevent aspiration

   − Harder to manage cuff volumes (Tight-to-Shaft (TTS) (TM)[1] cuff)[2]
   − Potential tracheal damage with overinflation

3. Low-Pressure/High-Volume Air Cuff Tracheostomy Tube
   + Minimizes tracheal damage
   + Cuff easy to manage (Shiley)
   + Helps prevent aspiration

   − More difficult to insert than cuffless or TTS
   − Potential tracheal damage with overinflation
   − Difficult to manage cuff volumes (Bivona)[2]

4. Fenestrated Tracheostomy Tube with Low-Pressure Air Cuff
   + Best for weaning purposes
   + Greater air leak with less resistance
   + Less resistance to breathing when plugged
   + Helps prevent aspiration

   − Potential for granulation tissue to grow into fenestration
   − Difficulty with placement of fenestration to facilitate phonation
   − Can be used with adolescents or adults only

5. Fome (TM)[3] Cuff Tracheostomy Tube
   + Least likely to cause tracheal damage
   + Easy to manage ventilation
   + Helps prevent aspiration

   − No oral communication with cuff maximally inflated
   − Air diffuses rapidly back into cuff when deflated
   − More difficult to insert and remove

6. Talking Tracheostomy Tube
   + Voicing with maximal cuff inflation
   + Can be switch operated
   + Helps prevent aspiration

   − Easily clogged with secretions
   − Always need independent air source (noisy and bulky)
   − Poor voice quality
   − Dries out mucosa
   − Requires port occlusion—finger or switch

[1]Tight-to-Shaft, or TTS, is trademark of Bivona.
[2]Silicone cuffs allow air to diffuse back into cuff over time.
[3]Fome cuff tube is trademark of Bivona.

Reprinted, with permission, from Driver and Hilker (17).

Appendix 2.   Tracheostomy Tube Decision Flowchart

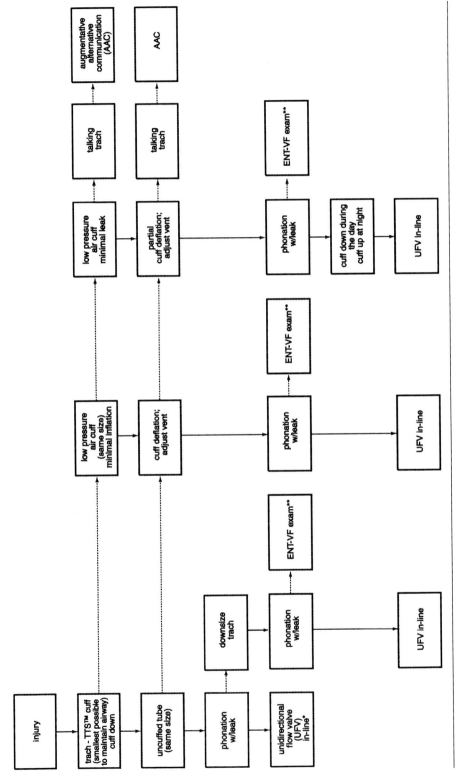

A solid line indicates optimal path (vertical). A dotted line indicates alternative paths (deviation from optimal) (horizontal). *See manufacturer's instructions regarding placement, restrictions, and contraindications. **The outcome of the otorhinolaryngology vocal fold (ENT-VF) exam dictates the next step in the process.

Reprinted, with permission, from Driver and Hilker (17).

Appendix 3. A. Talking Tracheostomy Tube

Indications for Use

1. Aphonic
2. No cuff deflation possible
3. Adequate articulation
4. Adequate vocal fold function
5. Adult size tracheostomy
6. Ability to occlude external speaking port
7. Minimal secretions

Benefits of Use

1. Phonation independent of the ventilator cycle
2. Phonation with maximal cuff inflation

Contraindications for Use

1. Bilateral vocal fold paralysis
2. Copious secretions
3. Severe dysarthria
4. Decreased alertness
5. Pediatric size tracheostomy

Troubleshooting

1. No voice—Clear excess secretions through irrigation of external air tubing, suctioning
2. Tickling/discomfort—Reduce air flow from external air source
3. Weak/hoarse voice quality—increase air flow from external air source; clear excess secretions
4. Dysphagia—Monitor cuff pressure closely to avoid tracheal injury, reduced sensitivity, and impingement on the anterior pharyngeal wall

Appendix 3.   B. One-Way Tracheostomy Speaking Valve

Indications for Use

1. Adequate tracheal lumen*
2. COMPLETE cuff deflation or cuffless tube
3. Acceptable O_2
4. Aphonia
5. Ventilator weaning

Benefits of Use

1. Allows phonation by redirecting air through vocal folds
2. Improves swallowing
    –normalizes pharyngeal pressure
    –assists with clearing of upper airway by allowing cough
3. Increases sense of smell and taste through increased air circulation through nose and mouth
4. Decreases secretions
5. Provides increased positive end-expiratory pressure or PEEP

Contraindications for Use

1. Cannula occludes tracheal lumen, preventing air passage
2. Inflated cuff
    –impedes air passage and results in air trapping, overinflation of lungs
3. Upper airway stenosis or obstruction
    –reduces air passage and results in air trapping, overinflation of lungs
4. Copious secretions
5. Permanent bilateral vocal fold paralysis (abducted)
    –prevents modulation of airstream
6. Laryngectomy
7. Anarthria
8. Unstable medical/pulmonary status

Troubleshooting

1. CO_2 retention—Check cuff deflation; if on ventilator, check PEEP settings
2. Patient anxiety—Use O_2 saturation monitor for biofeedback
3. Poor adaptation to breathing pattern—Teach intermittent glottic control to reduce airflow out mouth
4. High-pressure alarm on ventilator—Readjust settings to compensate for PEEP feature

*For children able to breathe spontaneously, this can be objectively assessed using manometry to measure inner tracheal pressure.

Reprinted, with permission, from Driver and Hilker (17).

Appendix 4. Speech Pathology Assessment Protocol for One-Way Tracheostomy Speaking Valve

1. Obtain physician referral

2. Obtain medical clearance
   a. Child is medically stable
   b. Upper airway is free from obstruction
   c. No contraindications for valve use are present[a]

3. Perform screening with respiratory care
   a. Child is adequately ventilated and safe without use of cuff
   b. Child is able to exhale adequately around the tracheostomy tube (use manometry, if appropriate)
   c. Child is able to achieve voicing

4. Perform assessment with respiratory care
   a. Deflate cuff completely if one is present
   b. Adjust ventilator settings, if necessary
   c. Monitor O_2, CO_2, and heart rate
   d. Place valve (over hub of tracheostomy tube if off ventilator, or in ventilator tubing)
   e. Use adapter to accommodate oxygen or metal tracheostomy tube, if needed
   f. Readjust ventilator settings, if necessary (e.g., compensate for autopeep feature of the valve)
   g. Coach the child as appropriate regarding relaxed breathing, speaking, and potential changes in ability to taste, smell, clear secretions, etc.
   h. Monitor O_2, CO_2, and heart rate, compare with prevalve measures
   i. Observe child for changes during different levels of activity[b]
   j. Have parents/caregivers observe child on their own (without monitors) for a period of time within the area (e.g., hospital cafeteria) until they feel comfortable

5. Provide patient, family, and staff education
   a. Determine wearing schedule and review with child and caregivers (e.g., gradually increase time wearing valve based on child's tolerance, assess child wearing valve during different levels of activity)
   b. Review precautions, potential difficulties, and proper care (e.g., never wear while sleeping, cuff always deflated, air trapping, etc.)
   c. Arrange for regular followup, including blood gases

[a]See Appendix 3 or manufacturer's literature for details regarding contraindications.
[b]If child tolerates valve during sitting, but not during increased activity, recommend increased period of wearing without activity prior to increasing activity; increase activity gradually. If continued difficulties, then refer to physician for further airway assessment.

Reprinted, with permission, from Driver and Hilker (17).

References

1. Bleile KM. Children with long-term tracheostomies. In: Bleile KM, ed. *The care of children with long-term tracheostomies*. San Diego: Singular Publishing Group, Inc., 1993:3–19.
2. Line WS Jr., Hawkins DB, Kahlstrom EJ, et al. Tracheotomy in infants and young children: the changing perspective 1970–1985. *Laryngoscope* 1986;96:510–515.
3. Albamonte S, Jerome AM. Pediatrics. In: Mason MF, ed. *Speech pathology for tracheostomized and ventilator-dependent patients*, Newport Beach: Voicing, Inc., 1993:383–422.
4. Hill B, Singer L. Speech and language development after infant tracheostomy. *J Speech Hearing Dis* 1990;55:15–20.
5. Singer LT, Kercsmar C, Legris G, et al. Developmental sequelae of long-term infant tracheostomy. *Dev Med Child Neurol* 1989;31:224–230.
6. Kaslon K, Stein R. Chronic pediatric tracheostomy: assessment and implications for habilitation of voice, speech and language in young children. *Int J Ped Otorhinolaryngol* 1985;9:165–171.
7. Gunn TR, Leporre E, Outerbridge EW. Outcome at school-age after neonatal mechanical ventilation. *Dev Med Child Neurol* 1983;25:305–314.
8. Simon BM, Fowler SM, Handler SD. Communication development in young children with long-term tracheostomies: preliminary report. *Int J Ped Otorhinolaryngol* 1983;6:37–50.
9. Kamper J. Long-term prognosis of infants with severe idiopathic respiratory distress syndrome: neurological and mental outcome. *Acta Paediatr Scand* 1978;67:61–69.
10. Morris SE. Development of oral motor skills in the neurologically impaired child receiving non-oral feedings. *Dysphagia* 1989;3:135–154.
11. Brodsky L, Volk M. The airway and swallowing. In: Arvedson J, Brodsky L, eds. *Pediatric swallowing and feeding assessment and management*. San Diego: Singular Publishing Group, Inc., 1993:93–122.
12. Schreiner MS, Downes JJ, Kettrick RG, et al. Chronic respiratory failure in infants with prolonged ventilatory dependence. *J A M A* 1987;258:3398–3404.
13. Senders CW, Muntz HR, Schweiss D. Physician survey on the care of children with tracheotomy. *Am J Otolaryngol* 1991;12(1):48–50.
14. Irving RM, Jones NS, Bailey CM, et al. A guide to the selection of pediatric tracheostomy tubes. *J Laryngol Otol* 1991;105:1046–1051.
15. Ramsey AM, Grady EA. Long-term airway management for the ventilator-assisted child. In: Driver LE, Nelson VS, Warschausky SA, eds. *The ventilator-assisted child: a practical resource guide*. San Antonio: Communication Skill Builders, 1997:9–23.
16. Levine SP, Koester DJ, Kett RL. Independent activated talking tracheostomy for quadriplegic patients. *Arch Phys Med Rehabil* 1987;68:571–573.
17. Driver LE, Hilker DF. Oral and written communication needs of the ventilator-assisted child. In: Driver LE, Nelson VS, Warschausky SA, eds. *The ventilator-assisted child: a practical resource guide*. San Antonio: Communication Skill Builders, 1997:69–83.
18. Beukelman DR, Mirenda P. *Augmentative and alternative communication*. Baltimore: Paul H. Brookes Publishing Co., Inc., 1992:309–370.
19. Yorkston K. *Augmentative communication in the medical setting*. Tucson: Communication Skill Builders, Inc., 1992:5–59.
20. Ross GS. Language functioning and speech development of six children receiving tracheostomy in infancy. *J Commun Dis* 1982;15:95–111.
21. Cox JZ, VanDeinse SD. Special needs of the prelinguistic ventilator-assisted child. In: Driver LE, Nelson VS, Warschausky SA, eds. *The ventilator-assisted child: a practical resource guide*. San Antonio: Communication Skill Builders, Inc., 1997:85–92.
22. Ahman E, Lipski K. Early intervention for technology dependent infants and young children. *Infants Young Children* 1991;3:67–77.
23. Pollack MM, Wilkinson JD, Glass NL. Long-stay pediatric intensive care unit patients: outcome and resource utilization. *Pediatrics* 1987;80:855–860.
24. Singer LT, Wood R, Lambert S. Developmental follow-up of long term infant tracheostomy: A preliminary report. *Dev Behav Pediatr* 1985;6(3):132–136.
25. Bennett FC, Robinson NM, Sells CJ. Growth and development in infants weighing less than 800 grams at birth. *Pediatrics* 1983;71:319–323.

26. Marsh R, Handler S. Hearing impairment in ventilator-dependent infants and children. *Int J Ped Otorhinolaryngol* 1990;20:213–217.

27. Simon BM, McGowan J. Tracheostomy in young children: implications for assessment and treatment of communication and feeding disorders. *Infants Young Children* 1989;1:1–9.

28. Simon BM, Handler SD. The speech pathologist and management of children with tracheostomies. *J Otolaryngol* 1981;10:6.

29. McGowan JS, Kerwin ML, Bleile KM. Oral-motor and feeding problems. In: Bleile KM, ed. *The care of children with long-term tracheostomies.* San Diego: Singular Publishing Group, Inc., 1993:89–112.

30. Morris SE, Klein MD. *Pre-feeding skills: a comprehensive resource for feeding development.* Tucson: Therapy Skill Builders, 1987:26–46.

31. Nash M. Swallowing problems in the tracheostomized patient. *Otolaryngol Clin North Am* 1988;21:701–709.

32. Dettelbach MA, Gross RD, Mahlmann J, et al. Effect of the Passy-Muir valve on aspiration in patients with tracheostomy. *Head Neck* 1995;7:297–300.

33. Arvedson JC, Rogers BT. Swallowing and feeding in the pediatric patient. In: Perlman AL, Schulze-Delrieu K, eds. *Deglutition and its disorders.* San Diego: Singular Publishing Group, Inc., 1997:419–448.

34. Rosenthal SR, Sheppard JJ, Lotze M. *Dysphagia and the child with developmental disabilities.* San Diego: Singular Publishing Group, Inc., 1995:15–75.

35. Tuchman DN, Walter RS. *Disorders of feeding and swallowing in infants and children.* San Diego: Singular Publishing Group, Inc., 1994:97–207.

36. Wolf LS, Glass RP. *Feeding and swallowing disorders in infancy: assessment and management.* Tucson: Therapy Skill Builders, Inc., 1992:63–252.

37. Arvedson JC, Brodsky L, eds. *Pediatric swallowing and feeding.* San Diego: Singular Publishing Group, Inc., 1993:130–144.

38. Puntil J, Mason MF, Scott M. Dysphagia. In: Mason MF, ed. *Speech pathology for tracheostomized and ventilator dependent patients.* Newport Beach: Voicing, Inc., 1993:479–519.

39. Thompson-Henry S, Braddock B. The modified Evan's blue dye procedure fails to detect aspiration in the tracheostomized patient: five case reports. *Dysphagia* 1995;10:172–174.

40. Tippett DC, Siebens AA. Reconsidering the value of the modified Evan's blue dye test: a comment on Thompson-Henry and Braddock (1995). *Dysphagia* 1996;11:78–81.

41. VanDeinse SD, Cox JZ. Feeding and swallowing issues in the ventilator-assisted child. In: Driver LE, Nelson VS, Warschausky SA, eds. *The ventilator-assisted child: a practical resource guide.* San Antonio: Communication Skill Builders, 1997:93–102.

42. Langmore SE, Schatz K, Olsen N. Fiberoptic endoscopic evaluation of swallowing safety: a new procedure. *Dysphagia* 1988;2:216–219.

43. Willging JP, Miller CK, Hogan MJ, et al. Fiberoptic endoscopic evaluation of swallowing in children: a preliminary report of 100 procedures. Paper presented at the Dysphagia Research Symposium Third Annual Scientific Meeting, McClean, VA, 1995.

44. Miller CK, Willging JP, Strife JL, et al. Fiberoptic endoscopic examination of swallowing in infants and children with feeding disorders. *Dysphagia* 1994;9:266.

45. Bach JR, Alba AS. Tracheostomy ventilation: a study of efficacy with deflated cuffs and cuffless tubes. *Chest* 1990;97:679–683.

46. Smith CD, Otherson HB, Gogan NJ, et al. Nissen fundoplication in children with profound neurologic disability. *Annals Surg* 1992;215(6):654–8.

47. Bosma JF, Donner MW, Tanaka E, Robertson D. Anatomy of the pharynx, pertinent to swallowing. *Dysphagia* 1986;1:22–33.

48. Kramer SS. Special swallowing problems in children. *Gastrointest Radial* 1985;10:242.

49. Finucane BT, Santora AH. *Principles of airway management.* Philadelphia: FA Davis, 1988.

50. Greenough A, Milner AD, Robertson NR, eds. *Neonatal respiratory disorders.* London: Edward Arnold Publishers, Ltd., 1996:40.

8

Transitioning the Client with a Tracheostomy from Acute Care to Alternative Settings

Beth C. Diehl, Louella K. Dorsey and Charnan L. S. Koller

Medical advances over the past two decades have resulted in the survival of individuals who may not have survived previously, specifically, those who have recovered from hospitalizations in intensive care and trauma units. Some of these individuals have residual healthcare issues related to their respiratory status, namely, the presence of tracheostomy with or without mechanical ventilation.

The penetration of managed care organizations has exerted tremendous influence on the ongoing management of these individuals. Lengthy hospital stays of an acute nature are strongly discouraged because of cost, therefore, alternative levels of care are explored for the postacute course. These alternative levels include skilled nursing facilities, alternative living units, or the individuals' home settings. An optimal environment not only controls cost, but also promotes high levels of well-being and satisfaction for the individual and the family. The complexity of care in both the acute and long-term phases can be overwhelming for the medical staff, individual, and family. Caregiver burden can be staggering in concert with the thrust for cost containment within managed care organizations. Given these factors, posthospitalization plans must be orchestrated carefully.

This chapter reviews medical stability and acute care hospital discharge, community reintegration, caregiver education, equipment needs, long-term case management/life planning, and financial considerations for individuals with tracheostomies and/or mechanical ventilation (hereafter referred to as clients). Community reentry may include school return, vocational skill training, resumption of recreation activities, and, of course, reintegration into the home and family. Legislative initiatives such as the Americans with Disabilities Act of 1990 (1) and

Tracheostomy and Ventilator Dependency: Management of Breathing, Speaking, and Swallowing. Edited by Donna C. Tippett, MPH, MA, CCC-SLP. Thieme Medical Publishers, Inc. New York © 2000.

the Education for All Handicapped Children Act of 1975 (2) have made a positive impact on community reentry.

Additional chapter content includes the design and content of the educational program to prepare clients and families for discharge. Goals, time lines, essential staff, and equipment needs are fundamental components. Financial issues are quite complex with various programs available according to the individual's place of residence. Both state and federal funds are occasionally blended with family financial resources to provide necessary services. Professional service requirements in terms of nursing visits, ancillary support services, and case manager function are reviewed. The role of the life care planner, a holistic and long-term coordinator for the family, is also discussed. Lastly, case studies of an infant, school-age child, and adult with a tracheostomy with or without mechanical ventilation synthesize the content.

Medical Stability and Acute Care Hospital Discharge

Individuals with tracheostomies, with or without mechanical ventilation, often have underlying medical conditions that interfere with their ability to breathe and/or clear and maintain their airway. These individuals may have:

- stridorous or noisy respirations,
- generalized muscle weakness or fatigue,
- the inability to lower the diaphragm to allow air to enter the lungs, or
- the inability to maintain adequate oxygenation and carbon dioxide levels.

Some of the accompanying medical diagnoses may include:

- tracheomalacia,
- tracheal stenosis,
- muscular dystrophy,
- Guillain-Barré syndrome,
- high spinal cord injury lesions, i.e., cervical,
- sleep apnea,
- bronchopulmonary dysplasia (BPD) in children, or
- chronic obstructive pulmonary disease (COPD) in adults.

The first initiative in the discharge process is determining medical stability and understanding why a particular client requires a tracheostomy and/or needs assistance with mechanical ventilation. Next, efforts are made to control or minimize, to the best of current technology, the progressive effects of the disease process. If the disease process cannot be halted, a clear plan regarding medical interventions must be developed that encompasses the client's and/or family's wishes related to resuscitative efforts. Once these two areas are addressed, then a coordinated discharge effort can begin.

Clients can be discharged to a variety of community settings depending on the degree of medical stability. For example, a client discharged to a subacute rehabilitative setting or skilled nursing facility, can have resolving medical issues, such as fine tuning of the ventilator settings or clearing of infection. The client who is discharged to the home setting without the supports of shift licensed nursing care (e.g., 8, 12, or 24 h/day), should have no signs of infection, vital signs within appropriate baselines, a stable medical regimen, and consistent ventilator settings on the type of ventilator to be used at home. In addition, caregivers should demonstrate competencies to provide all the necessary care for the client, including the maintenance and operation of all equipment. Regardless of the setting, the following criteria must be met before an individual can be discharged from the acute care setting:

- the tracheostomy tube is easily inserted and removed,
- suctioning the tracheostomy tube a minimum of every 4 h to an only as needed basis, and
- the tracheostomy site is healed and free from bleeding and granulation tissue formation.

The physician ultimately decides when and where the client will be discharged with input from the interdisciplinary team members and influences from the payor source.

Community Reintegration

Home Setting

In addition to medical stability, several factors influence discharge to home. First, the client is assessed to determine if he/she is capable of providing all the necessary care to optimize wellness and prevent complications. If the client is unable to provide the necessary self-care, then someone must be identified as the caregiver. At times, it is advisable to have a second or back-up caregiver, in case the primary caregiver is not available. The caregiver should be someone who is willing and capable of providing the necessary care, as well as someone the client wants to have take care of his/her overall ongoing needs. Second, the home is assessed to assure that the client is able to gain access, maneuver, and exit from the home. Occupational and physical therapists can be helpful in making recommendations for the home if structural changes are needed. The respiratory therapist and nursing agency help determine if the home's electrical supply is adequate to support all of the client's medical equipment. The ventilator should be on its own electrical circuit to prevent circuit overload and subsequent damage to the ventilator or other major appliances. Last, funding sources must be explored to determine the type of professional supports available to the client and caregiver in the home.

Findeis and colleagues (3) studied the burden of care, the impact of care, mastery of skills, and the satisfaction of providing care to loved ones using home mechanical ventilation. The authors found that for the caregivers the major burden of care was "negotiating with and coordinating home nursing services, equipment suppliers, and insurance companies" (p. 8) (3). These tasks were judged to be more difficult by the family than providing the actual physical care. Staffing, service coordination, and equipment supplier difficulties were distressing to caregivers because:

- the caregivers had not anticipated such problems,
- these problems had an impact on the caregivers' work schedules, their day-to-day routines, and personal finances, and
- the caregivers felt they should be able to rely on the home nurses to ease the work of caregiving.

Limitations on insurance policies, depletion of insurance benefits, and reimbursement time lags were areas that caregivers also identified as burdensome.

Regarding the impact of caring for a loved one on mechanical ventilation, caregivers felt their lives were negatively affected on a continuum from a "good deal" to "excessively." During the course of giving care, they were affected not only personally but socially and financially. Nevertheless, despite the problems the caregivers had, they would not consider institutionalizing the ventilator-assisted person.

In the mastery area, factors which aided the caregiver in coping and adjusting included:

- taking the initiative in acquiring information,
- developing a routine,
- sharing the caregiving responsibilities with a family member,
- receiving social support from family, friends, and church members,
- maintaining a positive attitude, and
- getting accustomed to the situation over time.

The last area the study addressed was satisfaction. "While most caregivers preferred to care for their ventilator-assisted family member (as opposed to having others do it), few were able to articulate specific satisfying aspects of caregiving" (p. 9) (3).

In summary, these authors found caregivers wanted information that would help them choose:

- nursing agencies that were reliable to ensure the adequate provision of competent nurses,
- respiratory and medical supply companies with which they could compare and contrast costs and services, and
- insurance policies with their respective restrictions and limitations.

School Setting

Two pieces of legislation that have influenced care issues for clients with tracheostomies with or without mechanical ventilation include the Education for All Handicapped Children Act of 1975 (2) and the Americans with Disabilities Act of 1990 (1). One aspect of the Americans with Disabilities Act of 1990 (1) mandates that all public buildings, including schools, be handicapped accessible. The Education for All Handicapped Children Act of 1975 (2) entitles all children ages three to 21 years to free public education and mandates that children with special education needs have an Individual Educational Plan (IEP). In 1986, the Education of the Handicaped Act Amendments (4) expanded education services to early intervention programs, stating that all children have a constitutional right to a publicly funded education in the least restrictive environment. Children with tracheostomies with or without mechanical ventilation may qualify for certain school services due to their individual limitations. For example, a child with muscular dystrophy and congential hypoventilation syndrome requiring night-time ventilation via a tracheostomy may qualify for occupational therapy, physical therapy, and speech–language pathology services provided by and funded through the public school system.

In 1990, Public Law 94-142 (2) was changed to the Individuals with Disabilities Education Act (IDEA) (5).

Disabilities listed in IDEA include (6):

- autism,
- hearing impairments, including deafness,
- mental retardation,
- orthopedic impairments,
- multiple disabilities,
- serious emotional disturbance,
- specific learning disabilities,
- speech or language impairments,
- traumatic brain injury, and
- visual impairments, including blindness.

If a child does not have one of the above disabilities, Section 504, an extension of IDEA (5), may offer assistance in meeting individual educational needs. Section 504 is a federal law which prohibits any agency that receives federal money from discriminating against a person on the basis of disability, and requires "reasonable accommodation" of a disability. An example of some issues that may not be covered by IDEA (5), but are covered by Section 504 are:

- the length of a child's school day (2 h, 4 h, etc.),
- the accessibility of the child's school building,
- services to parents with disabilities, or
- the educational treatment of children who have other disabilities not listed under IDEA (5), such as attention-deficit hyperactivity disorder.

Parents can obtain the federal regulations for these laws through the Superintendent of Documents, United States Government Printing Office, Washington, D.C. 20402 (telephone 202-783-3238). Parents may also want to contact their respective state departments of education and offices of special education, for a parent handbook on special education services.

Any child at risk can be referred for an evaluation of educational needs. For example, a premature infant with tracheomalacia, tracheostomy tube, and developmental deficits would be considered at risk for delayed speech and language

Table 8–1.   Time line of the evaluation process.

Stage	Time allowed between stages (calendar days)
Parent or other person requests screening Screening completed	30
Screening completed (ARD meeting held) Assessment ordered Assessment completed	45
Assessment completed ARD meeting held	30
ARD meeting held IEP written and approved by ARD	30
IEP written and approved by ARD IEP implemented	30
IEP implemented IEP reviewed for appropriateness	60
IEP reviewed for appropriateness Written report to parents	10
Annual Review	1 year (365 days)
Due processing hearing time line Local level hearing requested Local level hearing decision	45
Time line to appeal local level hearing decision State level hearing requested State level hearing decision	30 30
Time line to appeal state level hearing decision	180

Reprinted, with permission, from the Maryland Disability Law Center, Inc. (19).

production. Therefore, this infant and family would benefit from early intervention services from an infant and toddler program. The process is initiated by the parent, healthcare provider, or educational provider. Each state operationalizes the referral process differently. In some states, it may be accessed through the school board or other county agency. The intake is processed, then the child is evaluated for appropriate services. After the assessments are completed, an Admission, Review and Dismissal (ARD) meeting is held. It is essential for the therapists to be physically present and/or provide written assessment findings, and a list of goals with frequency and length of treatment needed. An Individual Education Plan (IEP) for ages three to 21 years or an Individualized Family Services Plan (IFSP) for birth to age three years is written and then implemented. The plan is periodically reviewed and changes are made as necessary. Specifically, an IEP is a document that describes the special education resources and related services a child is to receive. The IEP must contain:

- the current level of education performance,
- annual goals including short-term instructional objectives,
- when services will begin and the expected amount of time needed, and
- the ways that educational progress will be evaluated.

A time line of the evaluation process is provided (Table 8–1). An example of an IEP shell with a communication goal is included (Table 8–2).

Vocational Setting

The Americans with Disabilities Act (1), which was passed in 1990, is civil rights legislation which required changes in both the public and private sector. Employment, transportation, communication, and public accommodations must be equally accessible to the handicapped population as they are to the able-bodied population. Families and clients often are not aware of their rights and may need the assistance of social workers, case managers, life care planners, public health nurses, and/or teachers to be informed fully. A major issue for adults with tracheostomies with or without mechanical ventilation is employment options. These individuals cannot be discriminated against, and the employer must make reasonable accommodations for these employees.

Under the Rehabilitation Act of 1973 (7), amended in 1986 (8) and in 1991 (9), any state receiving federal funds is required to develop vocational assessment and training programs to persons who are disabled. Any individual with a physical or mental impairment that impedes employment, must receive an individualized written rehabilitation program. The program is developed in conjunction with the client and interdisciplinary team members to maximize the client's potential in reaching and maintaining employment. There are nine nationwide centers for comprehensive assessments and services (Appendix A). During the assessment, the rehabilitation and employment potential of each client is evaluated. These assessments can include a comprehensive evaluation of pertinent medical, psychiatric, and psychologic needs. An appraisal is made of the individual's work patterns, ability to acquire occupational skills, and the ability to integrate socialization skills in the work place.

Recreation

There are many activities in which the client with tracheostomy with or without mechanical ventilation can participate fully or with modifications. It is important for the client and family to be aware of appropriate recreational activities. Listed in Appendix B are some age-appropriate activities for the younger client. Promotion of normalcy for the client and family is the ultimate goal. The client's rehabilitative plan can be incorporated into ongoing recreational activities.

There are various organizations, (e.g., Girl Scouts, Boy Scouts, Camp Fire Girls) that provide an opportunity for peer interaction. The YMCA/YWCA have multiple recreational programs that serve children and adults with special needs. Other organizations have disease-specific emphasis (e.g., the Muscular Dystrophy Society, the Spinal Cord Injury Association) and provide modified activities for their respective populations.

Table 8–2. An IEP shell including communication goal.

Individual Education Program—Present Levels of Performance		

Student's Name _____   Public School _____   Date _____

Strengths	Weaknesses	Assessments (date adm)
A. Academic/cognitive B. General health/physical C. Perceptual functioning D. Speech/language	Unable to verbally communicate	Ability to communicate ideas using a combination of nonverbal (signing, facial expressions, etc.) skills and the Liberator (a communication device).
E. Social/emotional/behavior F. Prevocational attitudes/abilities		

Annual goal _____

Service provider(s) _____

Short-term objectives	Criteria for mastery	Evaluation procedures	Review schedules	Progress
1. Continue to keep all materials and mechanical assists organized and in good working order. 　A. Use care and responsibility in handling equipment 　B. Utilize assistive technology equipment to complete work tasks at school, and to communicate with peers and adults	100%	Teacher observation	Daily	

Some private agencies and service groups organize camps for disabled children. Camps provide the opportunity to be away from the home setting and foster self-esteem while providing socialization opportunities. Children with minimal disabilities can be mainstreamed into regular camps. To obtain information about camps in the client's geographic area, the family can check with local organizations, the primary care provider, the health department, or the local newspaper's camp edition. Parents should visit the camp and determine staff qualifications and ratio of care providers to campers. If possible, parents should talk to past and present campers and their parents regarding their camping experience. When mainstreaming a child in a standard camp environment, parents should speak with the camp director about the child's specific needs to determine if the camp is suitable. For a child with tracheostomy with or without mechanical ventilation, access to emergency medical services (EMS), experience of the staff with these types of children, and an adequate electrical power source are important considerations for parents evaluating a camp program.

Clients of all ages can participate in modified sports, such as therapeutic horseback riding. Adolescents and adults become involved through support groups, recreational therapists, or individual resources. Some professional organizations include the following:

- Brain Injury Association,
- National Head Injury Foundation,
- March of Dimes Defects Foundation,
- National Multiple Sclerosis Society,
- National Federation of the Blind,
- Pets on Wheels,
- Salvation Army Boys and Girls Clubs,
- Special Olympics,
- United Cerebral Palsy,
- United Way, and
- church and community organizations.

See Appendix C for additional resources.

Caregiver Education

The Hospital Educational Plan

Interdisciplinary team members are involved in providing the client and caregivers the necessary education and validation of their abilities to provide for all the needed care. As this has the potential to involve many people, a coordinated and well-developed plan for education must be devised. The primary nurse for the client is an ideal candidate to coordinate these efforts. The primary nurse has an understanding of the daily activities the client must accomplish and how much the client is able to participate in performing these activities. The nurse is also aware of the amount of rest time the client requires to maintain the highest level of function, as well as suctioning schedule, medication administration preferences, and what motivates the client to participate in therapies. The primary nurse has formal education regarding goal setting, developing a plan, implementing the identified measures, assessing their effectiveness, and then making changes to the plan as needed to obtain the goal. The nurse is usually the only member of the interdisciplinary team who is immediately available to the client and caregivers 24 hours a day, seven days a week. When unexpected changes occur with the client's condition or the educational plan, the nursing staff can implement immediate measures to protect the safety and welfare of the client. The primary nurse must be able to work in conjunction with the other interdisciplinary team members to develop a coordinated and systematic approach to caregiver education. In this way, the caregivers are less likely to become distraught, overwhelmed, and frustrated with the plan for taking their loved one home.

The first step of the plan is setting realistic goals of what can be accomplished in a given time period. The caregiver should be asked about the frequency and length of time he/she can devote to educational sessions. A caregiver who can commit to daily sessions lasting eight hours or more should move more quickly through the educational time lines, than a caregiver who can devote themselves to twice-a-week sessions lasting two hours in length.

Second, it is advisable to identify with the caregiver how he/she is able to learn best. A neuropsychologist or educational specialist can assist with this process if needed. Some caregivers prefer written material, others like to observe the skill being demonstrated, others would rather practice the skill in a simulated or practice station. Once the caregivers learn the information, the identified skills must be demonstrated at an independent level prior to discharge.

The third step in developing the plan is documenting all the skills the caregiver must perform prior to taking the client home (Table 8–3). This should be a comprehensive interdisciplinary team list. The skills can then be ranked from simple to complex. The list can be further categorized into identified milestones or subgoals. For example, if the caregiver would like to accompany the client off the nursing unit without nursing staff, the caregiver would need to be able to demonstrate certain skills. These milestones can be attached to motivational rewards for the client and caregiver such as an outing to a local restaurant or mall, with the ultimate goal of discharge home (Table 8–4). The list of skills is divided among the appropriate team members, and a schedule is formulated indicating who is going to be teaching specific content to the caregiver at any given time. A time line identifies various time intervals in which the skills should be accomplished. This allows the client and caregiver to feel a sense of accomplishment, as well as serve as an evaluation of whether the educational plan is appropriate or needs modifications.

Specifics to Teach Caregivers for Home Discharge

The more informed the client and caregiver are regarding the reason for the tracheostomy with or without mechanical ventilation, the more likely they are to be compliant with the performance of various aspects of care such as routine tracheal suctioning. It is vital that the client and caregiver understand how particular skills affect the maintenance of the client's optimal health. If adequate

Table 8–3.   Teaching plan.

Content	Method taught	Evidence of learning
1. Describe reason for the tracheostomy tube and mechanical ventilation		
2. State signs and symptoms of respiratory distress and appropriate interventions		
3. State reasons for and demonstrate ability to perform ambu bag ventilations via tracheostomy tube and face mask		
4. State indications for and demonstrate CPR techniques		
5. State frequency and demonstrate tracheostomy tube string or holder change		
6. Describe indications for tracheal suction and demonstrate appropriate technique		
7. State frequency and demonstrate tracheostomy tube change		
8. State appearance of normal/routine tracheal secretion color and consistency for client		
9. State signs and symptoms of possible stoma and pulmonary infection		
10. Describe conditions requiring notification of physician		
11. Describe frequency and how to clean and maintain suction equipment		
12. Describe frequency and method for cleaning and maintaining ventilator equipment		
13. Identify high pressure ventilator alarm and appropriate interventions		
14. Identify low pressure ventilator alarms and appropriate interventions		
15. Identify ventilator settings (IMV, date, total volume, etc.) and dial settings to prescribed levels		

Table 8–4. Skills checklist.

Skills to be demonstrated	Off the nursing unit	Trip out of the hospital	Discharged home
1. Suction the tracheostomy tube using portable suction	X	X	X
2. Routine and emergency tracheostomy tube changes	X	X	X
3. Troubleshooting the ventilator for high pressure alarms	X	X	X
4. Appropriate interventions for ventilator low pressure alarms	X	X	X
5. Ambu bag to tracheostomy ventilation	X	X	X
6. How to activate help within the hospital	X		
7. List of supplies to accompany the client always	X	X	X
8. How to transfer the client in and out of a car or lift van		X	X
9. How to secure the client in the car or lift van		X	X
10. Total understanding of how the ventilator works, appropriate settings the client is on, and how those settings affect the client's respiratory function		X	X
11. CPR		X	X
12. Performance of ADL skills and home therapy routines		X	X
13. Usage and maintenance of all equipment used in the home			X
14. How and when to order disposable supplies for the home			X
15. Who to call with problems (i.e. equipment company, home health nurse, primary care physician)			X

humidification is not present in the ventilator circuit, then the client may develop a mucus plug. Usually, the physician educates the client regarding the disease process and rationale for the tracheostomy tube and ventilator. The rationale may be reinforced by other team members. For example, the occupational therapist, who is educating the client and caregiver regarding bathing and dressing techniques, may reinforce how the ventilator helps the client reserve strength that was normally used for breathing, so the client can perform more of his own bathing and dressing.

The nursing staff, in conjunction with the respiratory therapist, educate the client and caregiver regarding routine tracheostomy tube care and stoma maintenance. Tracheostomy tube maintenance includes suctioning the tracheostomy tube, providing inner cannula care, performing tracheostomy tube changes, cleaning the stoma, and using humidity. Some tracheostomy tubes have inner cannulas. The purpose of the inner cannula is to prevent secretions from building up on the inside of the tracheostomy tube. The inner cannula is removed on a daily basis (or as needed), cleaned, or disposed of, and replaced with a cleaned or new inner cannula. Copious, tenacious secretions can be quickly eliminated from the tracheostomy tube by removing the inner cannula. The outside of the tracheostomy tube remains intact and patent, while the secretions are whisked away with removal of the inner cannula. Since the tracheostomy tube lumen is so small in children, pediatric size tracheostomy tubes do not have inner cannulas (see Chapter 7). Therefore, children may require more frequent tracheal suctioning than do adults who have tracheostomy tubes with inner cannulas.

Caregivers are taught clean (versus sterile) suction technique for the home setting. It is important for the client and caregiver to become familiar with the usual frequency of suctioning and consistency of secretions. An increase or decrease in the frequency of suctioning or a change in the consistency of tracheal secretions may indicate a deterioration of the client's medical condition. It is also vital for the client and caregiver to recognize that yellow, green, or bloody tracheal secretions require prompt physician notification.

The client and caregiver must be able to change the tracheostomy tube safely on a routine basis. This can vary from once a week to twice a month, depending on the client's risk for infection, granuloma tissue development, and physician preference. The client can perform his own routine tracheostomy tube change by placing himself in front of a mirror. First, the client removes the old tracheostomy tube. Then using hand-over-hand guidance from an assistant, the client places the tube into the stoma. With practice, the motivated client should be able to insert the tracheostomy tube in a controlled environment successfully, however, this is an unrealistic expectation in an emergency situation, such as in the case of a blocked or dislodged tube. The caregiver must also demonstrate competency in changing the tracheostomy tube. In addition, the caregiver must know the alternative steps to take if the same-size tracheostomy tube cannot be inserted. The first step is to insert a tracheostomy tube one size smaller. If that is not successful, either insert a suction catheter into the stoma until professional help arrives to dilate the stoma or cover the stoma and, if necessary, provide ambu bag and face mask ventilation or mouth-to-mouth ventilation.

Various devices are used to hold the tracheostomy tube in place, the most popular being a soft adjustable velcro collar, however, this may be inappropriate for some children or adults who may loosen the collar and dislodge the tracheostomy tube. In these instances, twill tape, ribbon, or shoe string attached to the tracheostomy tube, surrounding the neck and firmly knotted may be used to hold the tracheostomy tube in place (Fig. 8–1). These ties may become looser or tighter as either they become wet or the diameter of the neck changes with position changes and muscle tone. Close observation is needed to prevent skin breakdown around the neck or dislodgement of the tube. The caregiver should be able

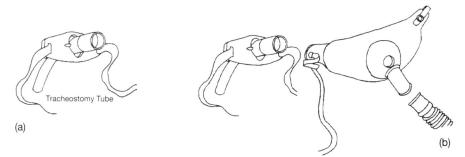

Fig. 8–1. (a) Tracheostomy tube with twill tape ties. (b) Tracheostomy collar surrounds the tracheostomy tube to connect supplemental oxygen and/or humidification.

to insert one or two fingers between the client's neck and the tracheostomy holder or ties. This is usually an adequate amount of tightness to hold the tube in place and prevent skin breakdown.

Stoma preservation includes cleansing the site at least daily with clean water or half-strength hydrogen peroxide. The site should be inspected daily for any signs of complications, such as extra tissue formation (granuloma), or bloody, green, or yellow drainage. The physician should be promptly notified if any of these complications occur. The stoma should look red and moist with pink healed edges. Small amounts of clear thin drainage are normal. Some clients prefer a split 2 × 2 absorbent pad under the tracheostomy tube to pad the area under the flange of the tracheostomy tube and help absorb secretions around the stoma.

Since the tracheostomy tube permits air entering the lungs to bypass the nose and upper airway, a humidification process must be utilized to moisten and, at times, warm the air entering the tracheostomy tube. There are many methods to accomplish this goal. The home care supply company should be able to help identify the most appropriate method to use in the home setting. Usually the client has two methods to provide humidity: one portable and one stationary. The stationary method usually requires a water reservoir attached to a compressor which is connected to the client via corrugated tubing (Fig. 8–2). A heater can be placed in or around the water reservoir if heated mist is needed. The portable method usually involves a small plastic hollow tube with filtering paper on the end. The plastic tube attaches directly to the tracheostomy tube. Both methods require routine cleaning or disposal of equipment to minimize the growth of bacteria.

The physician may prescribe certain medications that will open the airways, thin secretions, or help the client expectorate secretions. As with all medications, the client and caregiver should demonstrate knowledge of the name, dosage, rationale, and potential harmful side effects of each medication. In addition, the client and/or caregiver must demonstrate how to measure and appropriately administer the medication. This may include the use of a nebulization machine or metered dose inhaler (MDI) to administer inhalation medications.

Other interventions that may be used for certain clients include chest physiotherapy, postural drainage, tracheostomy tube cuff inflation and deflation, and

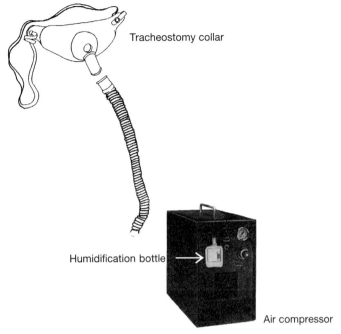

Tracheostomy collar

Humidification bottle ⟶

Air compressor

Fig. 8–2.   A humidification system that can be used in the home setting. The air compressor with attached humidification bottle creates humidified air, while the corrugated tubing connects the humidification bottle to the tracheostomy collar.

speaking valves. If these are utilized to maintain the client's optimum health, then the client and caregiver must demonstrate knowledge of why the intervention is used, how to perform related skills appropriately, and how to sanitize and maintain equipment.

Equipment

In the hospital, disposable equipment is used one time, then thrown away. This practice prevents the spread of infection. In the home setting, equipment such as suction catheters are often cleaned and reused. There are no standards to indicate how many times a suction catheter or tracheostomy tube can be reused and cleaned. Instead families ration the usage of supplies according to how many they are allotted from their payor source. For example, one state's medical assistance program may allow for two tracheostomy tubes of the ordered size per year. Families then clean and reuse the tracheostomy tubes throughout the year. Other states' medical assistance programs may pay for a new tracheostomy tube each time the tracheostomy tube is changed. Suction catheter replacement practices vary widely. Most payor sources provide an allotted number per month, and families use their own judgment of when to replace the catheter. With the standardization of home health agencies and equipment companies, some of these practices may become more uniform over the next few years.

If the client requires mechanical ventilation, then the client and caregiver must demonstrate competencies regarding the use and function of the particular type of ventilator. To begin the educational process, the client should understand the physiology of normal respiration, and how the client's disease process or disability affects normal respiration. Next, the client and caregiver must understand how the particular ventilator settings assist the client with breathing. The client and caregiver should know the purpose of each ventilator setting and the parameters in which to set alarm limits. The caregiver must know whether the ventilator is assisting the client with breathing, whether the client has some degree of spontaneous respiratory effort, or if the ventilator is doing all the breathing for the client (i.e., ventilator dependent). If the client is able to breathe on his/her own, then the caregiver may have more time to troubleshoot the reason for the ventilator alarm. If the client is ventilator dependent, the caregiver must be able to troubleshoot the ventilator alarm rapidly and, based on the client's physical appearance, provide ambu bag ventilation to the tracheostomy tube until the reason for the alarm is corrected. In addition to understanding how the ventilator functions, the caregiver must demonstrate how to change and clean the tubing (circuit) that connects the ventilator to the tracheostomy tube. The circuit is an excellent medium for bacterial growth. The ventilator circuit can be disposed of and then replaced, or cleaned and reused. If the cleaning method is used, two circuits are required. One circuit is attached to the client while the other one is soaking in cleaning solution and air drying. With either method, the tubing is disposed of or cleaned on a weekly basis.

Some clients may require supplemental oxygen. When oxygen is being used in the home, several precautions should be utilized. First, a sign should be posted on the outside of all doorways leading into the house indicating oxygen is in use and smoking is not permitted. Oxygen is highly flammable, therefore, no open flames or items causing sparks should be near the client receiving oxygen. This includes candles, matches, lighters, electric razors, and aerosol sprays (e.g., hair sprays that contain alcohol are highly flammable). The client should also avoid the use of petroleum-based products such as lip balm and hair ointment, as these products are highly ignitable. Clients and families must be instructed regarding these safe practices, and advised to have working flashlights in case of power outages to avoid the use of candles or kerosene lights.

The educational plan also must include all the techniques that are employed to help the client achieve an acceptable quality of life. One of the basic skills is aiding the client with a form of communication to express needs, wants, and desires. All clients with tracheostomy tubes need to adjust the way they communicate orally since the tracheostomy tube rests below the vocal folds. Several types of tracheostomy tubes, speaking valves, and ventilator settings can be employed to facilitate oral communication. Until oral communication is established, some type of communication system must be utilized. This could include eye movement for yes or no, a language board, or written communication. If oral communication is not an option, alternative communication systems must be established that can be understood by others outside the hospital and home arena (see Chapter 5).

Other interventions that may be included in the educational plan depend on the client's functional abilities. The occupational therapist (O.T.) may be involved in aiding the client and caregiver in completing activities of daily living, such as bathing, dressing, grooming, and self-feeding. Organizing and adapting the home, work, and/or school environment may be addressed to assist the client in establishing independence. The physical therapist (P.T.) may be involved in education regarding proper body alignment and positioning, range of motion exercises, and achieving a form of mobility in the home and community.

Finally, the educational plan must include an emergency section. A list of emergency supplies should be made. The supplies that should always be immediately available to the client or caregiver are:

- tracheostomy tube of the same size currently utilized,
- tracheostomy tube that is one size smaller than current size,
- water-soluble lubricant,
- scissors (to cut the tracheostomy tube holder),
- tracheostomy tube holder,
- suction catheters,
- suction machine,
- normal saline (to instill in the tracheostomy tube to thin secretions), and
- ambu bag.

Unless the client does not want to be resuscitated, the caregiver should be instructed in cardiopulmonary resuscitation including modifications for people with tracheostomy tubes. The emergency section should also include notification of local emergency medical providers (EMS) that a person with special needs will be discharged to the community. The electric company should be notified to place the client's house on a priority list to restore power in the event of an outage. If the client is taken to another hospital, "traveling papers" should be available. "Traveling papers" state the client's medical condition, reason for the tracheostomy tube and/or ventilator, size and brand name of the tracheostomy tube, ventilator type and current settings, list of medications, including dosage, frequency, and indication, and names and phone numbers of caregivers and the primary physician.

The educational plan can be overwhelming to the client and caregiver; therefore, the discharge plan should be clear with support and encouragement offered along the way. It is important to allow the caregiver and client time to practice the skills learned in a supportive and nonthreatening environment. In-house therapeutic leaves of absence (TLOA) is a term used to describe such a practice environment. In this setting, the client's hospital room is modified to resemble the home setting. All the equipment that the caregiver and client will be using at home is brought to the hospital room. The caregiver "rooms-in" with the client and provides all the care, while interdisciplinary team members are available to answer questions and evaluate the caregiver's abilities. Further education and practice sessions are encouraged until the caregiver and client are competent. A TLOA session at home is also helpful in providing the client and caregiver a realistic view of what life will be like once discharged home. These practice sessions are sometimes difficult to arrange if the client's home is distant from the discharging facility, or if multiple pieces of equipment must be transported back and forth. In these particular circumstances, community supports, such as 24-hour licensed nursing coverage, may be put in place to help ease the transition from hospital to home.

Long-Term Case Management and Life Care

As the educational plan is discussed and developed, the community plan should also develop simultaneously. The case manager is the optimal person to develop and coordinate the plan, because of his/her clinical background, knowledge of financial issues, and capability to act as a liaison with all health team members.

Case management is a description of a process rather than a structure or an outcome (10). It is more than a concern with an episode of illness, but rather the total continuum of care. This term is widely used in the insurance arena and hospital setting to facilitate the coordination and handling of complex clients. It is not a new practice. For example, mental health patients have been case managed for years. With the pressures of managed care, case management and the case manager now have become a necessity to control costs while providing optimal care for a variety of patient populations.

Most often, case managers have been social workers or advanced practice nurses. Nurses have the clinical expertise to articulate medical needs to business, insurance, and government health experts. Social workers are particularly sought out for those clients who have extensive psychosocial issues. According to Holt (11), nurses are already recognized as experts in managing individual clients' care across delivery settings. The focus on prevention and teaching is delegated routinely to nurses both within hospitals and in the community.

Case managers can attempt to meet the goals of managed care. Karen Zander of the New England Medical Center set forth the following goals of managed care in 1988 (12):

- achievement of expected or standardized patient outcomes,
- discharge within the appropriate length of stay,
- appropriate or reduced utilization of resources,
- collaborative practice directed toward attainment of patient outcomes,
- coordination and continuity of care involving patient and family, and
- professional development and satisfaction of hospital-based clinicians.

For clients with tracheostomies with or without mechanical ventilation, the utilization of a case manager is a necessity. These individuals have chronic medical conditions and may be frequently hospitalized, require expensive healthcare, and have multiple and/or complex diagnoses. They have complicated discharge needs and have been or are currently managed by a home care nurse and/or insurance company case manager. Psychosocial issues often plague these patients and their families.

The ideal flow of case management for these clients should cross the lifespan. In the case of an elective hospitalization, the case manager identifies resources for efficient quality care, potential discharge delays, and continuum of care issues. Specifically, they make telephone calls to the home or visit, schedule tests, contact the primary physician, and anticipate discharge needs on a preadmission basis.

During the acute care phase, the case manager interacts with utilization review staff, educates the family, determines if outcomes are being met, and continues communication with the primary care provider. At discharge, he or she may schedule follow-up appointments, continue educational efforts, assess medical/environmental resources, finalize and send the discharge summary, and ensure adequate social support. Post discharge, the case manager monitors client/family satisfaction, functional status, and outcome tracking as well as communicates with post-discharge caregivers.

For long-range planning, clients may require and benefit from a life care plan. A life care plan is a comprehensive assessment of needs over time and an attempt to match needs with resources. These plans are an extensive version of critical pathways or care maps that are commonly used in the inpatient hospital setting. Critical pathways identify critical or core events that need to occur to meet a patient's expected length of stay. The critical pathway includes functional health parameters (e.g., diet, activity, treatments, medications, patient education, assessment and monitoring of lines/drains, consults, standardized outcomes, and daily evaluation of those outcomes) (13). This results in decreased confusion regarding nursing and medical plans of care. The critical pathway is only helpful for the acute phase. Individuals with multiple needs require a life care plan. These documents are helpful for catastrophically injured clients who may have a lifetime cap on their health insurance policy. Any educated or experienced rehabilitation professional who is aware of the medical and therapy needs for a particular client can prepare a life care plan.

The life care plan is based on the medical history and current status of the client. Multiple areas should be considered, including projecting costs to determine feasibility. These areas are medical supervision, diagnostic studies, future procedures, complications, attendant/respite, therapeutic modalities, equipment, recreation, vocational planning, legal, residential placement, health insurance, and case management. Available financial resources are explored, such as public funding, private insurance, special programs and/or foundations, and family financial resources. After all areas are identified with assigned costs and coverage determined, the life plan can be implemented. A review of the plan should be undertaken periodically to reflect current clinical conditions and needs.

Financial Considerations

Multiple avenues exist to finance healthcare for clients with chronic conditions. Basically, coverage is sought through an insurance carrier if an individual is privately insured. Other avenues include publicly provided health insurance, such as Medical Assistance/Medicaid. Children can receive services from Services for Children with Special Care Needs. The family may have personal funds although these are frequently exhausted in a short time frame. Some foundations and/or community organizations may make funds available for certain pieces of equipment (e.g., specialized transportation). Resources vary tremendously from situation to situation, state to state, and at different points in time.

Private insurance carriers are based on either fee-for-service or prepayment. The fee-for-service approach is quickly vanishing as managed care penetration occurs which dictates enrollment of clients into a health maintenance organization (HMO). Since speciality services are fairly costly to the HMOs (which have limited funds in their organizations for all members), use of these services are controlled carefully.

Blue Cross/Blue Shield is an example of a fee-for-service model. These plans usually have a deductible and a co-pay. An 80% coverage/20% co-pay is a common distribution. An unfavorable feature of fee-for-service is that a maximum lifetime benefit of 1–2 million dollars may be dictated. For a client with multiple ongoing medical needs, even 2 million dollars is not adequate for care from "the cradle to the grave."

Health maintenance organizations are known primarily as prepaid health plans. They can be structured as individual practice associations, such as the Maryland Individual Practice Association (MDIPA) or group practices. An example of group practice in the State of Maryland is the Columbia-FreeState Health Plan. The advantage of an HMO is the emphasis that it places on primary care. Traditionally, these organizations do not exclude preexisting conditions and co-insurance/deductibles are minimal, if nonexistent. A disadvantage for the chronically ill client is the gatekeeper. This individual, usually the care manager or primary care physician, must authorize care by a specialist/subspecialist or out-of-plan institution. Gatekeepers must be accessed continually for the client to receive speciality services. Another disadvantage is that coverage for long-term physical therapy, speech–language services, occupational therapy, and durable medical equipment may be lacking. These therapies are vital to the care of ventilator-dependent individuals. Needless to say, caution must be exercised by the client and family concerning enrollment, transition, and access of healthcare benefits.

Some individuals are uninsured or drastically underinsured due to unemployment, part-time employment, employment with a small organization, or ineligibility due to preexisting conditions. In these cases, public healthcare programs such as Medical Assistance are administered by the federal government and individual states. This program, technically known as Medicaid, is Title XIX of the Social Security Act (14). For 30 years, this program has provided designated health services for eligible persons. Children with chronic conditions are often eligible if their family income status falls within a welfare category. The absolute financial criteria vary from state to state, so each family and/or client must complete a detailed application process. If approved, the family/client is able to receive a myriad of services from inpatient hospital care to home health. Clients, particularly children, who are technology dependent can be discharged from an inpatient hospital stay to a home setting under a waiver program. Individuals eligible for a waiver program are those who would not be able to be cared for in the community without intensive skilled nursing and other related health services. An agency, such as the Coordinating Center for Home and Community Care

(Maryland model), orchestrates the application for the waiver program. This organization assists the family in completing paperwork, provides ongoing case management services, and is a liaison with the healthcare agencies serving the client and family. Becoming a waiver client can take four to six weeks, so advanced planning is necessary. In some states, the patient must remain in the hospital while the waiver is being processed otherwise, they are not eligible for the waiver if they are discharged prior to acceptance.

Another federal-state program for children with special healthcare needs is Title V of the Social Security Act (15) which was established in 1935. Individual states receive funding via their respective health departments to assist mothers and children in need of services at the local level. Further enhancements to the Title V legislation were accomplished with the Maternal and Child Health Services Block Grant in 1981 (16) and 1989 (17). This provided for programs such as the Early Periodic Screening Diagnosis Treatment (EPSDT) program, Medicaid, and Women, Infants, and Children program (WIC). The EPSDT Program is operated differently by each state and supplies shift nursing without case management services. The EPSDT Program is more of a transitional program to carry the client through the acute rehabilitation phase, whereas the waiver program is able to blend private insurance coverage with medical assistance for those families who meet medical assistance criteria. Private insurers may also be willing to convert certain benefits into others (e.g., intermittent nursing visits into shift nursing coverage). This is very important for those individuals who do not qualify for medical assistance.

In 1981, with the passage of the Block Grant, the Supplemental Social Security Income (SSI) (Title XVI of the Social Security Act) (18), which covers adults and children with disabilities, was incorporated. The main emphasis is to help recipients become as self-sufficient as possible. It does not pay directly for the costs of healthcare for a child with a chronic condition, but it does make families eligible for Medicaid while the client is hospitalized. For example, if insurance provides 80% coverage, the remaining 20% is covered by Medicaid if the client is SSI eligible. As stated initially, various private funds and community foundations, such as Shriners, United Cerebral Palsy, and the Association of Retarded Citizens can augment these funding sources. Again, these vary tremendously from family to family and community to community.

Based on the various funding sources, the home care plan is developed. Interdisciplinary team members are encouraged to identify services necessary to help the client and caregiver be successful in the community. The home care plan includes a medical supply company that delivers and maintains the durable medical equipment as well as disposable items such as tracheostomy tubes and suction catheters. In-home nursing coverage may be involved if funding sources are available to pay for these services. Clients with tracheostomy tubes may require intermittent skilled nursing visits to the home and, depending on the school setting, a licensed nurse may need to accompany the child during school hours. The client on a ventilator may need shifts of skilled nursing care. More nursing care is generally required when the client is initially discharged and can be decreased once the client and caregiver settle into their daily routines. If the client is returning to the work setting, the employer and client must discuss what modifications need to be made to the work site and what reasonable accommodations the employer would need to provide to assist the client in the performance of the job. However, these reasonable accommodations are not defined and vary greatly from setting to setting.

Other service personnel that may be required in the community plan are a respiratory therapist, home health aide, a rehabilitative assistant, a physical and/or occupational therapist, and speech–language pathologist. The respiratory therapist usually is associated with the medical supply company. Monitoring of the client and the equipment is usually done at least once a month by either a certified or registered respiratory therapist. A home health aide works under the direction of a registered nurse, and usually assists the client and caregiver in performing activities of daily living and household maintenance. The registered nurse supervises the home health aide periodically. The frequency of this supervision, as well as what the registered nurse can delegate to the home health aide, is regulated by each state's Board of Nursing. A rehabilitation aide works under the supervision of a physical or occupational therapist. The rehabilitation aide assists the client and caregiver in performing daily exercises or activities that assist the client in becoming stronger or more independent. Again, the frequency of supervision and the delegated tasks are regulated by individual states and employment agencies. Educational and certification programs are available to provide basic instruction to the unlicensed home health and rehabilitation aide. Some states are also attempting to identify and track the performance of unlicensed healthcare providers in the home. This further defines the role of the unlicensed healthcare provider and protects the client and caregiver from fraudulent practices. Although these in-home services can appear costly, over the long haul, these ongoing arrangements demonstrate a cost savings from a traditional inpatient hospital stay.

In the future, healthcare will continue to offer new challenges in the management of these types of clients. Hopefully, with careful planning and case management utilization, these clients will receive optimal care.

Case Studies

Infant Case Study

S.W. was a full-term infant born at a small community hospital. The mother's pregnancy had been unremarkable. At birth, S.W. was noted to have a meningomyelocele, a left fractured clavicle, and periods of apnea or absence of respirations. She was transferred to a large academic medical center for further management.

Her hospital course included surgical repair of the meningomyelocele, a ventriculoperitoneal shunt placement, and surgical decompression of the foramen magnum. The latter procedure was performed to address with persistent apneic episodes related to the Arnold-Chiari malformation, however, the surgical decompression was not successful.

Other complications were lateral ventricle dilatation of the head, laryngomalacia, and gastroesophageal reflux. A sleep study revealed both obstructive and mixed apneas. To further manage her apnea, a tracheostomy was placed so that she could be ambu bagged during apneic episodes. Despite adminsitration of high calorie-formulas, a gastrostomy tube had to be placed for aspiration problems and suboptimal growth. Medication was required for seizure activity, bilateral hydro-nephrosis, and anemia.

From a social standpoint, her mother was 30 years old, married with two other children ages two and six years. She had worked as a phlebotomist prior to S.W.'s birth. Her husband was a long-distance truck driver who was emotionally and financially supportive, but away from home for substantial periods of time. The mother visited the neonatal intensive care unit (NICU) several times a week. This was a considerable hardship for her given her other children, geographic dis-tance from the hospital (two hours travel), and physical absence of her husband. S.W.'s hospital costs were covered through a private insurance company.

S.W. was transferred to a pediatric rehabilitation unit close to her home for in-tensive parent education, community reintegration, regulation of her seizure medications, and to achieve adequate weight gain.

Child Case Study

D.W. was a 6 year old, living in New York, who was struck by a motor vehicle after getting off the school bus and attempting to cross the street to his house. Cardiopulmonary resuscitation (CPR) was started at the scene by an off-duty po-lice officer. He was transported to the nearest hospital and found to be a C1 to C2 complete spinal cord injury. There were facial lacerations and a mild closed head injury. He was stabilized at the hospital with a shunt, a tracheostomy, and venti-lator support.

A month later, accompanied by his mother, he was transferred via air ambu-lance to the nearest pediatric rehabilitation hospital. His mother roomed in for approximately one month until D.W. became comfortable enough with the staff to be left alone. D.W.'s mother then rented a handicapped-accessible apartment close by so she could regularly participate in his care and later have a place to take him for therapeutic leaves of absence (TLOAs).

An interdisciplinary team worked with D.W. to obtain his optimal sitting po-sition, ventilator settings, mode of transportation, and communication skills. He learned how to operate his sip-and-puff wheelchair. The rehabilitation hospital had a home-based school program which assisted D.W. in maintaining his grade-level educational skills.

The patient's family had intense and ongoing skill training. This included:

- suctioning the tracheostomy tube and ambu bagging,
- tracheostomy tube changes, string changes, and tracheostomy site care,
- ventilator settings, maintenance and troubleshooting of alarms,
- signs and symptoms of infection,
- autonomic dysreflexia,
- signs of increased intracranial pressure associated with shunt dysfunction,
- clean intermittent urinary catheterization,
- skin care and proper positioning to maintain body alignment and prevent con-tractures,
- bowel evacuation program, and
- range of motion exercises, splint application, and removal.

After his family demonstrated competency in all these skills and D.W.'s motorized wheelchair was available, his mother took D.W. to her apartment every weekend for TLOAs. The TLOAs gave her the confidence she needed to care for her son fully, at which time he was transitioned back to his home, school, and community in New York.

Adult Case Study

J.W. was a 10-year veteran of the local fire company. One evening, his fire company was called to a local warehouse fire. While combating the fire, a large beam struck and injured J.W. He suffered extensive facial and inhalation burns, and back injuries. He spent several months in an intensive care unit (ICU) and had several procedures to attempt to restore his upper airway to regain normal breathing without a tracheostomy tube. J.W. was successfully weaned from mechanical ventilation, but required a tracheostomy due to large amounts of scarring tissue in the facial area and upper airway. His strength declined due to the prolonged ICU stay. He had multiple surgeries to correct his crushed vertebra at C3 and C4. When J.W. arrived in the rehabilitation program, he utilized a communication board on which he pointed to letters and phrases to indicate wants and desires. Although the MRI indicated the spinal column was intact, J.W. experienced numbness and, at times, loss of function in both hands. After intensive rehabilitation, J.W. transitioned to a day therapy and vocational program. At night, he was at home with his wife and 5-year-old daughter, who both helped him complete his daily care activities. J.W. remained tracheostomy dependent. He used a reuseable inner cannula tracheostomy tube as he was able to manipulate this type of tracheostomy device to clear secretions. Due to his residual limited fine motor hand function, J.W. was not able to perform deep tracheal suctioning. His wife performed this task for him as needed. There was also a nurse available at the day program to provide deep tracheal suction if needed. Besides working with an occupational therapist to help with fine motor function, a physical therapist helped J.W. with reconditioning and strengthening exercises to improve his distance with ambulation. The speech–language pathologist worked with J.W. to enhance his speech and ability to communicate because his vocal folds were damaged. The vocational assessments indicated that J.W. might be successful using a computer with adaptations. J.W.'s long-term goal was to find a job he enjoyed and provide sufficient financial support for his family. He investigated using a computer to develop layouts for the placement of fire sprinkler systems within buildings.

Case Study Summary

In all three cases, the individual needed to demonstrate medical stability such as adequate weight gain, a consistent medication regimen, and a stable airway whether they were mechanically ventilated or not. They achieved their rehabilitative goals and could participate in early-intervention (school or day rehabilitation) programs. Their respective families demonstrated satisfactory completion of their training programs.

At a minimum, each client was sent home with a tracheostomy tube of the appropriate size and a back-up tube one size smaller, a portable suction machine, suction catheters, and a compressor for humidification. Other supplies and equipment were dependent on individual needs.

A case manager or life care planner was utilized to secure the needed equipment and facilitate the discharge of the individual to home from a financial and logistical perspective.

Appendix A.   Comprehensive Assessment Centers

Carl D. Perkins Comprehensive Rehabilitation Center
5659 Main Street
Thelma, Kentucky 41260-8609
(606) 789-1440
(606) 789-6341

Hot Springs Rehabilitation Center
P.O. Box 1358
Hot Springs, Arkansas 71902
(501) 624-4411
(501) 624-0019

Michigan Career & Technical Institute
Pine Lake Development Office
11611 West Pink Lake Road
Plainwell, Missouri 49080
(616) 664-9230
(616) 664-5850

Roosevelt Institute
P.O. Box 1000
Warm Springs, Georgia 31830-0268
(706) 655-5001
(706) 655-5011

West Virginia Rehabilitation Center
Barron Drive, P.O. Box 1004
Institute, West Virginia 24112-1004
(304) 766-4696
(304) 766-4966

Maryland Rehabilitation Center
2301 Argonne Drive
Baltimore, Maryland 21218
(410) 554-9107
(410) 554-9222

Woodrow Wilson Rehabilitation Center
Box W-2
Fishersville, Virginia 22939
(540) 332-7265 (phone)
(540) 331-7132 (fax)

Hiram G. Andrews Center
727 Goucher Street
Johnstown, Pennsylvania 15905
(814) 255-6412
(814) 255-3406

Tennessee Rehabilitation Center
460 Ninth Avenue
Smyrna, Tennessee 37167-2010
(615) 741-4921 (phone)
(615) 355-1371 (fax)

Appendix B.   Age-Appropriate Activities

Age (years)		
1–3	Crawligators	Musical toys
	Adapted swings	Dolls
	Stuffed animals	Books
4–6	Tricycle	Board games
	Wheelchair sports	Blowing bubbles
	Puzzles	Computer games
7–12	Musical instruments	Arts & crafts
	Scouting	Special Olympics
13–17	Drawing	Driving
	Gardening	Table Tennis
	Fishing	Environmental control
	Photography	systems

Note: Activities in the lower age groups may be appropriate for older age groups, i.e., wheelchair sports, computer games, scouts, etc.

Appendix C.   National Organizations/Support Groups

American Lung Association
1740 Broadway
New York, New York 10019
(212) 245-8000

American Paralysis Association
4100 Spring Valley Road
#104, LB3
Dallas, Texas 75234
(800) 527-0321

Association for Children & Adults with Learning Disabilities
4156 Library Road
Pittsburgh, Pennsylvania 15234
(412) 341-1515

Association for the Severely Handicapped (TASH)
7010 Roosevelt Way, N.W.
Seattle, Washington 98103
(206) 523-8446

Guillain-Barré Syndrome Support Group
Box 262
Wynnewood, Pennsylvania 19096
(215) 649-7837

Muscular Dystrophy Association of America
810 Seventh Avenue
New York, New York 10019
(212) 586-0808

National Committee/Arts for the Handicapped (NCAH)
1825 Connecticut Avenue, N.W.
Washington, D.C. 20006
(202) 332-6960

National Easter Seal Society
2023 West Ogden Avenue
Chicago, Illinois 60612
(312) 243-8400

National Information Center for Handicapped
Children & Youth
Box 1492
Washington, D.C. 20013

National Library Service for the Blind & Physically Handicapped
Library of Congress
Washington, D.C. 20542
(202) 287-5100

National Maternal & Child Health Clearinghouse
3520 Prospect Street, N.W.
Washington, D.C. 20057
(202) 625-8410

National Spinal Cord Injury Association
369 Elliot Street
Newton Upper Falls, Maine 02164
(617) 964-0521

SKIP: Sick Kids Need Involved People
216 Newport Drive
Severna Park, Maryland 21146
(301) 647-0164

Society for the Advancement of Travel for the Handicapped (SATH)
26 Court Street
Brooklyn, New York 11222
(718) 858-5483

Spinal Cord Society
6203 Bellaire Avenue
North Hollywood, California 91606
(213) 761-2931

Travel Information Center
Moss Rehabilitation Hospital
12th Street and Tabor Road
Philadelphia, Pennsylvania 19141
(215) 329-5715

References

1. Americans with Disabilities Act of 1990. P.L. 101-336, 104 Stat. 327.
2. Education for All Handicapped Children Act of 1975. P.L. 94-142, 89 Stat. 773.
3. Findeis A, Larson JL, Gallo A, Shekleton M. Caring for individuals using home ventilators: an appraisal by family members. *Rehabil Nurs* 1994;19:6–11.
4. Education of the Handicapped Act Amendments of 1986. P.L. 99-457, 100 Stat. 1145.
5. Individuals with Disabilities Education Act. P.L. 91-230, 84 Stat. 121 § 601 et seq.; P.L. 101-476, 104 Stat. 1103, § 901.
6. NICHCY: News Digest. Questions and answers about the IDEA. *NICHY* 1993;3:1–15.
7. Rehabilitation Act of 1973. P.L. 93-112, 87 Stat. 355.
8. Rehabilitation Act Amendments of 1986. P.L. 99-506, 100 Stat. 1807.
9. Rehabilitation Act Amendments of 1991. P.L. 102-52, 105 Stat. 260.
10. Knollmeuller R. Case management: what's in a name? *Nursing Management* 1989;6:38–41.
11. Holt F. Managed care and the clinical care specialist. *Clinical Nurse Specialist* 1990;4:27.
12. Zander K. Personal communication via telephone. Baltimore, Maryland, 1995.
13. Ling K. On the scene: managed care at the Johns Hopkins Hospital . . . initiation and evaluation of managed care. *Nursing Administration Quarterly* 1993;17:54–79.
14. Title XIX Grants to States for Medical Assistance Programs. P.L. 89-97, 79 Stat. 343.
15. Title V Grants to States for Maternal and Child Welfare. August 14, 1935, c. 531, 49 Stat. 629.
16. Maternal and Child Health Services Block Grant. P.L. 97-35, 95 Stat. 818.
17. Maternal and Child Health Block Grant. P.L. 101-239, 103 Stat. 2273.
18. Title XVI Supplemental Security Income for the Aged, Blind and Disabled. P.L. 92-603, 86 Stat. 1465.
19. Maryland Disability Law Center Inc. Special education rights . . . and wrongs handbook. 3rd ed. Baltimore, Maryland, 1995.

9

Ethics and Ventilator Dependency

Dean S. Tippett

"... I will fulfill according to my ability and judgment this oath and covenant: ... I will keep them [the sick] from harm and injustice ... I will neither give a deadly drug to anybody if asked for it, nor will I make a suggestion to this effect ... In purity and holiness I will guard my life and my art ... Whatever houses I may visit, I will come for the benefit of the sick, remaining free of all intentional injustice ..." (1)

The Oath of Hippocrates, 400 B.C.

The Hippocratic oath has stood for more than two thousand years as a basis for the ethical practice of medicine. Some form of the original oath is used by 47% of all U.S. and Canadian medical schools (2). The classic Hippocratic oath specifically forbids euthanasia and abortion, and is believed to be the source for the more common and often used statement "First, do no harm" (3). Although 98% of all medical schools use an oath of some form, up from only 24% in 1928, only 14% have retained the prohibition against euthanasia and only 8% continue to forbid abortion (2). Some content, however, has not changed. All medical oaths refer to a covenant with patients and 97% continue to insist on confidentiality (2).

Just as the medical oaths have evolved, the practice of medicine has also changed. It is interesting that as the moral dimensions of medical practice have become more difficult, there is a return to the basic principles of ethics and morality. This is evidenced by a resurgence of interest in medical oaths and attempts to broaden them to include all healthcare providers (4).

Today, we increasingly find ourselves with complex medical decisions to make and, while we strive to provide the best patient outcomes, we face the real pos-

Tracheostomy and Ventilator Dependency: Management of Breathing, Speaking and Swallowing. Edited by Donna C. Tippett, MPH, MA, CCC-SLP. Thieme Medical Publishers, Inc. New York © 2000.

sibility of "doing harm." This may be in the form of prolonging an inevitable death or failing to honor a patient's wishes. The SUPPORT study, a large multi-center study of 9,105 patients with clearly identifiable life-threatening illnesses, found that only 47% of the doctors knew when their patients' preference was to avoid cardiopulmonary resuscitation (5). Additionally and sadly, the study found that after intensive attempts to increase physician-patient communication through education, there was no appreciable difference in understanding patients' wishes (5). The study raises questions about whether the time-honored practice of community and healthcare worker education is enough to promote the ideals of advance directive statutes.

Medical research has produced great advances in the last few decades. This has been especially true for patients requiring ventilatory care. Despite the hallmark development of the "iron lung" by Phillip Drinker and Louis Shaw in 1929 (6), the mortality of poliomyelitis patients requiring mechanical ventilation remained as high as 79% (7). In 1949, a positive pressure device was added to the tank respirator and reduced mortality to 17% (7). In 1964, only about 35% of general medical patients who required artificial ventilation survived (8). By 1985, 85% of patients ventilated survived (9). More recent advances in ventilatory and tracheostomy technology are described in earlier chapters of this book (see Chapters 3 and 4). These developments have, in many cases, given patients extended life and new opportunities. However, with these advances has come the possibility of prolonged suffering rather than well-being, of prolonged death rather than healing. By the 1970s, mechanical ventilation was being used with a wide variety of patients, as was renal dialysis and artificial alimentation. In a review of the history of mechanical ventilation, Snider observed that by the 1970s "ethical issues became a part of everyday life in the intensive care unit" (p. 55) (10). It is therefore our obligation as health professionals caring for patients with tracheostomy and ventilator dependency to step back and consider the options, present them to patients and families in an honest way, and allow informed autonomous decisions. Medical ethics decisions are difficult and call upon many areas of knowledge. The answers are not always clear. The decisions require the weighing of many variables. Therefore, it is important to understand ethical principles and have a process for ethical decision-making.

This chapter provides a review of the relevant ethical principles and a framework for helping patients and healthcare providers making these decisions. This includes advance directives, living wills, and appointment of a healthcare agent and surrogate decision maker. Ethics committees can be a valuable resource and in some situations may be a requirement. Although high-profile cases are often resolved in a court of law, the courts and lawyers are only occasionally needed to resolve ethical dilemmas.

The specific topics covered in this chapter include artificial nutrition and hydration, and communication and mechanical ventilation in patients with profound ventilatory failure and intact cognitive function. The very special and emotionally charged situation of an alert, competent person who wishes to be removed from the ventilator and allowed to die is examined. Training in ethical decision-making is discussed.

Conditions generally associated with impaired cognition (e.g., bilateral cerebrovascular accidents, end-stage Alzheimer's disease, profound closed head injury) are only briefly addressed. This book, and therefore this chapter, generally refers to patients with intact cognition. The causes of ventilatory failure may be classified as either profound neuromuscular impairment or severe pulmonary dysfunction. The causes can be further separated into two groups by onset type: acute and progressive. Acute conditions include high cervical spinal cord injury, pontine cerebrovascular accident (hemorrhagic or ischemic), and smoke inhalation. Guillain-Barré syndrome (acute inflammatory demyelinating polyneuropathy) may produce temporary ventilatory dependence, but is generally reversible. A similar although more chronic condition (i.e., chronic inflammatory demyelinating polyneuropathy) would be included in the slowly progressive group, as would some progressive forms of lung disease (e.g., cystic fibrosis, chronic obstructive pulmonary disease). Other progressive etiologies include amyotrophic lateral sclerosis (ALS), muscular dystrophy, brain stem mass, and progressive neurologic diseases (e.g., ponto-cerebellar degeneration). This distinction between acute and progressive conditions is important in that the progressive conditions afford the medical team with the opportunity to begin discussion of ethical issues months in advance of their need. Unfortunately, this is a luxury that many healthcare providers and patients do not utilize (5).

Case 1

Mr. Thomas is a 95-year-old resident of a nursing home. He has been living in the nursing home for the last five years after suffering a devastating cerebrovascular accident that left him paralyzed on his right side and unable to communicate. He was admitted to the hospital last night with a high fever, productive cough, and lethargy. A chest x-ray confirmed the admitting physician's clinical diagnosis of pneumonia. Mr. Thomas was given intravenous antibiotics and chest physical therapy. Early the next morning the nurse found Mr. Thomas with very labored breathing. He was taken to the intensive care unit, intubated, and placed on the ventilator. A nasogastric tube was placed. His family was notified of his worsened condition. Ten days later he could not be weaned from the ventilator and a tracheostomy was performed.

Mechanical ventilation and nasogastric alimentation were seen as requirements in this patient's care, the next logical step. No one considered any other options. The ventilator, the nasogastric tube, or both could have been withheld. The goal of treatment should be to honor the patient's wishes. An advance directive indicating the patient's wishes may have been available and utilized. The patient's family could have provided valuable information about his wishes. Since deterioration could have been foreseen upon admission, a discussion with the family should have been initiated.

Ethical Principles

Whether we know it or not, we are making ethical choices each day. Medical decision-making requires a step-by-step process. Even seemingly very simple medical acts follow these steps. Generally, symptoms or signs mark the onset of an illness. These are assessd by some form of examination. The results of the examination are processed into a diagnosis. From the diagnosis a plan of treatment is derived (Table 9–1, part A) (11). For example, the patient complains of feeling warm, a temperature is taken, a diagnosis of fever is made, and acetaminophen is given. Implicit in this simple interaction is the assumption of patient capacity (ability to make a decision) and the often unacknowledged consent to be treated (Table 9–1, part B). The issues of capacity and consent are generally only considered in the face of serious procedures (e.g., surgery). But these issues as well as other principles are present in each decision, if only implicitly.

Table 9–1. Medical decision-making model.

A. Symptoms	B. Symptoms
Examination	Examination
Diagnosis	Diagnosis
Treatment	*Capacity*
	Consent
	Treatment

A short review of ethical principles provides a foundation for the rest of the chapter. More in-depth reviews can be found in *Principles of Biomedical Ethics* by Beauchamp and Childress (3), and *Intervention and Reflection: Basic Issues in Medical Ethics* by Munson (12). A concise introduction is provided in *Introduction to Clinical Ethics* by Fletcher (13). A brief overview is sufficient for our purposes; however, each principle is much more complicated and rich in meaning. Many fine points have been and continue to be debated concerning these principles.

Autonomy

The principle of autonomy requires respect for the patient's right to make choices free of undue influence. This is the foundation of informed consent or informed refusal. An informed decision requires as full an understanding of all the related factors as possible. Incomplete information would therefore provide an undue influence over a decision. A free choice requires that others are not directing a decision. This does not mean a disregard for authority, but rather the freedom to follow an authority if desired (e.g., religious principles). Some individuals may be incapable of an autonomous decision because of decreased level of consciousness (e.g., coma), cognitive dysfunction (e.g., head injury), a psychiatric disorder (e.g., depression), or immaturity (child) (3).

Informed Consent

The elements of informed consent consist of competence/capacity, disclosure of information, understanding, voluntariness, and authorization. Competence is addressed more fully later. Disclosure of information is essentially the education of the patient about the procedure, risks involved both with and without the procedure, and the expected outcome. Understanding requires that the patient has processed the information and is able to reiterate it to the healthcare worker. Some believe that we can never be truly fully informed or have complete understanding. This has lead to the legalistic term, reasonable person standard. What would a hypothetical reasonable person be expected to understand? Voluntariness is the ability to act freely without control by another person or condition (e.g., drugs, depression) (3).

Nonmaleficence

The principle of nonmaleficence concerns the ideal of inflicting no injury upon the patient. This principle is contrasted with beneficence or the intention to produce good and prevent harm. Many ethical issues involve a balance between these two principles. Nonmaleficence is generally thought to be the more compelling principle in most situations. The principle of double effect is discussed later and requires the consideration and balance of these two principles (3).

Beneficence

The principle of beneficence involves the obligation to benefit the patient. This is at the heart of the healing professions. The goal of any patient interaction is to improve the patient's condition, whether through prevention of disease or the curing of disease. It is a principle that is so basic we sometimes think of it as a preeminent principle. This may lead to a paternalistic approach if patient autonomy is thought to be less important. Most believe that patient autonomy and beneficence must be considered together (3).

Justice

The principle of justice may be viewed broadly and with many nuances. However, only the concept of fairness is considered here. Some believe this principle is outside the realm of the healthcare provider and patient relationship and is better dealt with on a societal level (e.g., the allocation of healthcare resources). On an individual basis, it suggests that all patients should be treated equally, in a fair and just way. In a world and even a country where millions do not have adequate availability of healthcare, this clearly is not fully realized (3).

Truth-Telling

There is an obligation to provide the truth as we know it when interacting with our patients. We should never purposely deceive (3). This is expected by patients and is an essential part of the healthcare provider-patient relationship. There are times when the reporting of some specific information should be restricted to the attending physician (e.g., diagnosis, prognosis). These topics can be discussed with the patient further by other health professionals after discussion with the physician. For example, the prognosis concerning the future return of swallowing is best discussed by the speech-language pathologist and the most insight on the prognosis of walking can be offered by the physical therapist.

Privacy and Confidentiality

Patients have an expectation of privacy. They expect that access to their medical information is limited to their immediate healthcare providers (3). This is accomplished by the storage of medical records in safe locations where access is limited and controlled. Today, much information is maintained on computer systems. Adequate access controls are required. Confidentiality is the act of withholding information about a patient from others (e.g., family, community, employers, other healthcare workers not involved in the patient's care). If a computer hacker breaks into the hospital computer, he has violated your privacy; if a doctor discusses your diagnosis with your family without your consent, he has violated your confidentiality. These principles seem self-evident, but unfortunately are often violated. The limits of these rules are often tested. For example, what is your obligation when your HIV-positive patient refuses to admit the diagnosis to his wife?

Case 2

Mr. White has just been diagnosed with AIDS. Before ordering the HIV test, he completed a consent form where the risks of testing were discussed (*informed consent*). His HIV results are not displayed on the hospital computer (*privacy*) and his physician does not discuss his diagnosis with the patient's family (*confidentiality*). His physician provided the diagnosis to the patient as soon as they were available (*truth-telling*). Mr. White is weighing the treatment options as explained to him. Aggressive medication protocols may benefit him (*beneficence*), but may also produce severe side effects (*nonmaleficence*) and discomfort. His physician has explained each choice as fully as possible and Mr. White must make a decision (*autonomy*). He has full insurance coverage under his wife's insurance plan. He realizes that his coworkers could not afford these treatments (*injustice*).

The Principle of Double Effect

The principle of double effect means that an act with a harmful effect is not always prohibited if the same act has a beneficial effect as well. Giving a medication to cause someone's death is considered morally wrong. However, if the primary intention of giving that medication is pain control, then the secondary unintended effect of hastening death is acceptable. The intention of the act must be the good effect (pain control) not the bad effect (death). The bad effect may be foreseen or even expected. Some restrictions have been placed on this principle. Some insist that the action itself must be morally good or neutral. Therefore poisoning a patient to alleviate pain would be wrong. Others insist that the good effect cannot be achieved by way of the bad effect. For example abortion of a healthy child in an ill mother may not be allowed by some. As the principle is used here, it generally concerns giving medication to provide comfort at the end of life (e.g., morphine to decrease the sensation of air-hunger) (3).

Case 3

Mrs. Scott has end-stage ovarian cancer and has exhausted all treatment options. Her physician has discussed hospice care with her and she has agreed to it. Each day she must take morphine to control her pain. Over the last week, she has required increasing amounts and increased frequency of dosing to control her pain. She is lethargic and sleeps most of the day. Her family is concerned that at times she is unconscious and seems to stop breathing for several seconds. She cannot be aroused for her other medications. However, if they give her less morphine she is again in pain. They ask the hospice nurse for advice. The nurse explains that the primary intention of giving the medication is for pain control. A second unintended, although not unforseen, effect is respiratory depression. This may actually hasten her death, but it is not the intended purpose of giving the medication. The family continues to give the pain medication as instructed. Mrs. Scott goes into a coma and dies the following day. Her last day of life was pain free.

Competence and Capacity

In all patient interactions we must assess the patient's ability to participate actively in their medical care. We are assessing their medical decision-making capacity. Although we often refer to their "competence" or "incompetence," these are actually legal terms and technically can only be determined by a court of law. Physicians and other healthcare providers must determine medical decision-making *capacity* (13,14).

Patients in coma obviously do not have capacity. Patients whose wakefulness is waxing and waning may be considered to have capacity at specific instances and should be included in decision-making when possible. This is often difficult and reliance on surrogate decision-making is often required.

Children are generally not considered to have capacity. However, minors are increasingly involved in their medical decisions. Some states have passed laws allowing minors certain rights, such as treatment for pregnancy, sexually transmitted disease, and birth control. Some older children may be living on their own and are considered emancipated minors, having the full rights of adults in medical decision-making (13). Parenthood can emancipate minors in many states.

Many patients have clear cognitive deficits and cannot participate in medical decisions. However, many patients have mild cognitive problems and a more formal assessment is required. Physicians use various methods to determine capacity. There is no single universally accepted procedure or test. In broad terms, capacity requires the ability to understand the situation, evaluate the situation, and make an unhindered decision (14). These are also the basic components of informed consent. Initial information concerning mental status can be obtained from the patient's history or from family members (e.g., ability for self-care, financial management). The mental status examination is an integral part of capacity determination. This usually involves questions of orientation, memory, concentration, and judgment (15). There are several clinically useful tests of mental status. The most well-known is the Mini-Mental State Examination (16). Another very helpful test is the Short Test of Mental Status (17,18). Poor scores on these tests may suggest that the patient lacks medical decision-making capacity.

Patients may also lack capacity because of mental illness. A patient with a psychotic illness, like schizophrenia with unusual thoughts and delusional thinking, may be unable to make any decisions. With treatment, they may recover capacity and participate in their care. Severe depression may not allow patients to understand the chances of recovery and the hopefulness of treatment. They may only focus on what seems to them as inevitable disability, pain, or suffering. Not all patients with depression necessarily lack medical decision-making ability or capacity. For example, many patients with life-threatening illnesses or severe injuries may be depressed, such as the patient with quadriplegia after spinal cord injury (19,20). Only if the depression hinders their decision-making ability is the patient without capacity. Therefore, a psychiatric evaluation is imperative when making life and death decisions in this patient population (21).

Several standards have been used when determining capacity. The most widely accepted standard is the functional standard, which evaluates the patient's functional ability to make medical decisions (13). This standard was supported by the President's Commission for the Study of Ethical Problems in Medicine and Biomedical and Behavioral Research in 1982 (22). The determination of capacity is not a one-time determination but must be made independently for each important decision. A patient with full medical decision-making capacity can:

(1) understand the relevant information,
(2) consider alternatives, and
(3) explain the decision.

This can be demonstrated by having the patient repeat or paraphrase the information, discuss the alternatives and why they are or are not good options and, finally, explain the reasoning behind accepting or declining the medical treatment. Some have added that the decision must follow a rational manipulation of the information (23). Still others insist that the decision must be consistent over time. This is particularly important for decisions concerning life-sustaining treatments.

Lastly, some have suggested a sliding scale of capacity based on the seriousness of the decision at hand. For example, we would insist on a much higher level of capacity when deciding on a surgical procedure than on deciding whether to take a sleeping medication. Therefore, when the decision involves ending life-sustaining treatment, such as ventilation in a ventilator-dependent patient, we must insist on the highest level of medical decision-making capacity. Others have taken this further by allowing a lower level of capacity when the decision can be viewed as generally appropriate. For example, a mentally retarded man may be able to give consent for a procedure such as emergency appendectomy. A much higher level of capacity would be required for the same man to refuse treatment which is likely to result in his death. This last step is somewhat controversial as a theory, implying that as long as the patient agrees with the healthcare providers there is less question or concern about capacity. In reality, this is often how daily decisions are made, with only the disagreements finding their way to the ethics committees or courts (24).

Case 4

Mr. Malloy was admitted to the hospital 10 days earlier after falling 60 feet from a ladder in his yard. He is intubated and quadriplegic. When his physicians try to discuss the need for tracheostomy, Mr. Malloy closes his eyes and cries. Although he has learned to respond with eye movements to other questions from his nurses and family, he refuses to respond to his physicians' questions about surgery. His capacity to make decisions is in question. A psychiatric consultation is requested. He is placed on an antidepressant medication, his sedative medications are decreased, and other medications that may affect his cognition are discontinued. Several days later he is more interactive with his physicians. Through a series of yes and no questions he is able to demonstrate an understanding of the tracheostomy procedure, and the risks and benefits involved. He agrees to the procedure and is able to talk using a speaking valve a few days later.

Advance Directives

It is well established that if a patient has the capacity to make their own medical decisions, then they must be given the opportunity. When the patient is not able to participate in these decisions, we first refer to any advance directives the patient may have completed. This may be in the form of a living will, or appointment of a healthcare agent (medical power of attorney). If no advance directive is available, then a surrogate decision maker may be appointed (see next section).

The first living will legislation was passed in California in 1977, the "Natural Death Act" (12). It permitted a competent adult to direct physicians to withhold or discontinue medical treatment in the future if the patient was in a terminal condition. The federal Patient Self Determination Act (PSDA) of 1990 went into effect in December 1991 and required hospitals, nursing homes, and other facilities receiving federal funds (Medicare and Medicaid) to ask patients about the completion of advance directives, to record this information in the hospital chart, and to develop policies to follow the patient's wishes (25). However, it was noted at the time and with subsequent reviews that the law actually did little to directly promote the use of advance directives or the discussion of advance directives between the patient and physician (26,27). All states have now passed their own laws concerning advance directives and generally provide a sample document (Appendix A). Many of these documents are overly legalistic and intimidating to the public. An advance directive that is gaining in popularity is one termed "Five Wishes." This originated in Florida and is now spreading across the country. It is legal in 33 states and the District of Columbia, as determined by the American Bar Association's Commission on Legal Problems of the Elderly (28). The other states require a specific form or a mandatory notice when completing an advance directive. In October 1998, the Robert Wood Johnson Foundation provided a grant to the Aging with Dignity organization to provide copies of the 11-page document via the Internet and mail (see reference 28).

Maryland's living will form permits specific instructions when the patient is unable to participate in healthcare decisions and is in a terminal condition (e.g., cancer) or persistent vegetative state (Appendix A, pages 290–291) (29). A persistent vegetative state is a clinical condition of complete unawareness of the self and the environment. There often are preserved sleep-wake cycles and autonomic functions. Patients in a vegetative state show no evidence of voluntary behavioral responses or language. In addition, the condition must have been persistent for greater than one month (30,31). The living will form allows a patient to direct physicians to provide "all medical treatment" or to not extend life by life-sustaining procedures (e.g., ventilators, cardiopulmonary resuscitation, artificial nutrition and hydration). This form is applicable to only two end-of-life conditions. The appointment of a healthcare agent allows for more broad decisions to be made by the agent.

An advance directive with appointment of a healthcare agent allows the patient to name a specific person to act as a surrogate decision maker (Appendix A, pages 292–293) (29). That person is able to make all decisions concerning the patient's healthcare. Anyone may be appointed. For example, an elderly man may name his granddaughter because she works in healthcare, and he is concerned that his wife and children may be too emotional to follow his directions. In many ways, this is the optimal advance directive as it allows the patient to appoint a specific person and does not limit their decisions. The patient must be sure to discuss their wishes with the surrogate well in advance, preferably at the time the document is executed. If the appointed surrogate knows little about the patient's wishes, it is less useful.

The patient may choose to complete the healthcare instructions section of the advance directive to provide the healthcare agent with written direction in making decisions (Appendix A, pages 293–295) (29). Terminal conditions and persistent vegetative states are again addressed. Maryland allows a third condition to be included: end-stage condition. An end-stage condition is somewhat ambiguous but includes diagnoses that are not immediately terminal, such as end-stage Alzheimer's disease or end-stage liver disease. The same directives are allowed as noted above. In some ways, completion of this second part limits the decisions of the appointed healthcare agent. It may also provide needed direction when the directive is used. None of these forms can fully replace an in-depth discussion with the family and healthcare agent about the patient's values and concerns about care if one is cognitively impaired.

Some states have adopted an addendum to the advance directives allowing the intention of organ donation to be clearly documented. This is extremely important, as families have often not discussed this topic and have great difficulty in making this decision once faced with the medical tragedy that has lead to brain death (Appendix A, page 295) (29).

Lastly, some states (i.e., Maryland) allow for verbal advance directives. Statements generally made to the physician may be written into the patient's medical record and honored just as a more formal advance directive is honored. However, it is important to understand that these statements may be hard to obtain or recall when needed. A formal written advance directive with copies given to family members is the best assurance that the patient's wishes will be honored.

The forms referred to above are those used in Maryland. The laws in other states may differ. The patient should contact his or her state's Attorney General's office for specific regulations and copies of acceptable advance directives.

Case 5

Mrs. George was an active 59-year-old woman when she suffered a myocardial infarction (MI) and sudden cardiac arrest. Cardiopulmonary resuscitation was initiated by a co-worker within a few minutes. When paramedics arrived, she required a course of medication and two defibrillation attempts to recover a heart beat. She was transferred to a coronary care unit and stabilized. The diagnosis of a large MI was made. Two days later, she remained intubated and unresponsive. An electroencephalogram was consistent with diffuse brain damage. Mrs. George's children brought a copy of an advance directive she had completed two years earlier after the prolonged illness and death of her husband. The document stated that she wished aggressive care to be discontinued in the event of irreversible brain damage. The document went on to state that she wished to be considered for organ and tissue donation. On the third hospital day, the ventilator was discontinued and she died. The family consented to tissue donation (skin and bone) to honor her wishes.

Surrogate Decision Making

If no written or oral advance directive is available to the attending physician, a surrogate decision maker must be appointed. This is usually a close family member (i.e., the spouse). State laws may direct the healthcare team to an appropriate or legal representative. For example, in Maryland the healthcare team must first turn to a legal guardian if one has been previously appointed. Since this is a rare condition, the spouse is usually the surrogate decision-maker. If no spouse is available (i.e., deceased, incapable because of illness) then the healthcare provider next turns to the adult children (Table 9–2) (29).

Table 9–2. Surrogate hierarchy (Maryland) (29).

Court appointed guardian
Spouse
Adult Children
Parents
Adult Sibling
Friend or Other Relative

All persons at each level have equal weight in making decisions. If there is a disagreement among persons of equal weight in one hierarchy, then an ethics consultation should be initiated (see p. 281).

If no suitable surrogate can be located or surrogates refuse to accept the responsibility, then there is no choice but to go to court and have a guardian appointed. In the past, this was often a lengthy procedure, but many states now have expedited court proceedings. This can usually be arranged through the department of social work or the hospital attorney.

Substituted Judgment Standard

When a healthcare agent or surrogate decision maker is considering a decision, it is the intention that the surrogate is making a judgment just as the patient would if he was able. They are substituting their judgment based on their knowledge of the values and wishes of the patient. This is the reason that the surrogate should be someone that the patient knows well, trusts, and with whom he or she has discussed their values (12).

Best Interests Standard

Even when the surrogate is a close family member, specific situations may never have been anticipated or discussed. The surrogate may not have any knowledge upon which to base a judgment. In this situation the best interests standard is used. What does the surrogate think is in the best interest of the patient? The healthcare agent or proxy may consider the quality of life of the patient, likelihood of restoration of function, and the relief of pain (12).

Improper Surrogate

Occasionally, the identified surrogate decision maker, whether appointed by advance directive or state guidelines, is inappropriate. For example, the separated spouse who has been living away without contact with the patient may be the legally indicated surrogate, but obviously is not the appropriate one. Similarly, an abusive spouse would be inappropriate. If the surrogate is making decisions based on their own values and is ignoring the wishes of the patient, that surrogate may be inappropriate. These situations are best handled by a meeting and discussion with the surrogate. The long-ago separated husband may easily defer to the patient's adult children. However, there may be times when a court must be involved. It is the responsibility of the healthcare provider to assure that the patient's wishes are being honored to the best of their ability (12).

Futility

Occasionally competent patients or their surrogates demand a specific treatment that the healthcare team feels is not beneficial to the patient. Two main types of futility have been described. Medical futility concerns treatments that are not expected to benefit the patient in a physiological sense (e.g., nasogastric feedings in a patient with nonfunctional intestines, CPR in a patient with imminent demise) (32). Qualitative futility considers the patient's total condition (32). For example, nasogastric tube feedings for a patient in a persistent vegetative state are not expected to have any significant effect on the patient's cognitive state. Qualitative

Case 6

Mrs. Johnson is a 42-year-old patient with a history of asthma and diabetes. She is morbidly obese. She has been hospitalized on several other occasions for respiratory distress and once needed intubation for three days. She had a cold last week and became short of breath. This morning she called out to her family from bed because of difficulty breathing. She was brought to the hospital in respiratory distress. Once in the emergency room, she suddenly stopped breathing and had a cardiopulmonary arrest. Despite prompt treatment with intubation and CPR, she has not awakened. On the first day she developed myoclonic movements of her extremities. This resolved by day two. On day five she opened her eyes to stimulation, but did not look at the examiner or follow commands. Today, day ten, her examination results have changed very little. She continues to require the ventilator. The intensivist reports that the asthma is under control and the aspiration pneumonia requires a few more days of antibiotics. She feels that in the next few days the patient can be successfully removed from the ventilator. The neurologist describes her condition as hypoxic encephalopathy and feels that a persistent vegetative state is the likely outcome. He can not rule out some recovery of awareness, but reports that she will certainly still be very dependent.

Mrs. Johnson has no advanced directives. Her mother is 65 years old and has visited each day since admission. She feels that her daughter would not want to live this way and says "enough is enough." She wants to remove the ventilator now and let her daughter die "naturally." The patient's daughter is 17 years old, an "A" student in high school, and has also visited each day. She recalls her mother's last admission when intubated. Her mother hated and pulled at the endotracheal tube, and had to be sedated. Although her mother never clearly stated she didn't want to be intubated, she feels she would want it removed now. The patient's only adult child is 19 years old. He is incarcerated at a correctional facility and has been unable to visit his mother. He strongly disagrees with the withdrawal of care. He wants everything to continue, full code status, feeding tube placement, and chronic care if necessary. An ethics consult is initiated. Who is the appropriate surrogate decision maker?

futility is generally thought to be outside the realm of the healthcare team, but may be considered by the family. The American Medical Association's Code of Medical Ethics states, "Physicians are not ethically obligated to deliver care that, in their best professional judgment, will not have a reasonable chance of benefiting their patient" (p. 8) (33). However, futility has proven difficult to define (32,34). Is a treatment that has less than a one percent chance of success futile? . . . less than one chance in a thousand? Or must there be absolutely no chance of success to be considered futile? This has lead many to suggest less reliance on a determination of futility and more reliance on generally accepted standards of care (33,35). If a treatment would generally not be considered in a specific

Fig. 9-1. End-of-life medical decision-making algorithm. Adapted, with permission, from Silverman (36).

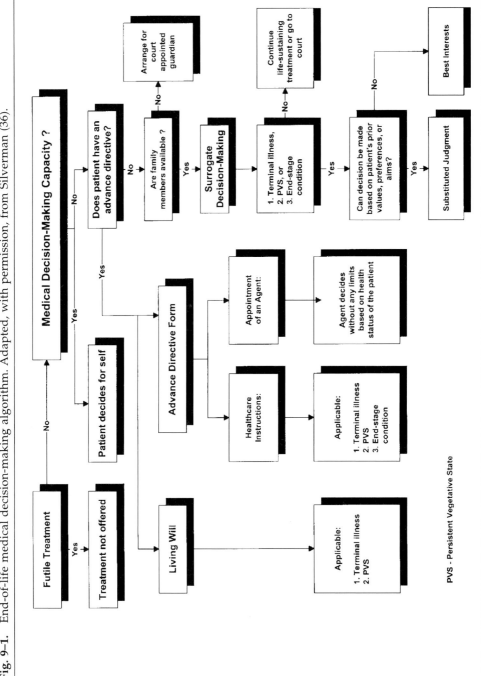

situation, then it need not be offered to a patient. A more thorough discussion of medical futility is beyond the scope of this chapter, but may be an important consideration when considering medical treatment options. Treatments that have no physiological benefit to the patient should clearly not be presented as an option. Treatments that have no qualitative benefits merit in-depth discussion, but ultimately must be left to the surrogate decision makers.

Many healthcare providers find the determination of surrogates, and when to use the advance directives, to be a confusing process with many nuances. An algorithm may help to show the logical steps taken when considering a medical decision. Figure 9-1 is a very helpful algorithm adapted from Dr. Henry Silverman's model for Maryland law (36). The first determination considers whether the intervention is futile or not. If it is determined to be futile, then there is no obligation to present it to the patient or the patient's surrogate. The patient's capacity is determined next. If the patient has medical decision-making capacity, then all of the healthcare decisions must be presented even if advance directive forms have been completed. The patient may, however, defer to a surrogate. If he or she has capacity, it is the healthcare provider's responsibility to make the patient aware of any treatments proposed and their risks. If the patient is without medical decision-making capacity, we would first look for any advance directives and consider their instructions. If there are no advance directives, we then look for an appropriate surrogate decision maker. Eventually the surrogate utilizes substituted judgment or best-interest standards in making medical decisions concerning the patient. It is often useful to discuss these two decision-making processes with the surrogate. Surrogates often feel that "they" are making a decision. It is helpful for them to understand that they are making a decision just as their loved one would have if they were able. This helps to minimize the responsibility a surrogate feels when making a difficult decision.

Ethics Committees

Occasionally there is a disagreement about a specific medical treatment. This may be between the patient and the physician, the surrogate and the physician, two or more surrogates, or two healthcare professionals. For example, a physician may question a patient's refusal of treatment for cancer when there is a question of depression. Another example may involve three adult children with equal weight as surrogates who disagree about resuscitation orders for their mother. Federal and state statutes have required the establishment of hospital clinical ethics committees to help resolve these conflicts (37).

Generally, the ethics committee consists of several diverse members of the hospital community, including but not limited to physicians, nurses, administrators, social workers, speech-language pathologists, chaplains, and ethicists. Some committees include community members to represent the values of the local area. Meetings are usually held ad-hoc for consultations. Consultations may be requested by any member of the healthcare team and should be available 24 hours a day (38). The goal of an ethics consultation is mediation between two parties that disagree.

After a call is placed to the ethics committee, there is generally a determination whether a true ethical question exists. Occasionally, people contact the ethics committee with concerns that are not ethical in nature (e.g., medical malpractice, poor communication between surrogate and physician). Once it is determined that an ethical question exists, then the ethics ad-hoc committee leader gathers information about the patient from the medical record, family, nurses, and physicians. A formal meeting is held during which the family, the patient (if possible), the treating physician, and the nurses attend. Everyone is given an opportunity to express their views. Frequently, the simple restatement and clarification of the medical options allow for a negotiation or mediation between the disagreeing parties. If no mediation can be achieved, then some advocate taking the disagreement to the courts for a decision (39). However, some suggest that the courts should really be used as a last resort and advocate a formal decision by the ethics committee (40). In fact, some state laws (i.e., in Maryland) encourage the committee not only to make a final recommendation, but also to notify the family of their right to appeal the decision through the courts (41). If a family has notified a healthcare institution of their intention to appeal a decision that may result in the death of a patient (e.g., removal of a nasogastric feeding tube), then that healthcare institution should maintain the patient's life until the appeal has been heard.

Case 7

Mr. Smith is an 64-year-old man with a long history of hypertension. He had a sudden severe headache, vomiting, and loss of consciousness. He fell to the floor, unable to move his right side. He was taken to the emergency room where he was intubated. A computed tomography scan revealed a large intracranial hemorrhage in the left basal ganglia with intraventricular blood. The neurologist met with the family—three adult children—and discussed his poor prognosis for recovery. The family wanted to know the possibility of recovery to a conscious state with the ability to communicate. The neurologist felt that it was very unlikely. The most likely outcome would be severe language problems and right hemiplegia. Two children wanted to discontinue the ventilator and allow him to die. The third child wanted to wait a week and see if he made any recovery. The family could not come to an agreement. An ethics committee consultation was requested by the attending physician. During the meeting, the third child reported that he and his father had conversations concerning medical care. His father always said, "don't let them stop too early." He had made clear indications that he wanted aggressive medical care. The ethics committee allowed all the children to discuss their father and what they knew of his wishes. The other two children admitted that they had not had similar discussions with their father and were unsure of his wishes. The committee mediated an agreement from the children and the attending physician to wait a week and re-evaluate his condition.

One week later he could open his eyes but was unable to communicate. The ventilator was discontinued and Mr. Smith was able to breathe on his own. He was transferred to a nursing home.

Pastoral Care

Pastoral care is often a source of comfort to the family and caregivers when difficult decisions are made (42). They may help the patient and family assess their values and focus on a patient's spiritual perspective (43,44). They are also an excellent resource for ethical principles and decision-making. In one study of hospital chaplains, 98% indicated that they had had continuing education in biomedical ethics within the previous two years (45).

Swallowing/Dysphagia

The ability to eat and swallow are taken for granted by the healthy. There is an automatic assumption of the desire for nourishment and drink. Numerous conditions may arise that impair a patient's ability to perform this function safely and adequately. Much controversy exists concerning the evaluation and treatment of disorders of swallowing. Patients and families often have great difficulty in understanding the risks involved and why such cumbersome interventions are required. Education is extremely important in obtaining compliance with various interventional strategies. There are times, however, when patients may find the strategies too burdensome. For them the benefit (often reducing the risk of aspiration and death) is not as great as the burden (reduced taste, unpalatable consistency, or not eating). When possible, we need to educate the patient and family concerning the various options and risks of various interventions.

In the past, the placement of a permanent feeding tube required major surgery. However, in the 1980s, the percutaneous endoscopic gastrostomy (PEG) was introduced. This could be performed by a medical physician using sedation only. From 1988 to 1995, the number of PEGs performed in the U.S. on hospitalized patients 65 years old or older almost doubled from 61,000 to 121,000 (46). In 1991, almost 1% of every hospitalized patient aged 65 years or older received a PEG or operatively-placed feeding tube (46). The most common primary diagnosis associated with a feeding tube was cerebrovascular disease (17.8%). "Some enterally-fed patients who do not have swallowing disorders are not dying because they lack nutrition, but rather lack the need to eat because they are dying" (p. 1976) (46). The overall mortality in this group is 23.9% at 30 days, 63.0% at one year and 81.3% at three years. The study did not look for differences among those that were able to survive for three years (46).

For example, the otherwise healthy patient who is undergoing an elective surgical procedure understands that eating and drinking restrictions are temporary and will minimize the risk of pneumonia post-operatively. The victim of a severe traumatic brain injury is not expected to be able to return to eating soon, but the potential for eventual recovery would suggest a course of nonoral feeding and early percutaneous endoscopic gastrostomy. But other situations may not be so clear cut. When a frail elderly woman with Parkinson's disease develops aspiration pneumonia, what are the chances that she will survive the pneumonia or return to normal eating? Many of these situations do not have clear answers.

Feeding tubes are generally placed to provide hydration and nutrition, and therefore prolong life. It is assumed that this goal is usually accomplished. However, some authors have questioned this assumption, as noted above. In another study, 64% of patients over age 70 years with chronic medical conditions, treated with a nasogastric tube, died in the hospital (47). It is also assumed that we are honoring the wishes of the patient. However, in many instances, the placement of a feeding tube is not discussed with the family. Oral or written consent was documented in the chart in only 4% of nasogastric tube placements (47). Another assumption is that nasogastric feeding tubes enhance the quality of life because they decrease a sensation of hunger. One aspect rarely considered is that in this same study, 53% of the patients required physical restraints to prevent them from removing the feeding tube. It is recommended that feeding tube placement be discussed with the family and that a balanced presentation of the benefits, risks, and expected outcome be given in advance of tube placement. This requires a longer discussion with families than is generally provided. Feeding tube placement should be considered a medical treatment and, therefore, informed consent must be obtained just as with any other procedure.

Many consider nutrition and hydration essential to patient comfort. Several studies, however, have demonstrated that patients in terminal states do not suffer pain or discomfort (48, 50). In fact continued intravenous fluids in these conditions may actually prolong discomfort (50).

Case 8

"We can't just let her starve. It's not legal" was the speech-language pathologist's reply to the acknowledgment that the physician was aware that Mrs. James was not receiving any nutrition. Mrs. James had suffered bilateral cerebrovascular accidents. Her heart, suddenly beating erratically in atrial fibrillation, had showered her arterial blood with small clots. Clots had gone to the brain, and lasted just long enough to produce severe and permanent damage. Mrs. James was mute and cognitively impaired. Although unconscious initially, she was now awake and able to look at her family. She was not able to participate in any decisions and was without medical decision-making capacity. She had been fed by a nasogastric tube until the day before, when it became dislodged and the family asked that it not be reinserted. A meeting consisting of the patient's family, nurse, and physician, was held to discuss the options, which included performing a percutaneous endoscopic gastrostomy (PEG), feeding the patient with the knowledge that aspiration was likely, or replacing the NG tube. The family explained how active and vibrant she had been and how she had always made it clear she would not want to live like this. She had completed a living will stipulating the withdrawal of food and water if her condition was determined to be an end-stage condition. Her condition was not expected to improve significantly and was consistent with an end-stage condition. The family chose not to reinsert the NG tube. They provided her with food and water when she appeared to want it. She would cough while eating. She became dehydrated, lapsed into a coma, eventually developed renal failure, and died with her family at her side.

Groher (51) advocates the development of institutional guidelines for artificial nutrition and hydration. He advises the development of guidelines that identify patients that are likely to need artificial nutrition, the development of a plan specifically for that patient, a mechanism that allows for the routine review of this plan, and the routine use of informed consent when a feeding tube is to be placed. As he points out, the development of institutional guidelines concerning artificial nutrition and hydration have not yet been carried out at most hospitals.

Communication

The ability to communicate is a fundamental necessity of human existence. Patients who loose the ability to communicate feel isolated. The restoration of communication through various devices is of significant importance to patients. Unfortunately, the importance of effective means of communication for ventilator-dependent patients is often overlooked in the intensive care unit setting (52). Burk (52) gives a description of his own frustrations with communication as a physician with Guillain-Barré. He states, "in the priority list of acute medical care needs, communication is not at the top" (p. 51). There are a variety of options available to the patient. These are described in Chapter 5 in this book. Effective programs to treat ventilator-dependent patients must have adequate methods of communication, from letter boards to sophisticated myoelectrically controlled switches (53). As Bernat (54) states, "clinicians have special ethical duties to attempt to enhance their disabled [ventilator-dependent] patients' communication abilities" (p. 206).

Ventilators

A brief history of the ventilator was described earlier in this chapter (also see Chapter 3). Much like the nasogastric tube or PEG, the decision to intubate a patient and place them on the ventilator is often an automatic response. When the patient is emergently short of breath or apneic and the diagnosis and prognosis are unclear, urgent intubation is appropriate. Therefore, the emergency use of ventilators will not be discussed further.

In many patients the need for a ventilator can be anticipated by hours, days, or even months. There is ample opportunity to discuss the benefits, risks, and expected outcomes with a patient or family. Patients that are acutely admitted to the hospital with a possible need for intubation should have this major medical intervention discussed at the first opportunity. The usual discussion includes only, "If you stop breathing would you like us to put you on the ventilator?" True informed consent should include the expected benefit in that particular patient, the risks including loss of communication and inability to wean, and the expected outcome. The latter is the most difficult to estimate upon admission. It requires a real understanding of the patient's diagnosis and prognosis. It is a difficult discussion to have with a patient. Do they really understand their diagnosis? Do they really want to hear the prognosis? Perhaps because we leave this discussion to the most junior physicians, we do the worst job of this most important component.

Patients with longer, more progressive illnesses should have the most oppor-tunity to consider intubation and ventilation (54). A patient with amyotropic lat-eral sclerosis (ALS) should be informed of the expected course of the illness and the definite progression to respiratory failure. In these patients there is ample time to provide examples of patients who have chosen long-term ventilation. Well known examples, such as Stephen Hawking and Christopher Reeves, are impor-tant symbols that patients with quadriplegia and ventilator-dependency can still lead a rich life with continued opportunities for accomplishment. However, per-haps the most effective examples are ordinary people living relatively common lives while ventilator-dependent (55).

Rational Patient Wants to Remove Ventilator

Many ventilator-dependent patients consider ending ventilatory support but few decide to do it. Some consider the removal of a ventilator, with the knowledge that death is near certain, to be suicide. However, as we will discuss it is not sui-cide and it has been upheld in numerous court decisions to be a refusal of a medi-cal treatment (54,56–58). It is important to differentiate this process from that of assisted suicide or even euthanasia. These are very different actions with very different moral implications.

In Table 9–3, a continuum of participation of a person in the death of another is proposed. At the far right is natural death with minimal involvement in the pro-cess of death, that is not to say that the physicians, nurses, and most importantly, the family, are not actively present and providing comfort. It only assumes that there is little involvement in the act of death itself. At the extreme opposite end is homicide with the active, involuntary, intended death of another. Other situa-tions are somewhere in between. Some would not agree with these assessments or the placement of "the line." Withholding or withdrawing treatment (e.g., ven-tilator, nasogastric tube, PEG) is considered essentially the same (59). The act is passive. It is done with the consent of the patient and the intention is comfort (e.g., the ventilator is considered burdensome by the patient). Although death can be foreseen, it is not the intention of the treatment withdrawal/withholding. Giv-ing a medication, such as morphine, to relieve air-hunger in a dying patient may be active, but again it is done with the consent of the patient or surrogate and with the intent of providing comfort. It is a form of palliative care (60). Therefore it is not morally wrong or "crossing the line." Once a medication is provided or given (e.g., potassium chloride) or an action is performed (e.g., suffocation) with the direct intention of causing death rather than the direct provision of comfort, many believe we have committed a morally wrong act, a homicide (i.e., active euthanasia). These were the actions and stated intentions of Dr. Jack Kevorkian, as evidenced on November 22, 1998 on national television. A video tape showed him injecting Thomas Youk, a nonventilator-dependent ALS patient, with lethal doses of three medications, none of which were pain medications (61). At the time of this publication, Dr. Kevorkian has been found guilty of first-degree murder and given a sentence of 8 to 15 years in prison (61).

Assisted suicide is the act of assisting someone with their own suicide. This may take the form of a healthcare professional prescribing a lethal dose of medi-

Table 9–3. Death with or without the participation of another person.

	Murder	Man-slaughter	Euthanasia	Assisted Suicide	Double Effect	Treatment Withdrawal	Treatment Withhold	Natural Death
Active/passive	Active	Active	Active	Active	Active	Passive	Passive	Passive
Consent/voluntary	No	No	No/Yes	Yes	Yes	Yes	Yes	N/A
Death intended	Yes	Yes/No	Yes	Yes	No	No	No	N/A
Comfort intended	No	No	No	No	Yes	Yes	Yes	N/A

(N/A, not applicable)

cation or providing specific instructions in how to complete a suicide. Dr. Kevorkian actually obtained the lethal medication, organized a delivery system, and assisted the patient in triggering the administration. Over 30 states have banned this practice (61). Oregon passed a physician-assisted suicide law in 1994 that went into effect in 1997. Later in 1997, the Supreme Court ruled that there is no constitutional right to die with the aid of a physician, effectively leaving the decision in the hands of state governments. In November 1998, Michigan defeated a ballot initiative to legalize physician-assisted suicide, apparently prompting Dr. Kevorkian's aforementioned nationally televised act (61).

This discussion is an attempt to place in perspective the action of a competent ventilator-dependent patient who has made the decision that the ventilator is too burdensome for him or her. The discomfort, the isolation or even the quality of life it provides is too much to bear for the patient. He or she may then make a request to have the ventilator disconnected. Death is expected and may even be considered a relief to this patient, but the intention is to relieve the burden of the ventilator and therefore remains to the right of "the line." The action can be justified as morally appropriate under a very specific set of circumstances.

Just as for informed consent, the patient must have capacity to make medical decisions, and must understand the risks of removing the ventilator (e.g., not just the obvious, death, but also the possibility of discomfort and air-hunger). The patient must also understand the possible future benefits of remaining intubated (57,58). This is where the educational component of chronic ventilator dependency becomes very important (54). From a hospital bed, life on a ventilator may seem bleak. The educational process must show patients the possibilities and probabilities of life on a ventilator. This should be an honest and straightforward presentation made by someone with knowledge of both the inpatient and outpatient realities. Visitation from a chronic ventilator-dependent patient should be encouraged. The patient must not be encumbered by psychiatric disease (e.g., depression). Therefore, a psychiatric evaluation is imperative. Lastly, we must be confident that this desire is constant over time (62). Therefore, the patient should be interviewed by more than one physician on more than one occasion. This is to assure the wish is not a whim (63) or a passing response to another setback in rehabilitation. Some have suggested that a ventilator-dependent patient cannot truly know what his life will be like until he lives it for several months (64). Others have even advocated waiting two years (65). There is debate about what the time requirement should be (66). A flexible time frame is probably best. Some patients may have very clear wishes. It may be inappropriate to impose a lengthy period of what they may consider suffering. Others may not have their thoughts and wishes clearly defined, as evidenced by their own statements (67). A longer period of time may allow these patients to either clarify their wishes or work towards rehabilitation and quality of life.

While we may desire that all patients chose to "fight" and remain ventilator-dependent, this clearly is not the choice for some. These patients need our understanding and commitment as well. There is a need for comfort care, including comfort medication after extubation (68–71).

Ventilator-Dependent Quality of Life

It must be pointed out that most ventilator-dependent patients choose rehabilitation and life. In a survey of 395 post-poliomyelitis ventilator-assisted individuals, respondents' mean satisfaction indices were greater than 4 (where 7 is for most satisfied and 1 for most dissatisfied) for all life domains except health. Healthcare professionals significantly underestimated patients' life satisfaction and overestimated the hardships associated with ventilator dependency (72). The obvious successes of other ventilator-dependent people are inspirational. Stephen Hawking continues to write best-selling books and Christopher Reeves continues to act, having starred in a 1998 made-for-television movie. Other ventilator-dependent patients hold jobs and are parents (73). In short, they continue to live.

Ethics Training

For those wishing further training in medical ethics, there are numerous opportunities. Each year, there are several national ethics conventions. Local universities often have courses or seminars each year. Most healthcare facilities have ethics committees and welcome new members. Ongoing education is increasingly a part of healthcare committees. At our health system, St. Agnes HealthCare, we have sponsored ethics retreats since 1996 and an annual ethics lecture since 1982. Every other month, we have combined medical-surgical ethics rounds, where the residents are encouraged to bring cases to present. The discussions become quite lively.

Conclusion

The tracheostomy and ventilator-dependent patient population presents a complicated and diverse set of ethical situations and questions. These patients often push ethical questions to the edge, from futility to autonomy, from pediatrics to the elderly. Understanding medical ethics enhances your ability to aid these special patients in making decisions. Your experience with these patients will further your knowledge and allow you to better care for all your patients.

> *One of the essential qualities of the clinician is interest in humanity, for the secret of the care of the patient is in caring for the patient.*
>
> Dr. Francis Peabody (1927)

Acknowledgment

My thanks to my wife Donna, without whose help and encouragement this work could not have been completed. Thanks also to Joanne Sullivan, the staff at the St. Agnes HealthCare Health Science Library, and to the many patients and colleagues that have shaped my understanding of ethics and have tested it daily.

Appendix A. Maryland Advance Directive Forms

Annotated Code of Maryland 5-601 5-618

LIVING WILL

(OPTIONAL FORM)

If I am not able to make an informed decision regarding my health care, I direct my health care providers to follow my instructions as set forth below. *(Initial those statements you wish to be included in the document and cross through those statements which do not apply.)*

A. If my death from a terminal condition is imminent and even if life-sustaining procedures are used there is no reasonable expectation of my recovery:

    _____ I direct that my life not be extended by life-sustaining procedures, including the administration of nutrition and hydration artificially.

    _____ I direct that my life not be extended by life-sustaining procedures, except that, if I am unable to take food by mouth, I wish to receive nutrition and hydration artificially.

    _____ I direct that, even in a terminal condition, I be given all available medical treatment in accordance with accepted health care standards.

B. If I am in a persistent vegetative state, that is, if I am not conscious and am not aware of my environment nor able to interact with others, and there is no reasonable expectation of my recovery within a medically appropriate period:

    _____ I direct that my life not be extended by life-sustaining **procedures,** including the administration of nutrition and hydration artificially.

    _____ I direct that my life not be extended by life-sustaining procedures, except that if I am unable to take in food by mouth, I wish to receive nutrition and hydration artificially.

    _____ I direct that I be given all available medical treatment in accordance with accepted health care standards.

C. If I am pregnant, my decision concerning life-sustaining procedures shall be modified as follows:

_____

_____

By signing below, I indicate that I am emotionally and mentally competent to make this Living Will and that I understand its purpose and effect.

_____   _____

           (Date)   (Signature of Declarant)

The declarant signed or acknowledged signing this Living Will in my presence and based upon my personal observation, the declarant appears to be a competent individual.

_____   _____
                (Witness)   (Witness)

_____   _____
                (Address)   (Address)

(Signatures and Addresses of Two Witnesses)

ADVANCE DIRECTIVE

PART A: APPOINTMENT OF HEALTH CARE AGENT

(OPTIONAL FORM)

(Cross through this whole part of the form if you do not want to appoint a health care agent to make health care decisions for you. If you do want to appoint an agent, cross through any items in the form that you do not want to apply.)

1. I, _____, residing at _____
    _____

    appoint the following individual as my agent to make health care decisions for me:

    _____
    _____

    (Full Name, address and telephone number of agent)

    Optional: If this agent is unavailable or is unable or unwilling to act as my agent, then I appoint the following person to act in this capacity:

    _____
    _____

    (Full Name, address and telephone number of back-up agent)

2. My agent has full power and authority to make health care decisions for me, including the power to:
    A. Request, receive, and review any information, oral or written, regarding my physical or mental health, including, but not limited to, medical and hospital records, and consent to disclosure of this information;
    B. Employ and discharge my health care providers;
    C. Authorize my admission to or discharge from (including transfer to another facility) any hospital, hospice, nursing home, adult home, or other medical care facility; and
    D. Consent to the provision, withholding, or withdrawal of health care, including, in appropriate circumstances, life-sustaining procedures.

3. The authority of my agent is subject to the following provisions and limitations:

    _____
    _____

4. If I am pregnant, my agent shall follow these specific instructions:

    _____
    _____

5. My agent's authority becomes operative *(initial only the one option that applies):*
    _____ When my attending physician and a second physician determine that I am incapable of making an informed decision regarding my health care; or

_____ When this document is signed.

6. My agent is to make health care decisions for me based on the health care instructions I give in this document and on my wishes as otherwise known to my agent. If my wishes are unknown or unclear, my agent is to make health care decisions for me in accordance with my best interest, to be determined by my agent after considering the benefits, burdens, and risks that might result from a given treatment or course of treatment, or from the withholding or withdrawal of a treatment or course of treatment.

7. My agent shall not be liable for the costs of care based solely on this authorization.

By signing below, I indicate that I am emotionally and mentally competent to make this appointment of a health care agent and that I understand its purpose and effect.

_____   _____
            (Date)   (Signature of Declarant)

The declarant signed or acknowledged signing this appointment of a health care agent in my presence and, based upon my personal observation, the declarant appears to be a competent individual.

_____   _____
          (Witness)   (Witness)

_____   _____
          (Address)   (Address)

(Signatures and Addresses of Two Witnesses)

PART B: HEALTH CARE INSTRUCTIONS

(OPTIONAL FORM)

(Cross through this whole part of the form if you do not want to use it to give health care instructions. If you do want to complete this portion of the form, initial those statements you want to be included in the document and cross through those statements that do not apply.)

If I am incapable of making an informed decision regarding my health care, I direct my health care providers to follow my instructions as set forth below. _(Initial all those that apply.)_

1. If my death from a terminal condition is imminent and even if life-sustaining procedures are used there is no reasonable expectation of my recovery:

    _____ I direct that my life not be extended by life-sustaining procedures, including the administration of nutrition and hydration artificially.

    _____ I direct that my life not be extended by life-sustaining procedures, except that if I am unable to take food by mouth, I wish to receive nutrition and hydration artificially.

2. If I am in a persistent vegetative state, that is, if I am not conscious and am not aware of my environment nor able to interact with others, and there is no reasonable expectation of my recovery:

    _____ I direct that my life not be extended by life-sustaining procedures, including the administration of nutrition and hydration artificially.

    _____ I direct that my life not be extended by life-sustaining procedures, except that if I am unable to take food by mouth, I wish to receive nutrition and hydration artificially.

3. If I have an end-stage condition, that is, a condition caused by injury, disease, or illness, as a result of which I have suffered severe and permanent deterioration indicated by incompetency and complete physical dependency and for which, to a reasonable degree of medical certainly, treatment of the irreversible condition would be medically ineffective:

    _____ I direct that my life not be extended by life-sustaining procedures, including the administration of nutrition and hydration artificially.

    _____ I direct that my life not be extended by life-sustaining procedures, except that if I am unable to take food and water by mouth, I wish to receive nutrition and hydration artificially.

4. _____ I direct that, no matter what my condition, medication to relieve pain and suffering not be given to me if the medication would shorten my remaining life.

5. _____ I direct that, no matter what my condition, I be given all available medical treatment in accordance with accepted health care standards.

6. _____ If I am pregnant, my decision concerning life-sustaining procedures shall be modified as follows:

    _____

    _____

7. I direct *(in the following space, indicate any other instructions regarding receipt or nonreceipt of any health care)*;

    _____

    _____

    _____

By signing below, I indicate that I am emotionally and mentally competent to make this Advance Directive and that I understand the purpose and effect of this document.

_____   _____
(Date)   (Signature of Declarant)

The declarant signed or acknowledged signing these health care instructions in my presence and, based upon my personal observation, appears to be a competent individual.

_____   _____
(Witness)   (Witness)

_____   _____
(Address)   (Address)

(Signatures and Addresses of Two Witnesses)

ORGAN DONATION ADDENDUM

PREPARED BY THE STATE OF MARYLAND OFFICE OF THE ATTORNEY GENERAL

(Note: If you want to be an organ donor, you can attach this page to your Living Will or Advance Directive. Sign it and have it witnessed.)

I direct that if I am brain dead, an anatomical gift be offered on my behalf to a patient in need of an organ or tissue transplant. If a transplant occurs, I want artificial heart/lung support devices to be continued on my behalf only until organ or tissue suitability of the patient is confirmed and organ or tissue recovery has taken place.

By signing below, I indicate that I am emotionally and mentally competent to make this organ donation addendum and that I understand the purpose and effect of this document.

_____   _____
(Date)   (Signature of Declarant)

The declarant signed or acknowledged signing this organ donation in my presence and based upon my personal observation, appears to be a competent individual.

_____   _____
(Witness)   (Witness)

(Signatures of Two Witnesses)

References

1. Temkin O and Temkin CL. *Ancient medicine: Selected papers of Ludwig Edelstein.* Baltimore: Johns Hopkins Press, 1967:6.
2. Orr RD, Pang N, Pellegrino ED, Siegler M. Use of the Hippocratic Oath: a review of twentieth century practice and a content analysis of oaths administered in medical schools in the U.S. and Canada in 1993. *J Clin Ethics* 1997;8:377–88.
3. Beauchamp TL, Childress JF. The principle of nonmaleficence. In: *Principles of biomedical ethics.* Oxford: Oxford University Press, 1989:120.
4. Hurwitz B, Richardson R. Swearing to care: the resurgence in medical oaths. *BMJ* 1997;315:1671–1674.
5. The SUPPORT principal investigators. A controlled trial to improve care for seriously ill hospitalized patients: the study to understand prognoses and preferences for outcomes and risks of treatments (SUPPORT). *JAMA* 1995;274:1591–1598.
6. Drinker P, Shaw LA. An apparatus for the prolonged administration of artificial respiration. I. A design for adults and children. *J Clin Invest* 1929;7:229–247.
7. Bower AG, Bennett VR, Dillon JB, Axelrod B. Poliomyelitis report: investigation on the care and treatment of poliomyelitis patients. Part I: Development of equipment. Part II: Physiologic studies of treatment procedures and mechanical equipment. *Ann West Med Surg* 1950;4:559–582, 686–716.
8. Bendixen HH, Egbert LD, Hedley-Whyte J, Larer MB, Pontoppidan H. *Respiratory care. Vol. 4.* St. Louis: Mosby, 1965.
9. Pontoppidan H. Respiratory failure: management and outcome. In: JE Parrillo, SM Ayres, eds. *Major issues in critical care medicine.* Baltimore: Williams and Wilkens, 1984;169–176.
10. Snider GL. Historical perspective on mechanical ventilation: from simple life support system to ethical dilemma. *Am Rev Respir Dis* 1989;140:S2–S7.
11. Petersdorf RG, Adams RD, Braunwald E, Isselbacher KJ, Martin JB, Wilson JD. Introduction to clinical medicine: the practice of medicine. In: *Harrison's principles of internal medicine.* New York: McGraw-Hill, 1983:1–5.
12. Munson R. *Intervention and reflection: basic issues in medical ethics.* Belmont: Wadsworth Publishing, 1992.
13. Fletcher JC, Hite CA, Lombardo PA, Marshall MF. *Introduction to clinical ethics.* Frederick: University Publishing Group, 1995.
14. Junkerman C, Schiedermayer D. *Practical ethics for students, interns and residents.* Frederick: University Publishing Group, 1994.
15. Cummings JL, Benson DF. *Dementia: a clinical approach.* Woburn: Butterworth Publishers, 1983.
16. Folstein MF, Folstein SE, McHugh PR. "Mini-mental state": a practical method for grading the mental state of patients for the clinician. *J. Psychiatr Res* 1975;12:189–198.
17. Kokmen E, Naessens JM, Offord KP. A short test of mental status: description and preliminary results. *Mayo Clin Proc* 1987;62(4):281–288.
18. Kokmen E, Smith GE, Petersen RC, Tangalos E, Ivnik RC. The short test of mental status. Correlations with standardized psychometric testing. *Arch Neurol* 1991;48:725–728.
19. Howell T, Fullerton DT, Harvey RF, Klein M. Depression in spinal cord injured patients. *Paraplegia* 1981;19:284–288.
20. Hancock KM, Craig AR, Dickson HG, Chang E, Martin J. Anxiety and depression over the first year of spinal cord injury: a longitudinal study. *Paraplegia* 1993;31:349–357.
21. Powell T. Consultation-liaison psychiatry and clinical ethics. Representative cases. *Psychosomatics* 1997;38:321–326.
22. President's commission for the study of ethical problems in medicine and biomedical and behavioral research. *Making Health Care Decisions* 1982; Volume 1.
23. Appelbaum PS, Grisso T. Assessing patients' capacities to consent to treatment. *N Engl J Med* 1988;319:1635–1638.
24. Roth LH, Meisel A, Lidz CW. Tests of competency to consent to treatment. *Am J Psychiatry* 1977;134:279–284.
25. Greco PJ, Schulman KA, Lavizzo-Mourey R, Hansen-Flaschen J. The Patient Self-Determination Act and the future of advance directives. *Ann Intern Med* 1991;115(8):639–643.

26. Emanuel EJ, Weinberg DS, Gonin R, Hummel LR, Emanuel LL. How well is the Patient Self-Determination Act working?: an early assessment. *Am J Med* 1993;95:619–628.

27. Silverman HJ, Tuma P, Schaeffer MH and Singh B. Implementation of the Patient Self-Determination Act in a hospital setting. An initial evaluation. *Arch Intern Med* 1995;155:502–510.

28. Aging with Dignity Website. October 24, 1998. http://www.agingwithdignity.org (P.O. Box 1661, Tallahassee, FL 32302–1661. Tel. (850) 681–2010; suggested donation, $4.

29. Annotated Code of Maryland 5-605.

30. The Multi-Society Task Force on PVS. Medical aspects of the persistent vegetative state (1). *N Engl J Med* 1994;330:1499–508.

31. The Quality Standards Subcommittee of the American Academy of Neurology. Practice parameters: assessment and management of patients in the persistent vegetative state (summary statement). *Neurology* 1995;45:1015–1018.

32. Brody BA, Halevy A. Is futility a futile concept? *J Med Philos* 1995;20:123–144.

33. Council on Ethical and Judicial Affairs. *Code of medical ethics.* Chicago: American Medical Association. 1997:8.

34. Weijer C, Singer PA, Dickens BM, Workman S. Bioethics for clinicians: 16. Dealing with demands for inappropriate treatment. *CMAJ* 1998;159:817–821.

35. Consensus statement of the Society of Critical Care Medicine's Ethics Committee regarding futile and other possibly inadvisable treatments. *Crit Care Med* 1997;25:887–891.

36. Silverman H. End-of-life decision-making algorithm. *Health Care Ethics* 1994;1(4).

37. Annotated Code of Maryland 19-370 to 19-374.

38. Puma JL, Schiedermayer D. *Ethics consultation: a practical guide.* Boston: Jones and Bartlett Publishers, 1994.

39. Spencer EM. The case consultation process. Concurrent session at Sustaining the Life of Your Ethics Committee, Bon Secours Spiritual Center, Marriottsville, Maryland, October 1998.

40. Tippett D. The case consultation process. Concurrent session at Sustaining the Life of Your Ethics Committee, Bon Secours Spiritual Center, Marriottsville, Maryland, October 1998.

41. Annotated Code of Maryland 19–374.

42. Thiel MM, Robinson MR. Physician's collaboration with chaplains: difficulties and benefits. *J Clin Ethics* 1997;8:94–103.

43. Simmonds AL. The chaplain as spiritual and moral agent. *Humane Medicine* 1994;10:103–107.

44. Fichtner CG, McKenny GP. Values interpretation: a new model for hospital ministry. *Journal of Religion and Health* 1991;30:109–118.

45. Simmonds AL. The chaplain's role in bioethical decision-making. *Healthcare Management Forum* 1994;7:5–10.

46. Grant MD, Rudberg MA, Brody JA. Gastrostomy placement and mortality among hospitalized medicare beneficiaries. *JAMA* 1998;279:1973–1976.

47. Quill TE. Utilization of nasogastric feeding tubes in a group of chronically ill, elderly patients in a community hospital. *Arch Intern Med* 1989;149:1937–1941.

48. Zerwekh JV. The dehydration question. *Nursing* 1983;13:47–51.

49. Printz LA. Is withholding hydration a valid comfort measure in the terminally ill? *Geriatrics* 1988;43:84–87.

50. Dresser RS, Boisaubin EV. Ethics, law, and nutrition support. *Arch Int Med* 1985;145:122–128.

51. Groher ME. Ethical dilemmas in providing nutrition. *Dysphagia* 1990;5:102–109.

52. Burk K. Communication and altered perceptions. *New Jersey Medicine* 1989;86:50–51.

53. Gryfe P, Kurtz I, Gutmann M, Laiken G. Freedom through a single switch: coping and communicating with artificial ventilation. *J Neurol Sci* 1996;139(S):132–133.

54. Bernat JL. States of profound paralysis with intact cognition. In: *Ethical issues in neurology.* Boston: Butterworth-Heinemann, 1994:201–220.

55. Gilgoff IS. Living with a ventilator. *The Western Journal of Medicine* 1991;154:619–622.

56. Maynard FM, Muth AS. The choice to end life as a ventilator-dependent quadriplegic. *Arch Phys Med Rehabil* 1987;68:862–864.

57. Bernat JL, Cranford RE, Kittredge FI, Rosenberg RN. Competent patients with advanced states of permanent paralysis have the right to forgo life-sustaining therapy. *Neurology* 1993;43:224–225.

58. Report of the Ethics and Humanities Subcommittee of the American Academy of Neurology. Position statement: certain aspects of the care and management of profoundly and irreversibly paralyzed patients with retained consciousness and cognition. *Neurology* 1993;43:222–223.

59. Luce JM. Withholding and withdrawal of life support: ethical, legal, and clinical aspects. *New Horiz* 1997;5:30–37.

60. Bernat JL. Physician-assisted suicide and voluntary active euthanasia. In: *Ethical issues in neurology*. Boston: Butterworth-Heinemann, 1994:313–332.

61. Shapiro JP. Dr. Death's last dance: Jack Kevorkian gets some jail time. *U.S. News and World Report* April 26, 1999:44.

62. Allen CMC. Conscious but paralysed: releasing the locked-in. *Lancet* 1993;342:130–131.

63. Kirschner KL, Smith J, Donnelley S. Case study: the tracheostomy tube with commentaries. *Hastings Center Report* March-April: 1994;26–27.

64. Gaul AL, Wilson SF. Should a ventilator be removed at a patient's request? An ethical analysis. *J Neurosci Nurs* 1990;22:326–329.

65. Patterson DR, Miller-Perrin C, McCormick TR, Hudson LD. Sounding board: when life support is questioned early in the care of patients with cervical-level quadriplegia. *N Eng J Med* 1993;328:506–509.

66. Edwards MJ, Tolle SW. Disconnecting a ventilator at the request of a patient who knows he will die: the doctor's anguish. *Ann Intern Med* 1997;117:254–256.

67. Bolin B. "I want to die, I think": a case study in clinical ethics and determination of truth. *Am J Crit Care* 1993;2:346–345.

68. Schneiderman LJ, Spragg RG. Sounding board: ethical decisions in discontinuing mechanical ventilation. *N Eng J Med* 1988;318:984–988.

69. Truog RD, Berde CB, Mitchell C, Grier HF. Sounding board: barbiturates in the care of the terminally ill. *N Eng J Med* 1992;327:1678–1682.

70. Gilligan T, Raffin TA. Withdrawing life support: extubation and prolonged terminal weans are inappropriate. *Crit Care Med* 1996;24:352–353.

71. Faber-Langendoen K. The clinical management of dying patients receiving mechanical ventilation: a survey of physician practice. *Chest* 1994;106:880–888.

72. Bach, JR, Campagnolo DI. Psychosocial adjustment of post-poliomyelitis ventilator-assisted individuals. *Ann Phys Med Rehabil* 1992;73:934–939.

73. Bach JR. Comprehensive rehabilitation of the severely disabled ventilator-assisted individual. *Monaldi Arch Chest Dis* 1993;48:331–345.

Index